WITHDRAWN
UTSA Libraries

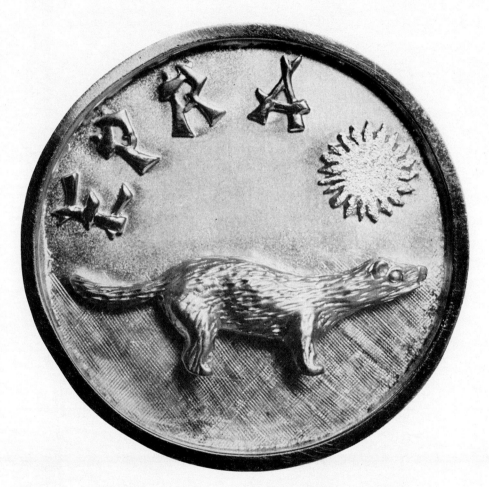

Eastern Psychiatric Research Association Gold Medal
(For explanation of Gold Medal, see Chapter 33.)

The greatest homage we can pay to truth
is to use it.

EMERSON

Expanding Goals of
GENETICS IN PSYCHIATRY

Edited by FRANZ J. KALLMANN, M.D.

Chief of Psychiatric Research, Department of Medical Genetics, New York State Psychiatric Institute; Professor of Psychiatry, Columbia University, New York

With the assistance of
L. ERLENMEYER-KIMLING, Ph.D.,
E. V. GLANVILLE, Ph.D., and
J. D. RAINER, M.D.

Anniversary Symposium of the Department of Medical Genetics, New York State Psychiatric Institute, October 27-28, 1961; and Proceedings of Sixth Annual Meeting of Eastern Psychiatric Research Association.

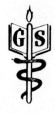

GRUNE & STRATTON   New York and London   1962

Library of Congress Catalog Card No. 62-15383

Copyright © 1962
GRUNE & STRATTON, INC.
381 Park Avenue South
New York 16, N. Y.

Printed and bound in U.S.A. (Conv-B)

Contents

Contributors

ALLEN, GORDON, M.D., Senior Assistant Surgeon, Research Branch, National Institute of Mental Health, Bethesda, Md.

ALTSHULER, KENNETH Z., M.D., Senior Research Scientist, Department of Medical Genetics, New York State Psychiatric Institute, Columbia University.

ATWOOD, K. C., M.D., Professor of Microbiology, University of Illinois, Urbana, Ill.

BAROFF, GEORGE, PH.D., Research Associate in Psychiatry (Medical Genetics), Columbia University; Chief Psychologist, The Training School at Vineland, N. J.

BEARN, A. G., M.D., Associate Professor, The Rockefeller Institute, New York, N. Y.

BENDER, LAURETTA, M.D., Director of Psychiatric Research, Children's Unit, Creedmoor State Hospital, Queens Village, N. Y.

BUCKMAN, CHARLES, M.D., Director, Kings Park State Hospital, Kings Park, N. Y.

DEMING, W. EDWARDS, PH.D., Consultant in Sampling Statistics, Department of Medical Genetics, New York State Psychiatric Institute, Columbia University; Professor of Statistics, New York University, New York, N. Y.

ERLENMEYER-KIMLING, L., PH.D., Senior Research Scientist, Department of Medical Genetics, New York State Psychiatric Institute, Columbia University.

FALEK, ARTHUR, PH.D., Senior Research Scientist, Department of Medical Genetics, New York State Psychiatric Institute; Research Associate in Psychiatry, Columbia University.

FERGUSON-SMITH, MALCOLM A., M.B., Ch.B., Lecturer in Medical Genetics, University of Glasgow, Glasgow, Scotland.

GLANVILLE, E. V., PH.D., Senior Research Scientist, Department of Medical Genetics, New York State Psychiatric Institute, Columbia University.

GLASS, H. BENTLEY, PH.D., Professor of Biology, Johns Hopkins University, Baltimore, Md.

GOLDFARB, CHARLES, M.D., Senior Research Scientist, Department of Medical Genetics, New York State Psychiatric Institute, Columbia University.

HABERLANDT, WALTER F., M.D., Dozent, Psychiatric University Clinic, Düsseldorf, West Germany.

HERNDON, C. NASH, M.D., Professor of Preventive Medicine and Genetics, The Bowman Gray School of Medicine, Winston-Salem, N. C.

HIRSCH, JERRY, PH.D., Associate Professor of Psychology, University of Illinois, Urbana, Ill.

HOCH, PAUL H., M.D., Commissioner of Mental Hygiene, State of New York; Professor of Clinical Psychiatry, Columbia University.

HOLT, WILLIAM L., JR., M.D., Professor of Psychiatry, Albany College, Albany, N. Y.

Horwitz, William A., M.D., Assistant Director, New York State Psychiatric Institute; Professor of Clinical Psychiatry, Columbia University.

Hurst, Lewis, Ph.D., M.D., Professor of Psychological Medicine, University of the Witwatersrand, Johannesburg, South Africa.

Impastato, David J., M.D., Associate Clinical Professor of Psychiatry, New York University College of Medicine, New York, N. Y.

Jarvik, Lissy Feingold, Ph.D., M.D., Senior Research Scientist, Department of Medical Genetics, New York State Psychiatric Institute; Assistant Clinical Professor of Psychiatry, Columbia University.

Jervis, George A., M.D., Director of Psychiatric Research, Letchworth Village, Thiells, N. Y.; Assistant Clinical Professor of Psychiatry, Columbia University.

Kallmann, Franz J., M.D., Chief of Psychiatric Research, Department of Medical Genetics, New York State Psychiatric Institute; Professor of Psychiatry, Columbia University.

Knox, W. Eugene, M.D., Visiting Professor of Biochemistry, American University, Beirut, Lebanon.

Kolb, Lawrence C., M.D., Director, New York State Psychiatric Institute; Professor and Chairman, Department of Psychiatry, Columbia University.

Kopac, M. J., Ph.D., Sc.D., Professor of Biology, New York University, New York, N. Y.

Lindegren, Carl C., Ph.D., Director of Biological Research Laboratory, Southern Illinois University, Carbondale, Ill.

Malamud, William, M.D., Professional and Research Director, National Association for Mental Health, New York, N. Y.

Merritt, H. Houston, M.D., Vice President in Charge of Medical Affairs and Dean, College of Physicians and Surgeons, Columbia University; Professor of Neurology, Columbia University.

Rado, Sandor, M.D., Dean and Professor of Psychiatry, The New York School of Psychiatry, New York, N. Y.

Rainer, John D., M.D., Associate Research Scientist, Department of Medical Genetics, New York State Psychiatric Institute; Assistant Clinical Professor of Psychiatry, Columbia University.

Roberts, J. A. Fraser, M.D., D.Sc., F.R.C.P., Director, Clinical Genetics Research Unit, Medical Research Council, Institute of Child Health, The Hospital for Sick Children, Great Ormond Street, London, England.

Sank, Diane, M.S., Senior Research Scientist, Department of Medical Genetics, New York State Psychiatric Institute, Columbia University.

Sarlin, Bruce, M.D., Lieutenant, Medical Corps, USNR; formerly Senior Research Scientist in Medical Genetics, New York State Psychiatric Institute.

Slater, Eliot, M.D., F.R.C.P., Director, Psychiatric Genetics Research Unit, Medical Research Council, Institute of Psychiatry, London, England.

Strömgren, Erik, M.D., Professor of Psychiatry, University of Aarhus; Medical Director, State Mental Hospital, Risskov, Denmark.

Tatum, Edward L., Ph.D., Professor, The Rockefeller Institute, New York, N. Y.

Preface and Acknowledgments

THE SPECIAL SYMPOSIUM, which gave its name to this *prima-facie* account of the proceedings, was designed as a triple-goaled event under multiple sponsorship. Held at the New York State Psychiatric Institute on October 27-28, 1961, it served, as may now be said in retrospect, its *threefold purpose* well.

In the first place, the program was planned as a report on the work of the Department of Medical Genetics over the past quarter of a century. However, while this particular goal meant a great deal to our own group, it seemed to be in need of some further attractions for clinical psychiatrists. We decided, therefore, to broaden the topic far enough to meet the criteria of a *general progress review* in the behavioral and mental health areas of human genetics.

The realization of this scheme required not only *strong reinforcements* from other research centers here and abroad, especially in the field of basic genetics, but also the funds for assembling them in New York at a strategic time and place. The long columns of able participants, financial backers and co-sponsoring organizations, listed in other parts of this volume, testify to the extraordinary degree of generosity and good will, with which our request for support was received. Obviously, a gathering of such an array of highly qualified experts in behavioral and population genetics could not have been accomplished either without the travel grants so liberally provided by the Division of Research Grants and Fellowships of the National Institute of Mental Health (United States Public Health Service) as well as the Rockefeller Foundation or without the decision of the Eastern Psychiatric Research Association to underwrite the planning and publishing of the proceedings within the limits of its financial capacity.

In line with this straightforward arrangement, *the second function* of the symposium was to serve as the sixth annual meeting of that still relatively young but extremely vigorous society. There is at least one bona-fide member of EPRA, the undersigned, who has derived nothing but benefits from this joint undertaking. For the same reason, it gives me great pleasure here to acknowledge the invaluable support received from all the other sponsors, co-workers, and friends of our department.

The *third goal* of the program was to substantiate its general theme by achieving immediacy and close relevance to the present and future of clinical psychiatry. Fortunately, the date of the symposium was only a few months after a series of regional, national and international psychiatric meetings, each of which had placed some pertinent research report of psychiatric-genetic interest on its agenda. Among the meetings were the symposium of the American Psychopathological Association on "The Future of Psychiatry" held in New York; the Third World Congress of Psychiatry in Montreal; the Fifth International Congress for Psychotherapy in Vienna; and the Second International Conference of Human Genetics as well as the Seventh International Congress of Neurology in Rome.

My personal impression formed at these conventions was that the previously tolerantly permissive attitude of mental health specialists toward the multitude of contributions, which genetics is able to make to their conceptual schemes and therapeutic programs, had undergone *a notable change*. Hence, one of the objectives of our symposium was seen in communicating to American psychiatrists the gist of what had transpired at the various scientific conferences held in the earlier part of 1961.

In keeping with this theme of the symposium, my earnest hope is that the five sections which follow will document concisely that the goals of genetics *have been expanded* in psychiatry, and that this trend has made some imprint on current psychiatric thought. What may at least be gained from these pages and would definitely seem to be to the credit of the slowly advancing phalanxes of the basic biological sciences is *the general tenet* that the goals achievable with modern genetic research methods can no longer be regarded as being too far away from the everyday concerns of the clinical and demographic disciplines dealing with the complex problems of mental health and mental illness.

With psychiatry finally being able to derive full benefit from a clearer understanding of molecular and chromosomal disarrangements in the genetic building blocks of the body, I am glad to have this occasion to express my thanks for all the help and good will that have come our way during the past 25 years. Whatever may be accomplished during the next quarter of a century, I should like to reaffirm that even in my least optimistic moments I never wavered in the belief that planners of research in mental health genetics were working toward something of real significance in this crucial field.

It is a matter of great satisfaction to me that the present and previous members of this department are no longer alone in holding that view.

FRANZ J. KALLMANN

SECTION I: PROGRESS IN BEHAVIORAL AND PSYCHIATRIC GENETICS

1

Introduction

PAUL H. HOCH, M.D.

LOOKING OVER THE EXCELLENT PROGRAM of this anniversary symposium of the Department of Medical Genetics, one is struck by the variety of investigative pursuits and the highly diversified yet clearly convergent spheres of interest that furnish the tools for studying the genetics of human behavior variations in their over-all biological setting. The roster of outstanding contributors to this well balanced symposium volume is a truly impressive one. Not only do Dr. Kallmann and his staff deserve credit for having conceived the scheme for this comprehensive anniversary account of the activities of their department, but, in furnishing the theatre of operations for a gathering of experts from the many different subdisciplines of human genetics, they succeeded in converting their provocative ideas into the fully documented pages of this fruitful research report.

What emerges from these pages is the inspired message that psychiatric genetics is undergoing a revolution within a framework of evolution. Previously largely confined to descriptive-statistical approaches to the problems of clinical psychiatry, genetic research has now moved to the technically more advanced stage of direct cytological exploration. By scrutinizing and micromanipulating the cellular (chromosomal) elements through which the transmission of genetic regulation takes place, many remarkable contributions have been made to our current body of knowledge regarding the biological components of human life and behavior, as reviewed in this symposium. There is little doubt that in the very near future illuminating discoveries will come out of this highly active field of research.

A wide array of front line reports on genetic subjects are presented in this volume: the biochemistry and function of DNA, the basic carrier of genetic information from one generation to the next, and those of other cellular components; the molecular changes underlying mutation and gene action, and the micromanipulation of chromosomes; and the more peripheral biochemical, metabolic and clinical effects of mutated genes and disarranged chromosomes.

Other reports are concerned with clinical genetics, including the various methodological problems arising in sampling design and in the investigation of genetic carriers, as well as the application of these methods to genetic studies of neurological disorders, mental deficiency, and deafness. With good reason,

1

the symposium begins and ends with reviews of studies on the possible role of genetic factors in the etiology of mental illness and behavior disorders, and on various demographic aspects of these conditions in the United States and abroad.

Many of the ideas which have reached crystallized form in this symposium have been reflected in the fine research work of Dr. Kallmann and his staff during the past 25 years. While it is not possible here to enumerate all the contributions to psychiatric genetics made by them during that period, the following general statement can be made: The Department of Mental Hygiene is most appreciative of the achievements of its Department of Medical Genetics at the Psychiatric Institute, and is looking forward with considerable pride to the work of this research unit in the years to come.

2

Studies in the Genetics of Disordered Behavior:

Methods and Objectives

JOHN D. RAINER, M.D.

In this introductory account of genetic investigations of disordered behavior, the main emphasis will be placed on reviewing *the methods and objectives* of such studies in a deliberately narrowed historical perspective; namely, in relation to the research program of the Department of Medical Genetics during the past 25 years. In line with this conceptual scheme, all varieties of physiodynamic interactions, implied in current notions of heredity as a determinant of human behavior potentials, will be viewed in the perspective of essential links in *the chain of biological processes* which may lead to the end product of disordered behavior as observed by the psychiatrist.

It is well known that the hereditary components of mental illness have been pondered by physicians from Hippocrates on. Only for the past 60 years, however, has a more exact conceptual basis been provided for the formulation of verifiable genetic hypotheses. More recently, refined research methods and new investigative approaches in psychiatry and its allied disciplines have brought the behavioral sciences much closer to that crucial stage where their joint attention can be devoted to exploring the primary etiological and developmental problems of disordered behavior.

If as a result of these advances it has finally become feasible to view any and all variations in physical and mental health as products of genic action and developmental processes, then the goals of genetics in psychiatry have indeed been expanded. This propitious trend was clearly anticipated by Kallmann's description of unusual behavior as "an extremely complex and continuous chain of events in the individual's adaptive history, rather than the automatic expression of a fixed congenital error in metabolism."[6]

Working at the molecular, chemical, physiological, psychological and demographic levels, and welding together psychodynamic and physiodynamic considerations, genetics can become the finest vehicle for an integrated approach to psychopathology. Patently, any comprehensive appraisal of the human organism in a temporal framework is bound to deal first with the fertilized ovum and the potentialities contained therein.

When Dr. and Mrs. Kallmann began their work in this department of the Psychiatric Institute in 1936, the way was already paved for the careful quantitative study of the genetics of well defined psychiatric syndromes. This work was quite different from previously existing pre-Mendelian, hence pre-

3

Kraepelinian case reports — descriptive family histories which sought to confirm the popular notion that "psychoses" tend to run in families. Studies of this kind were of little merit since they were usually limited to pedigrees selected because they contained large numbers of mentally ill persons. Since no individual pedigree could distinguish genetic from other familial influences, the statistical value of such collections was limited.

By 1916, a group of psychiatrists in Munich, headed by Rüdin, realized the necessity for studying the heredity contribution to schizophrenia in statistically representative and clinically homogeneous samples. In the contingency method of statistical prediction that they perfected, the objective was to compare the expectancy of the condition developing among relatives of affected individuals with that in the general population.

The definition of that aim calls for certain clarifications. To begin with, the possible genetic transmission of, for example, a schizophrenia-predisposing factor cannot be evaluated without allowing for the fact that not all persons in the group of relatives studied who are found to be free of schizophrenic symptoms will necessarily remain so if they live to an older age. Those under age 15 have not yet entered the period of risk; those in the 15 to 45 age range still have a risk, the younger the age the more so; and only after the age of 45 can the risk period clinically be deemed over. For the relatives, therefore, one cannot simply consider the prevalence of schizophrenia, but has to obtain a corrected figure known as the expectancy rate.

A number of methods were developed for making this correction, some involving the use of empirical risk figures for each age. More simple and shown to be sufficiently accurate is Weinberg's *abridged method*[4,8,9] whereby the absolute number of actually observed cases is related to the number of persons in the total population who have survived the given period of manifestation, increased by one-half the number of persons who, at the end of the study, are still within the age limits of this period. Persons who did not reach (because of death), or are too young to have reached, the beginning of the manifestation period are not counted as part of the base. This method yields morbidity rates that denote the average expectancy of developing the disease by persons who remain alive through its manifestation period. The range of this period is chosen on the basis of clinical experience, and for adult schizophrenia is taken as 15 to 45 years of age.

It was the relatives of schizophrenics for whom this expectancy rate was computed. The earliest studies of Rüdin,[8] Luxenburger[7] and Schulz[9] considered siblings as well as half-siblings; others studied children; still others, nephews, nieces and first cousins. Kallmann's first survey, conducted in the late 1920's and reported in 1936 and 1938, dealt with the expectancy of schizophrenia in a large group of descendants of schizophrenics and their sibs.[3,4]

Of prime importance is the requisite that the original group of patients whose relatives are to be investigated be a consecutively reported group, representing either a 100 per cent ascertainment or a random sample thereof. Only then can the members of this group be called *index cases* or *probands*. In practice, they will usually represent all admissions to a given hospital or hospital system over a certain period of time, or a properly selected sample of such a list.

Finally, in this scheme of investigation the expectancy figures for the various groups of relatives studied can be compared with one another, but they should also be compared with expectancy rates for the general population. They are available only as the result of careful demographic studies of the total population of small areas or of unbiased samples of the population of larger districts. Most studies of schizophrenia throughout the world yield an expectancy rate varying from just below one per cent to about two per cent.

By comparison, the rates in the various categories of relatives that have been investigated are significantly higher, the more so as they approach the schizophrenic index case in degree of genetic similarity. The *minimum expectancy rates* obtained in many different studies fall close together in the following ranges:

	Percentage Expectancy of Schizophrenia
General population	0.85
Half-siblings	7- 8
Full siblings	5-15*
Parents	5-10
Children (of one index case)	8-16
Children (of two index cases)	53-68

*Most investigators agree that the expectancy is greater than 10 per cent.

The contingency method of genetic investigation can be fruitfully extended in a number of directions. The results of some of these studies, representing current research projects of this department, are reported in this volume. One of the reports is part of an extensive psychiatric investigation of *the deaf,* using as index cases schizophrenic patients who have also been totally deaf since birth or early childhood. The findings regarding the morbidity rate for schizophrenia among their deaf and hearing siblings can be expected to throw light on the interacting roles and relative effects of genetic predisposition and extreme communication stress on the development of schizophrenia.

Another investigation, part of a study of changing *marriage* and *fertility* rates among schizophrenics, is designed to focus on the children of two schizophrenic parents. With a 53 to 68 per cent risk of developing schizophrenia, these children may furnish important data for research work on preclinical manifestations associated with biochemical or cytological irregularities. Such data, aside from their basic value in the areas of etiology and development, will be of considerable help in prevention and counseling.

One of the most refined extensions of the contingency method is the *twin-family method,* developed and utilized in the United States at this institute,[4] and abroad by Essen-Möller, Slater and others. It has been applied not only to schizophrenia, but to manic-depressive and involutional psychoses as well. In this method, the index cases represent one particular sample of a consecutive series of affected individuals, namely, all the twins among them. It is then possible to determine risk figures not only for their single-born siblings, parents and children, as before, but also for their co-twins. This group of co-twins can be independently divided into identical or one-egg twins and fraternal or two-egg twins, with separate risk figures to be obtained for each of these two groups.

In the most extensive twin series, reported in 1946 by Kallmann[5] on work carried on during the first decade of this department's existence, the expectancy rates were 14.5 per cent for dizygotic co-twins and 86.2 per cent for monozygotic co-twins of *schizophrenic* index cases. The expectancy among the dizygotic twins of schizophrenic probands was approximately the same as that of other sibs (14.2 per cent), despite the fact that they usually shared the same environment at a comparable age. By comparison, the schizophrenia risk of one-egg co-twins represented by far the highest expectancy rate in any group studied. The given data agreed with the results of the earlier family study and were confirmed by the work of other twin investigators. None of them could explain the increased risk of schizophrenia in the various categories of relatives of schizophrenics without assuming the existence of some genetic factor.

Debates over the *mode of inheritance* of this factor have lost their crucial quality with the advances in genetic theory embodying the concepts of penetrance, expressivity and modifying genes. Also, it is rather clear by this time that until the enzymatic substrate of the inherited vulnerability factor is identified, theories as to the exact mode of its inheritance will remain inconclusive.

Operating by means of a long series of interactions and feedback mechanisms, the development of schizophrenia most certainly includes biochemical, neurological and psychological alterations. Therefore, it is to specialists in these fields that one turns for further elucidation of the problems of specificity and pathogenesis in this disorder.

It may be remembered that in Kallmann's earlier studies,[4] fairly consistent variations in resistance to *pulmonary tuberculosis* among relatives of schizophrenics pointed to a nonspecific, probably multifactorial constitutional defense mechanism related to mesodermal tissue elements. This work was representative of tentative approaches to old cellular theories relating the metabolic deficiencies in schizophrenia to the immunological or detoxifying functions of the reticuloendothelial system. The search for the toxic metabolite itself goes on in many parts of the world, with abnormalities in adrenalin metabolism, in serotonin production, and in a plasma protein fraction variously implicated.

Parenthetically, it may be noted that a similar statement can be made with respect to the results of such other twin-family studies carried out in this department as those on *preadolescent* forms of schizophrenia, *manic-depressive psychosis* and *involutional psychosis*.[6] Each of these studies revealed highly significant increases in concordance with closer genetic similarity to the index case.

An important recent advance in genetics, foreshadowed by twin studies conducted here, related to the etiology of an equally obscure developmental anomaly, *Down's syndrome*. With improved techniques for visualizing, distinguishing and counting human chromosomes, observations on concordance for this defect in one-egg twins, as well as on the role of advanced maternal age, were explained by the discovery of a supernumerary chromosome of a given size, a trisomy, in persons with this condition. This trisomy appeared to result from a nondisjunction in the reduction division forming the ovum in the mother.

Similarly, various defects in *sexual development* were previously observed here in sibships and individual twin pairs and were believed to be the result of chromosomal disarrangement. This surmise was also confirmed by recent work, especially that dealing with Klinefelter's syndrome, Turner's syndrome and similar conditions. On the other hand, chromosomal mechanisms responsible for male homosexuality have not yet been identified despite suggestive evidence for some genetic basis as shown by observations on a consecutive series of twins. Here one may have to unravel a more complex series of interactional stages, with the initial defect being of a less apparent nature.

While one major line of investigation proceeds in the direction of the identification of changes at the biochemical and cellular levels, twin studies have also given impetus to the comparative study of individual development, including *behavioral* and *psychodynamic* components. As pointed out by Shields and Slater, "The modern trend in twin research recognizes the value of detailed individual analysis, in addition to mass statistics."[10] In particular, strong clues may come of the extension of twin research to the comparatively rare cases, in which a pair of one-egg twins is dissimilar with respect to a major sensory, motor or behavioral characteristic. For one thing, such investigations may throw light on the nature of threshold components, that for want of more precise information are grouped under the heading of "penetrance" or "expressivity."

Generally, it may be assumed that the genic structure in identical twins is likewise identical. However, the pathway from the postulated molecular structure to the trait's manifestation in later life is a tortuous one. Modern genetic theories do not preclude changes in gene action due to subtle shifts in the balance of forces in the total chromosomal or nuclear structure, which thereafter may perpetuate themselves via divergent biochemical pathways.

At the same time, interactional patterns during *embryonic life* leading to gross phenotypic differences can only be broadly subsumed under the heading of expressivity. Other threshold components include age, sex, and physical, social and familial environment. A spiral-like development toward marked behavioral dissimilarity may arise in the chromosomal, prenatal and postnatal stages. Among the innumerable determinants conceivable in a total biological approach are comparative studies of cellular reaction, endocrine function, protein synthesis or interpersonal relations. Various techniques from intensive chemical analysis to intensive psychoanalysis of both members of selected pairs of discordant twins may provide illuminating hypotheses.

Regarding such hypothetical schemes, one may quote Ernest Jones's prediction[2] that by *psychoanalytic methods* ". . . one is enabled to dissect and isolate mental processes to an extent not previously possible." Inevitably, the given procedure will ". . . bring us nearer to the primary elements, to the mental genes in terms of which genetic investigations can alone be carried out."[2,p.160] The next study to be applied, Jones predicted, ". . . would be one in the field of heredity."[(1,p.134)] Today, psychodynamic attention can be directed not only through the classical methods of introspection, free reporting and dream analysis, but also through psychological testing, observation of children and controlled experimental studies of humans and animals.

Therefore, the resurgence of *behavioral genetics* as a science, while pursuing the elucidation of cause, effect and interaction in the major deviant forms of behavior and psychopathology, goes beyond this particular goal. It addresses itself as well to the study of normal growth, including the description of behavior development for an entire species, determining the role of genic, chromosomal, cytoplasmic, biochemical, embryologic, nutritional, experiential and social factors, and the phenomena of individual differences within the species. The latter task has been given impetus by current work defining identifiable categories of infant behavior in earliest life. Studies of this kind have been aided in theoretical formulation and research design by work in experimental genetics using such animals as fruit flies and dogs.

Of course, it would be a mistake to leave the impression that the only goals of genetic research in psychiatry are related to the study of etiology and mechanism. A guiding principle of this department has been that genetic concepts can be incorporated into clinical management in a *psychotherapeutic* setting. It is certainly essential in that form of psychotherapy required by persons seeking genetic counseling in the psychiatric sector. Here only a combination of adequate genetic knowledge, good judgment, and awareness of the profound emotional significance of such momentous decisions as marriage and childbearing can make for beneficial patient care.

The framework provided by genetics is no less effective in the areas of *child psychiatry* and advice on *child-rearing,* and in general in the keener understanding of a patient within his *family constellation.* A child's development, including neurotic and psychopathic behavior patterns, is affected by the genetic constitution of both parents and himself. From the moment the mother first sees her baby, both react to the behavior of the other.

To individualize therapy, it is necessary to understand the role of individual differences in *psychological* reaction patterns, in response to *psychopharmacological* agents, in *psychosomatic* and *psychosexual* predispositions, and in *mood responses* and *stress vulnerability.* While much is unknown in these spheres, their investigation acquires meaning when pursued in an atmosphere of a unitary biological orientation which includes genetics as an important basic science.

Just as biological and social trends of evolution intertwine and together furnish a framework in which to understand human biology in historical perspective, so individual human development is the resultant of many forces along the axis originating in the person's *genetic structure.* It is for this reason that the many biological disciplines represented by the participants in this symposium and their diverse endeavors, all bearing on the genetic aspects of human development and disorders, form a solid groundwork for our scientific and professional efforts. One has the good feeling in psychiatry that somehow, now that we have both feet on the ground and no longer have to wear blinders either on the right side or the left, we can make truly rapid strides.

REFERENCES

1. JONES, E.: Mental heredity (1930). In Jones, E., Ed.: Essays in Applied Psycho-analysis. London, Hogarth Press, 1951.
2. ———: Psycho-analysis and biology (1930). In Jones, E., Ed.: Essays in Applied Psycho-analysis. London, Hogarth Press, 1951.
3. KALLMANN, F. J.: Erbprognose und Fruchtbarkeit bei den verschiedenen Formen der Schizophrenie. Allg. Ztschr. Psychiat. 104: 119, 1936.
4. ———: The Genetics of Schizophrenia. New York, Augustin, 1938.
5. ———: The genetic theory of schizophrenia. Am. J. Psychiat. 103: 309, 1946.
6. ———: An appraisal of psychogenetic twin data. Dis. Nerv. System (suppl.) 19: 9, 1958.
7. LUXENBURGER, H.: Psychiatrisch-neurologische Zwillingspathologie. Zentralbl. ges. Neurol. Psychiat. 56: 145, 1930.
8. RÜDIN, E.: Zur Vererbung und Neuentstehung der Dementia Praecox. Berlin, Springer, 1916.
9. SCHULTZ, B.: Zur Erbpathologie der Schizophrenie. Ztschr. ges. Neurol. Psychiat. 143: 175, 1932.
10. SHIELDS, J., AND SLATER, E.: Heredity and psychological abnormality. In Eysenck, H. J., Ed.: Handbook of Abnormal Psychology. New York, Basic Books, 1961.

3

Genetic Variations in Disease Resistance and Survival Potential

LISSY FEINGOLD JARVIK, Ph.D., M.D.

SCIENTIFIC SCRUTINY OF GENETIC VARIATIONS in *disease resistance* and *survival potential* is of relatively recent origin compared with the traditional emphasis on inherited susceptibility to specific disease entities. The long-standing tendency to stress the life-shortening effects of certain genic components is readily understood. By and large, it is easier to investigate abnormalities resulting from single major gene mutations than to demonstrate graded variations in disease resistance which depend on the interaction of several or many genes with each other and with a variety of environmental factors.

Awareness of the intricately interacting forces leads to the realization that attempts at classifying the outcome of these complex processes as the result of either hereditary or environmental influences introduce an artificial distinction. An example of current interest is the etiology of Down's syndrome (mongolism), a disorder which can now be attributed to heritable chromosomal changes. Consequently, the classification of this disorder as a hereditary disturbance would seem to be justified. Yet, the stimuli initiating the genetic aberration, through nondisjunction or translocation, remain unknown. It has been suggested that maternal exposure to radiation may represent one such stimulus, thus placing the syndrome into the category of "environmentally" produced disorders. The situation becomes even more confused when we consider that some maternal genotypes may exhibit greater resistance than others to this type of radiation injury. Of interest in this connection is the reported derivation of radiation-resistant strains from mass cultures of certain mouse cells.[51]

Despite the complex interplay of pathogenic agents in the causation of disease, constantly increasing refinements of experimental techniques may be expected to facilitate progress toward the evaluation of specific contributions made by various interacting etiologic factors. A promising approach in this direction is that of *pharmacogenetics*. Pharmacologists have long been familiar with the observation that drugs which are therapeutic for most people may have detrimental and even fatal effects in others. The aberrant individual reactions have been designated as idiosyncratic.

Some of these *idiosyncrasies* have recently been shown to occur in specific genotypes, including reaction to such widely used drugs as barbiturates and primaquine. Commonly used doses of barbiturates may be lethal if admin-

10

istered to a patient with porphyria,[13] and a deficiency in the enzyme glucose-6-phosphate dehydrogenase predisposes primaquine-sensitive individuals to hemolytic anemia.[40] Genetic variations have also been reported in reaction to such other drugs as salicylates and isoniazid.[17] Although the corresponding metabolic changes still await identification in various instances, at least some knowledge has been accumulated concerning the metabolic dysfunctions underlying scores of hereditary diseases.[22] Many of them are reviewed in other sections of this symposium, as are recent advances in cytogenetics. For this reason, it may be sufficient here to point out that in addition to Down's syndrome, chromosomal changes have been described in a number of sexual anomalies and in certain types of congenital malformations.

Evidence of this sort has not yet been obtained for any graded character such as resistance to infection. Although individual differences in response to infection have been known since the time of Hippocrates, they were long overshadowed by the dramatic discoveries of microbiologists. For many decades, therefore, attention was focused upon the etiological role of specific infective agents rather than upon host resistance factors. Only now are epidemiologists beginning to reassign equal weight to the study of each of the three crucial factors that interact in disease production — causative agent, environmental conditions and host resistance.[15,56]

This renewed interest in host factors may be ascribed, at least in part, to the remarkable control achieved over known infectious diseases. As a consequence, other types of disorder have assumed major epidemiological importance. Cardiovascular and neoplastic diseases are prominent examples of conditions for which no distinct causative agents have been identified. This failure has stimulated inquiries into individual differences in reaction patterns.

Although present knowledge regarding the mechanisms of host resistance and immunity (natural or innate) is limited, the perspicacity and pioneering efforts of two recent Nobel laureates, Medawar and Burnet, portend rapid advances in this area.[6,44] It was the experimental production of immunological tolerance that has opened up new vistas for the study of host defense mechanisms and is virtually certain to lead to the elucidation of processes by which morphological and functional integrity is maintained in higher organisms. Aside from providing confirmation for the true genic uniqueness of the individual,[43] this novel approach to immunology re-emphasized the importance of the interaction between environmental variables and differences in host genotypes.

Various difficulties are encountered in an attempt to unravel the complicated interplay of multiple causes of the phenotypic differences which characterize both disease resistance and survival potential. This statement holds true especially for differences in natural life span, which can be expressed only after the individual has successfully overcome the numerous forces challenging his survival from the moment of birth and even before birth. Attainment of senescence implies that a person has demonstrated his ability to resist a variety of deleterious endogenous and exogenous influences. Only then can differences become manifest in the physical, physiological and psychological decrements, which are associated with the aging process. A detailed study of

these changes may provide information which will prove to be useful not only
for prophylaxis of morbidity, but also for the identification of basic mechanisms responsible for the mounting mortality with advancing age.

Attempts to clarify some of these underlying mechanisms have been made
by comparing the changes attributed to normal aging with the biochemical,
physiological and genetic effects of radiation injury.[47] In his recent review
of the subject, Handler[20] concluded that the analogy is warranted. He considered it a matter of personal choice, however, "whether the resemblances or
the differences are to be emphasized . . . at the present time."

In drawing this type of analogy one should be mindful of the restricted
repertoire available to the human organism for responding to a variety of stimuli. This limitation becomes progressively more pronounced as we descend
from the total organism to cellular and subcellular structures where widely
divergent stimuli may produce identical responses. Parenthetically, it may be
said that identity of response represents a judgment that is largely a function
of our lack of sophistication in a given area. A good example is that of hemophilia where deficiency of several distinct factors seemingly produces the same
disease.[50] Thus, as Li[37] has pointed out, "Even when an apparently homogeneous condition is attained, it is no guarantee that we are dealing with a
single trait."

How much more complex, then, is the situation with respect to the graded
characters that form "the bulk of the genetically conditioned variability observed in either health or disease."[46] Despite some question concerning the
modes of inheritance, considerable information has been accumulated on the
expression of genetic differences in several of these continuous traits. Three
of them have been selected for more detailed review here: tuberculosis, cancer
and total length of life. This selection has not been made because the three
are the only or the most important examples, but because they illustrate the
type of research initiated by Dr. Kallmann and carried out in this department
during the past two and a half decades. Incidentally, they may be of historical interest since Dr. Kallmann is inclined to believe that studies of this
sort lack the depth that can now be achieved by means of the more refined
techniques available to the human geneticist.

Investigations of twins and their relatives have served to demonstrate that
genic elements exert a measurable influence upon variations in host resistance
to *reinfection tuberculosis*. The morbidity risk figures provided by the twin-
family method[34] lent support to the clinical observation that mere exposure
to Koch bacilli often proves insufficient to produce manifest disease.

The age-corrected morbidity rates (fig. 1) indicate that resistance to tuberculosis increases in inverse proportion to the degree of blood relationship to a
tuberculous index case rather than in consistent relation to the length or extent of exposure to a known index case. All sibship groups were shown to
have far higher expectancy rates than the general population, and the rates
were distributed in such a way as to preclude any simple correlation between
degree of consanguinity and similarity in exposure to infection. While one-
egg co-twins had a morbidity risk (87.3 per cent) more than three times as
high as that for two-egg twin partners, the risk for two-egg co-twins did not
differ from that for single-born siblings (25.6 and 25.5 per cent, respectively). Extended follow-up studies confirmed these differences.[49]

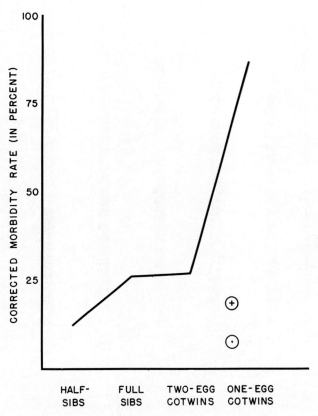

Fig. 1. Tuberculosis risk (adapted from Kallmann and Reisner, 1943). Dot in circle indicates mates; cross in circle indicates parents.

Between 1936 and 1957, the results of four other serial twin studies were reported. The average uncorrected concordance rate (fig. 2) based on a total of 698 twin pairs (186 one-egg and 512 two-egg), from five separate institutions, was 53.8 per cent for one-egg and 16.2 per cent for two-egg pairs.[32] Inasmuch as the given studies, conducted in five different populations (three European, one North American, one South American) were derived from samples of unequal size, ethnic composition and social stratification, they were not strictly comparable. Moreover, clinical data were obtained at different times and may have conformed to different diagnostic standards. In the light of these considerations, the findings corresponded remarkably well.

Corroborative data on gene-controlled differences in resistance to tuberculosis have been provided by animal experiments. Detailed studies of resistant and susceptible strains of rabbits showed marked differences in host reaction to the same concentration of pathogens. While susceptible animals could not inhibit the profuse multiplication of tubercle bacilli, and ultimately succumbed to the disease, the resistant group responded with a localized pathological process. Revealing neither lymphogenous nor hematogenous spread, it was arrested after a time. Although much work remains to be done in this area, the experimental approach to the pathogenesis of tuberculosis[38] still holds a great deal of promise for the eventual clarification of the basic mechanisms responsible for graded variations in host resistance to tuberculosis.

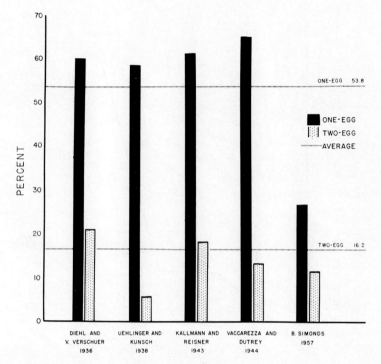

FIG. 2. Twin concordance rates for tuberculosis.

Similarly, studies of susceptible and resistant animals, mice in particular, have yielded valuable clues to further investigations into the complex interaction between host defense mechanisms and *tumor-inducing agents*. Mammary cancer in mice is perhaps the best-known example of this sort. It was observed 25 years ago[4] that a milk-borne factor, subsequently identified as an infectious agent or virus, was transferred in the milk of females from cancerous stocks. This factor was long assumed to be necessary and sufficient to produce mammary cancer in mice. Literally hundreds of papers were subsequently published on the subject to prove or disprove this view, although the current balance of evidence favors the interaction of several causative factors in the usual type of spontaneous mammary cancer in mice. Prominent among them are the milk-borne factor (mammary tumor agent), hormonal stimulation of the mammary glands, and inherited susceptibility to spontaneous mammary cancer. According to one theory, the mammary tumor agent itself may be of genic origin and "operate in the individual through enzymelike control of hormonal metabolism and/or production or through other processes."[5] There is little evidence for a relationship between mammary cancer in mice and human breast cancer, but the experiences gained by animal research are certain to be helpful in exploring the etiology of cancer in man. Considering the difficulties encountered in defining the role of genetic factors in tumor production under circumstances where hereditary as well as environmental factors could be varied at the experimenter's whim, it is not surprising that the results of the comparatively few human studies are still in the realm of controversy.

Apart from lack of control over a multitude of environmental conditions, investigators are confronted with the relatively low incidence of malignant neoplastic disease, a factor which is not conducive to the use of the twin-study method in this trait.

Hence, only five serial twin studies of cancer are available for comparing concordance rates for one-egg and two-egg pairs (fig. 3). They yielded in-

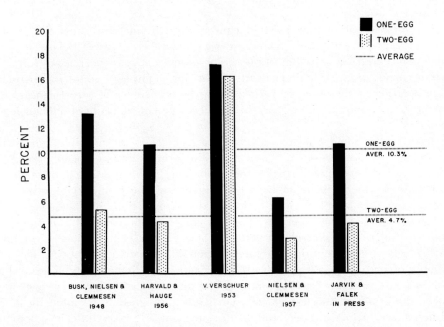

FIG. 3. Twin concordance rates for cancer.

formation about 948 twin pairs from three different countries (Denmark, Germany, United States). Although the data were collected by means of different sampling procedures, the concordance rates (uncorrected for age) show a considerable degree of correspondence, with the rates varying from 6.5 to 13.5 per cent for one-egg pairs, and from 2.8 to 5.3 per cent for two-egg pairs.[7,21,26,45] The exception was the German follow-up study,[61] which yielded somewhat higher figures for both groups (17.4 and 16.1 per cent if only cases collected prior to 1940 are used). The over-all incidence of cancer among the twin subjects of the American series was found by us to be no higher than that for the comparable general population. If anything, the cancer rates in twins tended to be slightly lower than those for the population at large.[25]

The average concordance rates based on all five studies were 10.3 per cent for 252 one-egg pairs, and 4.7 per cent for 696 two-egg pairs. This difference between the two groups of twins may be relatively small, but the trend toward a higher one-egg concordance rate is so uniform that it can hardly be ignored. In fact, the difference in concordance is statistically significant at the 0.01 level of confidence.

Irrespective of this difference between the zygosity groups, the concordance rates for one-egg twins are consistently low. A plausible explanation might be that genetic factors tend to be of limited importance in cancer, with exogenous agents bearing the major etiological weight, just as they do in tuberculosis. Obviously, exposure to tubercle bacilli is a necessary condition for the acquisition of tuberculous infection, and yet it is not sufficient for the development of tuberculous disease.

A similar situation may exist in cancer, even if one disregards the possibility of a direct relationship between cancer and tuberculosis.[8] Relatively low concordance rates are in line with the assumption that cancer cases form a heterogeneous group. Genic elements might, for example, account for the major proportion of the observed variability in the occurrence of breast cancer,[12] but may have only a minor share in the development of acute childhood leukemia.[59]

Apart from some such relatively rare conditions as multiple intestinal polyposis,[16] retinoblastoma,[39] and a certain form of basal cell carcinoma,[11] which may depend upon single-gene mutations, symptomatic manifestations of malignant disease seem to be a consequence of the complex interplay between exogenous agents (viral, toxic or otherwise noxious in character) and endogenous defense mechanisms.[54] Since the final outcome of this interaction is a function of the relative strength of each, the combination of several etiologically distinct entities — forced upon investigators by the insufficient number of twin pairs with a given type of cancer — is bound to obscure the expression of specific genetic components. In crudely analogous terms, one might think of the hopelessness of twin studies designed to examine the role of hereditary factors in susceptibility to skin rashes. It takes little imagination to foresee the conflicting results of such studies. Their outcome would depend primarily on the relative number of cases with, for example, infectious diseases, allergic reactions, deficiency states, lesions induced by toxic agents (physical or chemical), metabolic dysfunctions or changes associated with advancing age.

This comparison is not as far-fetched as it may appear at first glance, since every one of the conditions mentioned has been implicated in the etiology of neoplastic disease.[23] Moreover, genetic variability has been shown to exert a measurable influence upon the development of morbid changes falling into each of these categories. The mutagenic effects of physical and chemical agents (radiation, nitrogen mustard, etc.) have been as universally accepted as the responsibility of major mutant genes for inborn errors of metabolism. The list of infectious diseases which can be cited, in addition to tuberculosis, includes such well-known examples as malaria, rheumatic fever, and poliomyelitis. [2,3,56,58]

Single gene differences have been demonstrated in certain *deficiency states,* e.g., vitamin D resistant rickets,[62] nephrogenic diabetes insipidus[9] and virilizing adrenal hyperplasia.[10] Not yet clearly defined are the possible genetic factors operating in a number of *allergic conditions,*[55,57] while a great deal of evidence has been accumulated in support of genetically conditioned variations in *senescent decline* and *longevity potentials*.

The inference that hereditary factors may be among the determinants of longevity stems from a number of statistical investigations conducted since the beginning of this century. Despite the application of various statistical techniques to different population groups, all of these studies demonstrated a positive relationship between parental age and filial life span.[33] The consistent finding of a relatively longer life span for children of long-lived parents pointed to the expression of genetic influences in survival. Supportive evidence for these data was provided by a longitudinal study of aging twins, organized here in 1936.[18,28,30,31,35]

Over 2000 twins who were 60 years old or older were ascertained in New York State and then followed for a period of 12 years. At the time of the final analysis, both members of 75 one-egg and 88 same-sex two-egg pairs had died of verified natural causes after the age of 60. Two-egg co-twins survived, on the average, 6.2 years after the death of their twin partners, while the corresponding mean intra-pair difference for monozygotic twins was 4.9 years.

Mean intra-pair differences decreased with increasing age (fig. 4) as would be expected from the asymptotic nature of the survival curve: the older the pair at the time of the first twin's death, the fewer the years of life remaining to the cotwin. A centenarian's partner, for example, is destined soon to follow his twin's demise, making it impossible for the pair, regardless of zygosity, to exhibit more than a minor difference in ages at death. No matter how inconvenient this trend has proved to be for research in aging twins, it is merely an expression of the fact that unfortunately, or perhaps fortunately, the human life span is limited—for twins as well as for single-born people. It was remarkable, therefore, that even after the age of 80, the average differences in survival of two-egg twin partners were still found to exceed those of one-egg twins.

Greater mean intra-pair life span differences in dizygotic than in monozygotic pairs were observed with respect to both sexes and all five age groups above 60 years. This consistent difference would be expected by chance less than once in a thousand times so that we have concluded that gene-specific elements significantly affect man's natural life span.[28] It may be noted, however, that no information has as yet been obtained concerning the mechanisms of action by which these genic influences exert their effect.

The *multifactorial* type of inheritance, postulated for graded variations in survival potentials, appears to be the most plausible one at the present stage of knowledge. It implies the cumulative action of a great number of genes which individually produce only minor effects. In various combinations, these polygenes yield the continuous distribution curves characteristic not only of disease resistance and total life span, but also of stature, intelligence and fingerprint patterns. A new method for locating polygenes has recently been applied to Drosophila data,[60] calling our attention to the fact that polygenic systems represent theoretical constructs, devised for the sake of mathematical simplicity. Conceivably, a finite number of causes, some with and others without a genetic basis, may ultimately be identified as giving rise to normal distribution curves.[37]

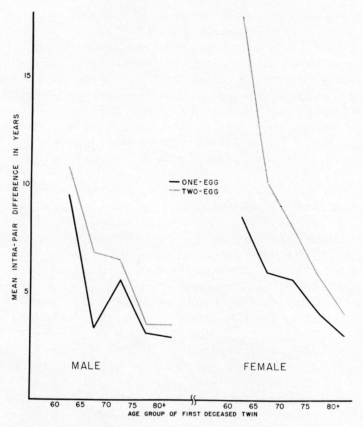

Fig. 4. Mean intra-pair life span differences for 163 same-sex pairs. (Both partners died of natural causes over age 60.)

With respect to longevity, we may assign some of the genetic effects to the category concerned with resistance to specific degenerative diseases. The difficulties encountered by investigators in this area have already been discussed in relation to neoplastic processes and may be further exemplified by the group of *cardiovascular diseases*. There are several disorders with extensive cardiac involvement, which apparently are due to single-gene mutations.[41] The incidence of diseases of this kind which seem to be manifested under most environmental conditions may be relatively low. However, the total number of cases reported in a rare condition such as familial cardiomegaly[48] probably increases in direct proportion to the dissemination of genetic information. With single major genes being implicated in the etiology of certain types of atherosclerosis[1,24] and hypertension,[14] too, resistance to these more common forms of cardiovascular disturbances would seem to represent the complex interaction of several genes with appropriate environmental components as has recently been suggested by McKusick[42] as well as by Roberts.[52]

Although *decreased resistance* to specific diseases may eventually prove to account for a large proportion of the observed variations in length of life, it is by no means certain that differences in host resistance factors will be sufficient to explain the total variability in natural life span. Yet a genetic mechanism (be it uni-, bi-, or multifactorial) directly concerned with longevity lacks meaning in the evolutionary scheme where postreproductive effects are not subject to the forces of natural selection. It may be postulated, however, that there is some pleiotropic system with major actions upon other attributes which coincidentally modify the life span.

One such relationship has been suggested by animal experiments. Apparently, genes affecting litter size also affect the life span of female mice.[53] In humans, the possibility of another association has been considered, that between intellectual performance and length of survival.[27,29] Evidence for this type of association was tentatively derived from longitudinal psychometric data on a sample of same-sex twin pairs over the age of 60. Aside from demonstrating, for the first time, that hereditary differences in certain intellectual functions persist to a measurable degree into senescence,[19] the data have revealed a tendency toward higher test scores in twins who survived than in those who died during the follow-up period.

The final evaluation of these results requires much further work, on a larger scale and extending over a longer period than that covered in our pilot study. The lower mean scores of the earlier deceased subjects, for example, may have been a function of the limited period of life remaining to them, or an expression of the "imminence of death factor." Such a factor was assumed in a longitudinal study of aged men[36] to explain the observed acceleration in decline of performance on certain intellectual tasks prior to death. The given factor seemed to be relatively independent of age, and its effects were found to precede death by intervals varying from a few months to several years. The complexities of this interesting problem cannot be disentangled without longitudinal data on a representative sample of individuals followed from childhood into adult life and through the senium.

If such a study were designed to include a representative sample of twins, it would assist also in identifying environmental factors conducive to enhancement of, or reduction in, the degrees of intellectual deterioration associated with aging. In previous investigations it was the consistently observed expression of genotypic similarity in the face of considerable environmental diversity which necessarily focused attention upon the genetic components.

The marked degree of similarity seen in monozygotic twins is illustrated in figure 5 by the scores of a female pair separated for a period of 47 years. One of the twins married a local farmer at the age of 18, raised a large family, and continued to live within 10 miles of the small rural community where she was born. Her co-twin entered a Bible school, was sent as a missionary to the Orient, and remained there until her retirement at the age of 65. After she had rejoined her sister who had meanwhile become a widow, the twins lived together until death intervened. Their deaths occurred at the ages of 92 and 94, respectively, with the missionary dying first. The degree of their intellectual resemblance is illustrated by the test scores which were obtained when the twins were 88 years old. At that time, differences in theoretical and aesthetic values were the only reflections of their diverse experiences.

Although environmental differences of this magnitude are exceedingly rare

for twins in both zygosity groups, marked similarities in test scores are typical
only of one-egg pairs. By contrast, dissimilar two-egg pairs do not tend to become alike even under very similar conditions of life.

The twin sisters whose psychometric scores are shown in figure 6 spent their
entire lives together, except for a three year period in their early twenties. Twin

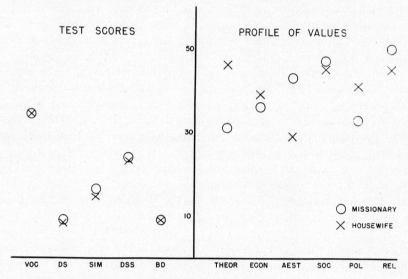

FIG. 5. One-egg female twins separated 47 years.

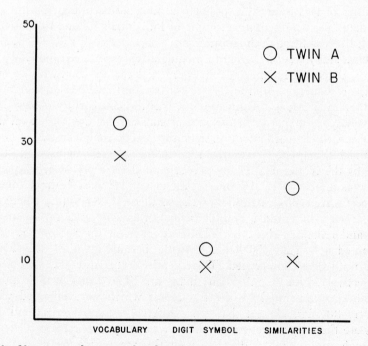

FIG. 6. Nonseparated two-egg female twins.

A had always been brighter; she had a complete college education, while twin B failed to go beyond high school. The differences observable at the age of 80 were considerably reduced in comparison with those which presumably were present before the age of 72. At that time, twin A suffered a cerebrovascular accident with resulting hemiplegia.

Of course, significant environmental differences could have led either to a further divergence or to a closer approximation of the test scores. Had the brighter twin been exposed to circumstances conducive to maximum development and the maintenance of potential intellectual abilities, including protection from disease, and had her sister been handicapped by grossly inferior environmental constellations, accentuation of their differences in scores would have been the predicted outcome. A reversal of opportunities might have had the opposite effect, although such factors as may result in optimal performance during later life are still largely unknown. Detrimental effects are generally conceded for a few constellations such as those connected with institutionalization, while beneficial stimuli await definition. Utilization of the co-twin control method would be certain to furnish crucial information for the identification of pertinent variables.

The potential merits of studies designed to determine both relatively advantageous and relatively deleterious conditions need not be stressed at a time when patients with senile deterioration demand a major share of psychiatric attention. The fact that hereditary components tend to exert a measurable influence upon individual resistance to senescent decline does require emphasis. Too often, the demonstration of genic elements has been equated with "predestination" toward disease, defect, deficiency, and demise. It may be true that a significant portion of human disability is attributable to heritable imperfections. In fact, it may be argued that immortality as such is precluded by man's genetic make-up as constituted at present. However, it is equally probable that fortuitous combinations of genes were responsible not only for the musical genius of Toscanini, but also for his longevity and comparative resistance to senile decline.

In conclusion, it may be stated that comprehensive investigations of genetic variations in disease resistance and survival potential are of fairly recent origin and relatively few in number. Resistance to a large number of diseases may be assumed to require the presence of the specific "normal" allele for a given trait. Occasionally, a single major mutant gene may have protective value. For the most common varieties of degenerative diseases as well as for significant variations in the potential life span, the complex interactions of different gene products with each other and with diverse exogenous factors have not as yet been disentangled. Observations of changes in similar phenotypes under varied outside influences (controlled twin studies) are certain to provide valuable clues to the recognition of disease-producing or disease-inhibiting agents which could not easily be obtained in any other manner.

Hence, it is justified to say that through the identification of individuals with potentially decreased resistance to specific diseases and through properly applied techniques of prophylactic and therapeutic management, significant reductions in both morbidity and mortality might be achieved for a considerable segment of the population. In general, the human organism, given the appropriate assortment of genes and adequate life conditions, possesses remarkable abilities to adapt itself to the manifold stresses of its ever changing surroundings.

REFERENCES

1. ADLERSBERG, D.: Hypercholesteremia with predisposition to atherosclerosis: An inborn error of lipid metabolism. Am. J. Med. 11:600, 1951.
2. ALLISON, A. C.: Protection afforded by the sickle-cell trait against subtertian malarial infection. Brit. M. J. 1:290, 1954.
3. ——, AND CLYDE, D. F.: Malaria in African children with deficient erythrocyte glucose-6-phosphate dehydrogenase. Brit. M. J. 1: 1346, 1961.
4. BITTNER, J. J.: Some possible effects of nursing on the mammary gland tumor incidence in mice. Science 84: 162, 1936.
5. ——, Genetic concepts in mammary cancer in mice. Ann. New York Acad. Sc. 71: 943, 1958.
6. BURNET, F. M.: Immunological recognition of self. Science 133: 307, 1961.
7. BUSK, T., CLEMMESEN, J., AND NIELSEN, A.: Twin studies and other genetical investigations in the Danish Cancer Registry. Brit. J. Cancer 2: 156, 1948.
8. CAMPBELL, A. H.: The association of lung cancer and tuberculosis. Australasian Ann. Med. 10: 129, 1961.
9. CARTER, C. O., AND SIMPKISS, M.: The "carrier" state in nephrogenic diabetes insipidus. Lancet 2: 1069, 1956.
10. CHILDS, B., GRUMBACH, M. M., AND VAN WYK, J. J.: Virilizing adrenal hyperplasia: A genetic and hormonal study. J. Clin. Invest. 35: 213, 1956.
11. COLETTE, A. T., AND LINSEMANN, K.: A family pedigree of basal cell carcinoma of the skin. Second Internat. Conf. Hum. Genet. (Rome 1961). Amsterdam, Excerpta Medica, 1961.
12. CRITTENDEN, L. B.: An interpretation of familial aggregation based on multiple genetic and environmental factors. Ann. New York Acad. Sc. 91: 769, 1961.
13. DEAN, G., AND BARNES, H. D.: The inheritance of porphyria. Brit. M. J. 2: 89, 1955.
14. DOYLE, A. E., AND FRASER, J. R. E.: Essential hypertension and inheritance of vascular reactivity. Lancet 2: 509, 1961.
15. DUBLIN, T. D., AND BLUMBERG, B. S.: An epidemiologic approach to inherited disease susceptibility. Pub. Health Rep. 76: 499, 1961.
16. DUKES, C. E.: Familial intestinal polyposis. Ann. Eugenics 17: 1, 1952.
17. EVANS, D. A. P., AND CLARKE, C. A.: Pharmacogenetics. Brit. M. Bull. 17: 234, 1961.
18. FALEK, A., et al.: Longevity and intellectual variations in a senescent twin population. J. Gerontol. 15: 305, 1960.
19. FEINGOLD, L.: A psychometric study of senescent twins. Unpublished doctoral dissertation. New York, Columbia University, 1950.
20. HANDLER, P. (ED.): Radiation and aging. Fed. Proc. 20 (no. 2, suppl. 8), 1961.
21. HARVALD, B., AND HAUGE, M.: A catamnestic investigation of Danish twins. Danish M. Bull. 3: 150, 1956.
22. HERNDON, C. N.: Basic contributions to medicine by research in genetics. J.A.M.A. 177: 695, 1961.
23. HIEGER, I.: Carcinogenesis. New York, Academic Press, 1961.
24. HIRSCHHORN, K., AND WILKINSON, C. F.: The mode of inheritance in essential familial hypercholesterolemia. Am. J. Med. 26: 60, 1959.
25. JARVIK, L. F., AND FALEK, A.: Cancer rates in aging twins. Am. J. Human Genet. 13: 413, 1961.
26. ——, and ——: Comparative data on cancer in aging twins. Cancer, in press.
27. ——, et al.: Changing intellectual functions in senescent twins. Acta Genet. 7: 421, 1957.

28. ———.: Survival trends in a senescent twin population. Am. J. Human Genet. 12: 170, 1960.

29. ———.: Longitudinal study of intellectual changes in senescent twins. Fifth Internat. Congr. Geront. (San Francisco, 1960), in press.

30. KALLMANN, F. J.: Genetic factors in aging: Comparative and longitudinal observations on a senescent twin population. In Hoch, P. H. and Zubin, J., Eds.: Psychopathology of Aging. New York, Grune & Stratton, 1961.

31. ———, ASCHNER, B., AND FALEK, A.: Comparative data on longevity, adjustment to aging, and causes of death in a senescent twin population. In Gedda, L., Ed.: Novant'anni delle Leggi Mendeliane. Rome; Istituto Gregorio Mendel, 1956.

32. ———, AND JARVIK, L. F.: Twin data on genetic variations in resistance to tuberculosis. In Gedda, L., Ed.: Genetica della Tubercolosi e dei Tumori. Rome, Istituto Gregorio Mendel, 1958.

33. ———, and ———: Individual differences in constitution and genetic background. In Birren, J. E., Ed.: Handbook of Aging and the Individual. Chicago, Univ. Chicago Press, 1959.

34. ———, AND REISNER, D.: Twin studies on the significance of genetic factors in tuberculosis. Am. Rev. Tuberc. 47: 549, 1943.

35. ———, AND SANDER, G.: Twin studies on aging and longevity. J. Hered. 39: 349, 1948.

36. KLEEMEIER, R. W.: Intellectual changes in the senium or death and the I. Q. Presidential address, Division on Maturity and Old Age. Am. Psychol. A., Sept. 1, 1961.

37. LI, C. C.: Genetic methods for epidemiological investigations: A synthesis. Ann. New York Acad. Sc. 91: 806, 1961.

38. LURIE, M. B., ABRAMSON, S., AND HEPPELSTON, A. C.: On the response of genetically resistant and susceptible rabbits to the quantitative inhalation of human type tubercle bacilli and the nature of resistance to tuberculosis. J. Exper. Med. 95: 119, 1952.

39. MACKLIN, M. T.: Inheritance of retinoblastoma in Ohio. A.M.A. Arch. Ophth. 62: 842, 1959.

40. MARKS, P. A.: Biochemical aspects of red cell aging and drug-induced hemolytic anemia: A review. Nouv. Rev. Hemat., in press.

41. McKUSICK, V. A.: Genetic factors in cardiovascular diseases. II. Disorders of primarily genetic etiology. Mod. Concepts Cardiovasc. Dis. 28: 547, 1959.

42. ———: Genetic factors in cardiovascular diseases. J. Am. Geriat. Soc. 9: 465, 1961.

43. MEDAWAR, P. B.: The Uniqueness of the Individual. New York, Basic Books, 1957.

44. ———: Immunological tolerance. Science 133: 303, 1961.

45. NIELSEN, A., AND CLEMMESEN, J.: Twin studies in the Danish Cancer Registry, 1942-55. Brit. J. Cancer 11: 327, 1957.

46. OSBORNE, R. H.: The "host factor" in disease: Genetic and environmental interaction. Ann. New York Acad. Sc. 91: 602, 1961.

47. OSTER, I. I.: Genetic aspects of mutagen-induced life-shortening. Second Internat. Conf. Hum. Genet. (Rome, 1961). Amsterdam, Excerpta Medica, 1961.

48. PARÉ, J. A. P., et al.: Hereditary cardiovascular dysplasia. Am. J. Med. 31: 37, 1961.

49. PLANANSKY, K., AND ALLEN, G.: Resistance to pulmonary tuberculosis. Am. J. Human Genet. 5: 322, 1953.

50. RANNEY, H.: Abnormal hemoglobins. Paper presented at 110th annual meeting of Am. Med. Assoc., Section on Experimental Medicine and Therapeutics, June 27, 1961.

51. RHYNAS, P. O. W., AND NEWCOMBE, H. B.: A heritable change in radiation resistance of strain L mouse cells. Exper. Cell Res. 21: 326, 1960.

52. ROBERTS, J. A. F.: Multifactorial inheritance in relation to normal and abnormal traits. Brit. M. Bull. 17: 241, 1961.

53. RODERICK, T. H., AND STORER, J. B.: Correlation between mean litter size and mean life span among twelve inbred strains of mice. Science 134: 48, 1961.

54. SAXÉN, E., AND PENTTINEN, K.: Host factors in cell culture: Further studies on the growth controlling action of fresh human serum. J. Nat. Cancer Inst. 26: 1367, 1961.

55. SCHNYDER, U. W.: Family allergies and antibody formation. Second Internat. Conf. Hum. Genet. (Rome, 1961). Amsterdam, Excerpta Medica, 1961.

56. SCHWEITZER, M. D.: Genetic determinants of communicable disease. Ann. New York Acad. Sc. 91: 730, 1961.

57. SHERMAN, W. B., AND KESSLER, W. R.: Allergy in Pediatric Practice. St. Louis, Mosby, 1957.

58. SINISCALCO, M., et al.: Favism and thalassaemia in Sardinia and their relationship to malaria. Nature 190: 1179, 1961.

59. STEINBERG, A. G.: The genetics of acute leukemia in children. Cancer 13: 985, 1960.

60. THODAY, J. M.: Location of polygenes. Nature 191: 368, 1961.

61. v. VERSCHUER, O.: Die Bedeutung der Erbforschung für die praktische Medizin. Regensburger Jahrb. Aerztl. Fortbild. 3: 1, 1953.

62. WINTERS, R. W., et al.: Genetic study of familial hypophosphatemia and vitamin D resistant rickets with a review of the literature. Medicine 37: 97, 1958.

4

The Contribution of Behavior Genetics to the Study of Behavior

JERRY HIRSCH, Ph.D.

IT IS INDEED AN UNUSUAL PLEASURE for me to participate in this symposium. For a psychologist this is a very special occasion. It represents a milestone which signifies the winning in two branches of science of a most important battle against nescience and misunderstanding. Dr. Kallmann, the chairman of this anniversary symposium, has played a key role in dispelling the cloud of misinformation and misconception that shrouded large areas of both psychiatry and psychology. In very uncritical fashion, unfortunately, the majority of workers in these two fields for too long accepted a point of view dogmatically summarized in 1924 by John Broadus Watson, the father of the behaviorist movement, when he proclaimed "Our conclusion, then, is that we have no real evidence of the inheritance of traits . . . I am going beyond my facts and I admit it, but so have the advocates of the contrary and they have been doing it for many thousands of years."[8]

All of us know how Dr. Kallmann and his associates have been unravelling the story of the role that inheritance plays in many behavioral malfunctions. For those of us in cognate branches of science, this anniversary symposium provides an opportunity to take both a retrospective and prospective look at our own fields. My assignment is to examine the implications for the experimental analysis of behavior, the traditional province of academic psychology, of the recent developments in behavior genetics.

A large part of the hard core subject matter of experimental psychology is to be found under the rubrics that categorize its two major methodologies: psychophysics and conditioning. Psychophysical methods are used to study the relations between variations in responding and variations in the stimuli to which an organism is responding. A typical problem in psychophysics is the study of discrimination: How does the size of the interval between stimuli which are just noticeably different along dimensions like heaviness or loudness vary as a function of the magnitude of the physical stimulus. Conditioning describes a set of procedures for the study of the modification of behavior by manipulating previous experience.

There are, of course, many other ways in which psychologists study behavior; for example, by building mathematical models of behavior, administering

The author wishes to express his indebtedness for the financial assistance, which he received in this study in the form of grant-in-aid No. G13595 from the National Science Foundation.

drugs, manipulating the nervous, endocrine and other physiological systems, and so forth. Most of these approaches are, by and large, the application to the study of behavior of methods from other disciplines. Since the number of parameters influencing behavior is probably unlimited, it is reasonable to expect that the psychologist will borrow investigative procedures from many sources.

The application of methods to the study of problems calls for certain assumptions about the nature of the material under study. The assumption most widely made in psychophysical and conditioning studies is that repeated observations represent observations of the same thing. Regardless of whether a given procedure for observing behavior is applied to a single organism on different occasions or to different organisms on either the same or different occasions, within the limits of both sampling and experimental error, not only is it expected that the same response will be observed, but also it is assumed that the same mechanism must underlie the observed behaviors. Hence, any variation that occurs in the observed behavior can be ascribed to sampling and experimental error and, so the argument goes, if sufficiently rigorous controls are applied to the conditions of observations, variation might either be eliminated or greatly reduced.

In an earlier discussion of individual differences in behavior and their genetic basis,[3] an attempt was made to explain why behavioral variations among organisms are expected to occur under most conditions, no matter how pure the methods of observation. In fact, contrary to widespread conviction in psychology, the more refined and sensitive the method of observing behavior, the less likely is it that members of any biparental species will behave exactly alike.

Since similar assumptions about the uniformity of the material under investigation are often made in physiology—the field of biology which has exerted a particularly strong influence on academic psychology—our understanding may be improved by an analysis of the difference between the organisms whose behavior is studied by the psychologist and the systems whose functioning is studied by the physiologist.

In the study of physiological systems such as the adrenals, gonads or any of the other endocrines, or any of the segmental reflexes of the central nervous system, anatomical verification is made, either pre- or post-experimentally, of the normality of the material whose functioning has been under study. Ostensibly, psychologists do the same thing in the study of behavior. Normal organisms are observed, such as rats, monkeys, flies or college sophomores.

However, there is a critical difference in the meaning of normality as operationally determined in the two disciplines. The physiologist chooses a normal animal; that is to say, one that looks healthy and in no way appears unusual. He then makes anatomical or even histological and biochemical verification of the normality of the particular system studied, and not infrequently of some related or adjacent systems to boot. The psychologist chooses a normal appearing animal for behavior study, too. However, he rarely performs anatomical examinations or autopsies, unless he happens to have a specific physiological interest, in which case he may operate in a manner very similar to the physiologist.

It is important to recognize the difference between the types of system with which the two disciplines are concerned. For example, the nerve physiologist may be engaged in a study of the properties of a particular subsystem in a complex integration of a large number of subsystems. The accumulated evidence shows how the form and function of these systems tend to vary among the members of a population. However, the variance in any one of the systems studied by the physiologist may be considered as relatively homogeneous in comparison with the kind of variation to be taken into account by the student of behavior who observes individual differences.

In the study of behavior, we deal with the integration of all the systems in the physiologist's lexicon. Even if we postulate that every one of those systems is distinguished by homogeneous variation of the kind that the statistician would call "in control" on the quality control chart for a manufacturing process, [7] the many possible combinations and integrations of those systems, that go to make up the members of a population, cannot be assumed to yield a homogeneous distribution of responses with respect to any behavioral measures. In fact, purely logical analysis points to negative deviates from some of those distributions, which will combine with positive deviates from others. Both kinds of extreme deviates are likely to combine with centrally located ones from still others no less frequently than will deviates of similar algebraic sign and magnitude combine from all distributions.

This state of affairs would not complicate matters unduly if there were only a single physiological system underlying every form of behavior. For instance, if mating behavior were solely dependent on the gonads, or escape behavior on the adrenals, then the same kind of distribution might be expected for both the behavior and the underlying system. There is a strong conviction among some militant students of behavior that the "real" explanation must be reductionistic.

In its most extreme form, this point of view asserts that a given bit of behavior cannot be understood until its physical basis has been worked out and the search for the physical basis proceeds along physiological, biochemical and/or genetical lines, depending on the skills and predilections of the investigators. During the last few decades, however, extensive work on the biological correlates of behavior has made it increasingly clear that behavior is the integration of many of the systems comprising the organism rather than the expression of any one of them. Hence, an organism that is richly endowed with the components of one subset of systems, and poorly endowed with those of another, is not likely to behave in the same manner as another organism with an entirely different balance of endowments. The obviousness of this fact is well illustrated by the various breeds of dogs and horses.

In laboratory experiments, some rats learn their way through mazes readily on the basis of visual cues while others do better on the basis of predominantly kinaesthetic ones. A series of studies of domestication in the rat[5] revealed the kinds of differences in organization that can co-exist as alternative forms within a species. The same experiments disclosed some of the relations between behavior and the component subsystems that are alternative possibilities. In domesticated rats, activity as measured in a revolving drum was found to be controlled by the gonads. Normal rats registered a daily activity score of about

18,000 revolutions, while gonadectomized rats scored only a few hundred revolutions. Cortisone therapy was sufficient to maintain a high activity level in the gonadectomized rats. However, when the same experiment was performed on wild rats, the presence or absence of gonads made no detectable difference in measured activity.

Further study of the differences between laboratory and wild rats revealed that wild rats have much larger adrenals, and laboratory rats have much larger gonads. So it appears that activity may be under the control of adrenal output in the one case, and gonadal output in the other.

Here we see how *behavior genetics* contributes to the study of behavior in two of its most fundamental aspects: *methodology* and *conceptualization*. Its methodological contribution is simply breeding as a technique for fashioning and refashioning the very organisms whose behavior is studied. Never before has the student of behavior had available a technique powerful enough to influence, without insult, every cell in the body of the behaving organism.

The example of the relations between activity and the endocrines serves to illustrate some consequences of reproductive isolation and selective breeding. Actually, the application of breeding techniques of this kind brought to light three relationships among three variables: the dependent variable, activity, proved to be correlated with two independent variables, adrenal function and gonadal function. Furthermore, these two independent variables appear to be mutually interdependent in that they interact in their relations with measured activity.

Conceptually, behavior genetics brings to the study of behavior the idea of heterogenic, biparental populations with the manifold multivalued dimensions of allelic variation that comprise their gene pools. It has also contributed the realization that under a given set of environmental conditions, the composition of each organism in a population is determined by the random sample of allelic values and genic combinations, that nature's meiotic lottery deals to that organism at anaphase segregation and gametic recombination.

Empirically, behavior genetics has accumulated from diverse sources an impressive body of evidence demonstrating that wherever it has been sought, a correlation has been found between genotypic variations and individual differences in behavior. In their excellent review of the literature on heredity and behavior, Fuller and Thompson[2] call attention to "the ubiquity of genetic effects." According to these investigators, "quantitative measurement of behavior combined with genetic techniques finds an influence of heredity in insects, rats, and men, both in behavior which is relatively unmodifiable . . . and in behavior which is the outcome of a long period of development . . ." (p. 137). Their conclusion is that a "significant contribution of behavior genetics is its documentation of the fact that two individuals of superficially similar phenotype may be quite different genotypically and respond in completely different fashion when treated alike" (p. 318). In other words, behavior genetics furnishes the student of behavior with advance information both about the material on which he must make his observations and about some features of the distribution of those observations.

Obviously, this is a major advance over that unhappy state of affairs which generated a discouragingly large number of attempts to explain behavior by building elaborate models to account for the performance of "organisms that can be considered identical at the start of an experiment . . . " (p. 3).[1]

By combining and attempting to integrate various features of evolutionary genetics, population genetics and physiological genetics, the discipline of behavior genetics brings a radically new perspective to research on behavior and its biological correlates. The key to this new approach lies in the breeding techniques of classic genetics for selection, inbreeding, hybridization and test-cross analysis. Technically, these procedures have long been known. Nevertheless, their implications for the study of behavior seem to have escaped the notice of all but a few people like Stockard in the previous generation and Benson Ginsburg in the present generation. It appears that most thinking about behavior tends to be cross-sectional, normative and static, rather than in terms of the ontogeny of behavior in organisms that can only exist as members of populations, all of which follow their own unique paths of evolutionary divergence.

Thinking in the behavioral sciences has for the most part shown the tendency to be both ontogenetically and phylogenetically static. Rigorous study of behavior is usually prosecuted by the method of group differences, with the influences of both environmental conditions and physiological mechanisms on the behavior of normal organisms being assessed experimentally by comparing behavior patterns in the presence and in the absence of a given condition. For example, the progress of learning is studied in the presence and absence either of reinforcement or of one of the lobes of the brain. As a rule, individual and population differences are considered irrelevant, if only because their study would divert attention from the central problem of analyzing the mechanisms controlling behavior. Conveniently, the assumption is made that the same mechanisms must be involved wherever and whenever the behavior occurs. Promising exceptions to this practice in our time have been the ethology movement in zoology and some recent work on early experience in psychology.

Just as the parsing of a sentence provides an understanding of the sentence in terms of its elementary units and their organization, so, by means of the Mendelian techniques of hybridization and testcrossing, can behavior genetics accomplish an elegant dissection of the total organism under study and a subsequent re-assembling of its component parts into an array of alternative organizations. The understanding to be achieved through such analyses will give us an urgently needed insurance against the inferring of causal connections from nonessential correlations.

According to research started by Krech, Rosenzweig and Bennett in 1953, differences in the concentration of the enzyme cholinesterase (ChE) in the brain were found to be correlated with differences in behavior between two strains of rats. High ChE concentration seemed to be associated with better learning. This report was followed by a spate of publications, doctoral theses and symposium contributions, all of which described various aspects of the presumed relationship (cf. ref. 6).

The discovery of this relationship was announced as a very important advance. After all, the processes in the brain underlying learning have to be chemical in nature, and here was the first real breakthrough into the brain chemistry of learning. From the psychologist's standpoint, the establishment of a relationship between such a basic neurochemical system as the choline acety-lase-acetylcholine-cholinesterase system and behavior implied that the physical basis of behavior was finally being unravelled at a fundamental level.

Six years later, however, indications of the opposite relationship between ChE concentration and learning were observed in both the progeny of hybrids between the two strains in which the originally positive relationship had been found and in new strains developed by selective breeding for enzyme concentration.[4,6] From the point of view of behavior genetics, the operations necessary to pinpoint the nature of such an apparent relationship are simple and straightforward.

Is such a correlation essential or fortuitous? The geneticist would hypothesize that two distinct phenotypic variables were found to be correlated, one chemical and the other behavioral. Genetically speaking, a phenotypic correlation means one of two things: either the pleiotropic effects of a single genetic system or the linkage of two or more genetic systems. The distinction between these alternatives in the rat requires a simple experiment and less than one year's work: hybridization of the strains showing the correlation, interbreeding of their F_1 hybrid progeny at sexual maturity, and measurement of the correlation in the F_2 progeny. If more than a single locus is involved, and not a small number of very closely linked loci, the implicated genes will assort independently and their original phenotypic correlations will break up. On the other hand, if the correlation is the result of pleiotropy, it will reappear in the F_2 generation.

Thus, the pursuit of the will-o-the-wisp, called the physical basis of behavior in the name of causal analysis, can now be looked at in a much broader perspective. Many distinguishable systems exist in the body, whose integration and coordination make up the behaving organism. In order to be understood in relation to behavior, each system should be studied with respect to its own internal dynamics. It is also essential that the dynamics of the behavior be fully described and that the particular functional balance achieved by the integration of the relevant systems as well as their coordination with the behavior be worked out for each organism or group of organisms to be studied. We cannot understand the behavior of an organism without understanding the organism not only as an integrated and coordinated system responsive to its environment, but also as a member of a population with a unique evolutionary history adapting it to the niche it presently occupies.

It is fair to state, therefore, that behavior genetics represents the first attempt at studying behavior, which has achieved an explicit formulation of these questions and provides us with an empirically validated methodology for performing the appropriate analyses.

REFERENCES

1. BUSH, R. R., AND MOSTELLER, F.: Stochastic Models for Learning. New York, Wiley, 1955.
2. FULLER, J. L., AND THOMPSON, W. R.: Behavior Genetics. New York, Wiley, 1960.
3. HIRSCH, J.: Individual differences in behavior and their genetic basis. In Bliss, E. L., Ed.: Roots of Behavior. New York, Hoeber, 1962.

4. McGaugh, J. L.: Some neurochemical factors in learning. Unpublished doctoral dissertation, Berkeley, Univ. of California, 1959.
5. Richter, C. P.: The effects of domestication and selection on the behavior of the Norway rat. J. Nat. Cancer Inst. 15: 727, 1954.
6. Rosenzweig, M. R., Krech, D., and Bennett, E. L.: A search for relations between brain chemistry and behavior. Psychol. Bull. 57: 476, 1960.
7. Wallis, W. A., and Roberts, H. V.: Statistics, a New Approach. Glencoe, Ill., Free Press, 1956.
8. Watson, J. B.: Behaviorism. New York, Norton, 1924.

5

Some Statistical Principles for Efficient Design of Surveys and Experiments

W. EDWARDS DEMING, Ph.D.

SKILLS AND RESOURCES for research are always limited. Hence, an ever-present problem in the planning stages of any investigation is how to use the available skills and resources to the best advantage. To the statistician, this is the problem of efficient design, namely, to maximize the amount of information per unit cost, or per man-day, within any restrictions imposed. Statistical theory is the statistician's tool for design.

AIM AND SCOPE OF THE REPORT

It may be pointed out that *sample design* is much more than a procedure for the selection of cases for investigation. Sample design includes, in the planning stages, organizational assistance to the experts in the subject matter (human genetics, biochemistry, agricultural science, etc.). The aim is to formulate the problems of the survey in statistical terms so that the information to be obtained from the survey will be maximally useful.

Sample design includes the choice of sampling units as well as the search for procedures and formulas for calculating estimates of whatever characteristics constitute the aim of the survey. It requires, moreover, plans of selection and estimation that will permit, without undue labor and expense, calculation of standard errors and tests of significance. It includes tests to measure the biases of nonresponse, tests to detect and measure the effects of human errors in carrying out the prescribed procedures, including the recording, coding, punching, and tabulating.

Finally, statistical theory and experience are helpful in the interpretation of results. At the completion of the study, the investigator wishes to draw whatever conclusions seem warranted. Statistically, it will have to be determined, therefore, whether certain hypotheses are apparently confirmed, or left in doubt, or require re-examination.

The prescription of aims for a study is never statistical. No amount of statistical knowledge will indicate the need of an investigation in medical, research, nor in any other kind of research. The perception of a problem and the initial prescription of aims for the survey come from substantive knowledge in such fields as medicine in general or one of its specialities. The statistician's part in a study is to maximize its utility and to protect it from unwarranted and uneconomical expenditures—in short, to obtain the most possible information for the skill and resources that are available.

This report gives two illustrations of the use of statistical theory directed toward efficient design. The illustrations will come from work in several departmental research projects. However, the theory and principles have wide application to other studies in medical research, as well as to demography, sociology, current government statistical series, censuses, and to other problems that the statistician encounters. The wide applicability of statistical theory comes from its abstract nature, as the symbols in any theory are unmindful of the uses that man may make of them.

The first illustration will deal with the design of an *enumerative* study[1,ch.7] where the aim is to count the number of people that have certain characteristics. The second illustration will deal with the design of an *analytic* study[1] where the aim is to detect causes of differences, and to measure their effects. Both illustrations will bear on the problem of allocation of skill and of other resources.

ILLUSTRATION OF ALLOCATION OF RESOURCES IN AN ENUMERATIVE STUDY

As stated before, in an enumerative problem, the aim is to count. Let us take for illustration the study of the fertility of schizophrenics which we are now working on. One enumerative aim of the study, for example, is to estimate the number of schizophrenics by sex and age in the hospital population admitted (or readmitted) during 1934-36. Another enumerative aim is to estimate the number of children born to schizophrenics before onset, before first admission, before second admission; likewise for admissions during 1954-56.

The frame in the study is the hospital admissions recorded in mental hospitals in the State of New York during the years 1934-36, and during the years 1954-56. The sampling unit is the hospital admission. The admissions in any hospital have serial numbers; hence, one may draw from any hospital, by random numbers, any desired number of admissions.

Any hospital admission may be schizophrenic, or may not be. If we were to study a 100 per cent sample of all hospital admissions in the years 1934-36 (or 1954-56), and discard those that are not schizophrenic, the remainder would be all the schizophrenics that were admitted (or readmitted) to hospitals over that period. Hence, to draw a sample of one in eight schizophrenics of any age or sex, admitted during the years 1934-36, it is only necessary to draw a sample of hospital admissions for that period; then to study each admission by means of hospital records to decide whether the case was schizophrenic or otherwise. If the case is schizophrenic, retain it for investigation; if not schizophrenic, reject it as a blank, as it does not fall within the scope of this investigation.

As the definition of schizophrenia is a medical and not a statistical problem, the examination of each case requires the proficiency of a psychiatrist. The rules for examination would be the same whether we were to use sampling or a complete coverage. It may be mentioned in passing that, for medical reasons, first admissions 60 years old or over at the time of admission were not eligible for the study, nor cases 14 years or under.

Formula for the Sampling Variance of the Mean in an Enumerative Study

Assume that there are $\bar{N}$ schizophrenics in each hospital, and that we draw with random numbers, without stratification, a sample of $\bar{n}$ schizophrenics from each of m hospitals, the m hospitals themselves being drawn at random from the M mental hospitals in the State of New York. On page 38, a simple modification of the formula takes care of variation in size. Let $\bar{x}$ be the average of some characteristic per sampling unit. Then the formula for the variance of $\bar{x}$ will be

$$\text{Var } \bar{x} = \frac{M-m}{M-1} \frac{\sigma_b^2}{m} + \frac{\bar{N}-\bar{n}}{\bar{N}-1} \frac{\sigma_w^2}{m\bar{n}}$$

The symbol σ_w^2 is the average variance between the $\bar{N}$ sampling units within a hospital, and σ_b^2 is the variance between the means of the sampling units in the M hospitals. For example, to illustrate numerical values of σ_w and σ_b, we may work with the number of children ever born to schizophrenic females ever married and in the age group 20-39. The number of children will vary from 0 to possibly 7 or 8 per patient in any one hospital. The standard deviation σ_w between patients[2,p.260] would then be about .24 $\times$ 8, call it 2 for the sake of simplicity. A few women might have more than eight children, but their effect on the variance may be neglected, as their number is small. The mean number of children per schizophrenic female in the various hospitals in New York State might range normally from perhaps 1.5 to 2.5; σ_b would then be about 1/6. These numerical values will be used later on.

The multiplier $(\bar{N} - \bar{n})/(\bar{N} - 1)$ in the above equation reduces the second term on the right to 0 if the sample includes all the $\bar{N}$ patients in each of the m hospitals, for then $\bar{n} = \bar{N}$, and $\bar{N} - \bar{n}$ will be 0. The multiplier $(M - m)/(M - 1)$ reduces the first term to 0 if all M hospitals are put into the sample, for then m = M, and M — m will be 0.

A Simple Cost-Function

Whatever be the numerical values of σ_b and σ_w, we may derive with little effort a very important principle of sampling for enumerative purposes. We start with an oversimplified assumption concerning costs, namely, that the cost of drawing one more schizophrenic into the sample will be c dollars, regardless of which one of the M hospitals the case comes from. This assumption is about right for some kinds of surveys, although we can improve on it for the present study (see next section). We proceed with it here, nevertheless, because it leads unmistakably and with ease to a very important principle of sample design, namely, to disperse the sample, even in circumstances where costs are not so simple to represent.

The problem is to find the optimum values of $\bar{n}$ and m. The total sample will be

$$n = m\,\bar{n}$$

On the simple assumption just described, the total cost of the study will be

$$C = c\,n = c\,m\,\bar{n}$$

regardless of which hospital any of the n cases may come from.

The question is how to vary m and ñ so as to minimize Var x̄ while keeping the cost C constant. The variance of x̄, for a fixed cost C, will now be

$$\text{Var } \bar{x} = \frac{\sigma_b{}^2}{m} + \frac{c\sigma_w{}^2}{C}$$

because $m\bar{n} = C/c$. We observe that the second term is constant; it neither increases nor decreases as we vary the number m of hospitals in the study. This is so because if m increases, ñ must decrease to keep the cost C constant. The first term, however, decreases as m increases. The only way to decrease Var x̄ is obviously to add more hospitals to the study, i.e., to make m big and ñ small. In fact, the best possible sample, under the cost-function assumed, would be to take ñ = 1. In other words, we should take only one schizophrenic from each hospital, and go into enough hospitals (i.e., make m big enough) to reduce Var x̄ to the level desired.

Stated simply, what our theory tells us is to disperse the sample, rather than concentrate it into a few hospitals. A refinement in the cost-function, as we shall soon see, leads to the same principle.

Refinement in the Cost-Function

Our assumption about costs may be refined by taking account of the fact that, in the study of schizophrenics, it costs less to admit a new case into the study if it is drawn from a hospital where we are already working, rather than from a hospital not yet in the study. It should be borne in mind that, in this study, there will be the cost of adding a hospital. To arrive at a workable rule, we assume that it costs c_1 dollars, on the average, to bring into the sample one more hospital, and that this cost c_1 will be the same whether we draw one schizophrenic or 10 or 100. The cost c_1 is the average cost of paying a visit to the director of a hospital to describe the purpose of the study, to meet the supervisor who will later on assist our fieldworkers when they come to draw the sample of admissions; and to study the hospital records; and to discover, in advance, any special problems with respect to the records or use thereof.

We may further suppose that it costs c_2 dollars, on the average, to study one more admission in a hospital, once the hospital is in the sample. The cost c_2 will be chiefly the average cost of studying the hospital records to decide whether a case is schizophrenic or not, plus the average cost of transcribing the information required for an admission, and of carrying out any fieldwork that may be necessary to complete the records on a patient. The cost c_2 also includes the costs of tabulation. The total cost of the study will now be

$$C = mc_1 + m\bar{n}c_2$$

Compared with the previous cost-function, the special feature of this one is that it divides the cost into two parts: one part for the m hospitals in the study, and another part for the mñ cases within these hospitals.

The question arises again how to minimize Var x̄ by varying m and ñ while keeping the cost C constant. For an answer to this question, one may show by the ordinary methods of the calculus that the optimum value of ñ is

$$\bar{n} = \frac{\sigma_w}{\sigma_b} \sqrt{\frac{c_1}{c_2}}$$

This formula was first given simultaneously by W. A. Shewhart[3,p.389] and by L. H. C. Tippett[4,p.177] in 1931. As before, the optimum number m of hospitals to take into the study is whatever number reduces Var $\bar{x}$ to the level desired, or which consumes the allowable budget C. Thus, in summary, the procedure of allocation would be the following:

1. Calculate $\bar{n}$, based on plausible values of $\sigma_w : \sigma_b$ and of $c_1 : c_2$.

2. Substitute this number $\bar{n}$ into the cost-function $C = mc_1 + m\bar{n}c_2$ to find what number m of hospitals will consume the allowable budget C, or substitute $\bar{n}$ into the formula for Var $\bar{x}$ to find what number m will yield the precision desired.

Application to an Enumerative Survey

For a numerical example of the equation under discussion, we may return to the proposed values $\sigma_w = 2$ and $\sigma_b = 1/6$ as plausible standard deviations for the number of children ever born to married female schizophrenics. Suppose further that $c_1 = \$225$ and that $c_2 = \$25$. Then

$$\bar{n} = \frac{2}{1/6} \sqrt{\frac{225}{25}} = 36$$

The meaning of this finding is that, for any age group for which we require separate estimates, we should take about 36 women from the average hospital, and enough hospitals to build up the total sample required.

With this procedure, our refined assumption leads us to almost the same conclusions that we derived from the very simple cost-function assumed in previous paragraphs, but not to the extreme recommendation that $\bar{n}$ should be 1.

Some characteristic other than the number of children ever born would possibly have a different ratio for $\sigma_w : \sigma_b$, and might lead to some $\bar{n}$ slightly different. What one does in practice is to estimate in advance what $\sigma_w : \sigma_b$ might be for several important characteristics: then to observe by a number of such calculations, what appears to be a reasonable number for $\bar{n}$. The important point is the principle that comes forth; namely, that we should take a fairly small sample of cases from each hospital, and disperse the sample to enough hospitals.

This is a very important principle. Where it is used, it saves thousands of dollars every day in research and in industrial and agricultural production. It tells us that if the variability within a hospital is large, compared with the difference between hospitals, then we should take a fairly large sample from each hospital. On the other hand, as is more usual, hospitals are considerably different in character, for various reasons. They are under different directors. Some hospitals are located in metropolitan districts, while others are located in rural areas with distinct cultural and religious backgrounds. These differences between hospitals enlarge the denominator σ_b, reduce $\bar{n}$, and enlarge m, the optimum number of hospitals in the sample.

Let us consider how costs affect the allocation in an enumerative design. Our equation for $\bar{n}$ contains the factor $\sqrt{(c_1 : c_2)}$, which tells us that if it costs a great deal to go into a hospital to open it up for investigation (that is, if c_1 is large), then we should increase $\bar{n}$ and reduce the number m of hospitals in the sample to hold the cost C to the allowable budget. Converse remarks hold for the quantity c_2, the cost of investigating a single case. If the cost c_2 is fairly large, then we care not so much where the additional case is located, which means that we reduce $\bar{n}$ and go into more hospitals.

In short, the foregoing theory tells us what to do and, more specifically, what statistical characteristics of the sampling units we need to know approximately in the planning stages in order to design an efficient sample. It tells us that we only need to know the ratios $\sigma_w : \sigma_b$ and $c_1 : c_2$.

Parenthetically, it may be mentioned that a very helpful principle applies in the statistician's efforts to achieve efficiency. It so happens, as further theory shows, that rough values for the ratios $\sigma_w : \sigma_b$ and $c_1 : c_2$ are as good as exact values for allocation of skills and resources. The explanation comes from the fact that the graph of Var $\bar{x}$ against these ratios is very flat in the neighborhood of the optimum value of $\bar{n}$. This statement is especially true with respect to the ratio $c_1 : c_2$, because $c_1 : c_2$ occurs under the root-sign.

Thus, where our calculations lead to $\bar{n} = 36$, any size of sample between 28 and 50 would yield almost as much precision for the same cost for this characteristic as $\bar{n} = 36$. This wide range of acceptable size of sample usually takes care of the fact that different characteristics lead to slightly different optimum values of $\bar{n}$. Choice of some number over such a range is a lot different from taking $\bar{n} = 100$ or 150, as one might be tempted to do without the aid of statistical theory.

Two remarks may be interjected at this time. First, calculations like those that we have just made almost always lead to much smaller samples ($\bar{n}$) from each hospital than people are in the habit of taking, when they fail to use theory. Thus, suppose that without the aid of statistical theory, one were to draw a sample of 125 schizophrenics in an age group, instead of some number in the range 28 to 50. The loss of information would then be perhaps as much as 50 per cent. In other words, half the skills and resources expended on the study would be wasted.

Second, good research requires one to abide by the recommendations of theory. To do otherwise is to throw away some portion of the skills and physical resources available for the study. If the results of calculations lead to values of $\bar{n}$ and m that seem strikingly different from the values that one might have prescribed without the aid of statistical theory, then he must choose between two alternatives: (a) look carefully at his arithmetic and at the ratios $\sigma_w : \sigma_b$ and $c_1 : c_2$ that he used in his calculations; and possibly repeat the calculations with new ratios; or (b) resign his conscience, if possible, to accept a lower degree of precision in his estimates and comparisons than would be possible with values of $\bar{n}$ and m closer to optimum. There is no third possibility.

When the hospitals are not all the same size, the optimum allocation is embodied in the equation

$$\frac{n_i}{N_i} = \frac{\sigma_{wi}}{\sigma_b}\sqrt{\frac{c_{1i}}{c_{2i}}}$$

Here the subscript i refers to Hospital i. Usually the standard deviations σ_{wi} and the costs do not vary appreciably from one hospital to another, in which case, as in this study, the equation simplifies to

$$\frac{n_i}{N_i} = \text{constant}$$

indicating proportionate allocation of the sample. Thus, if we take a sample of 1 in 10 admissions in one hospital, we should take a sample of 1 in 10 admissions in another hospital.

ILLUSTRATION OF ALLOCATION OF RESOURCES IN AN ANALYTIC STUDY

The aim in an analytic study is to discover causes or sources of variation, or to learn whether some treatment or environmental condition produces an effect, and if so, how much.

Formula for the Sampling Variance in an Analytic Study

The general formula for the variance of the difference between two means $\bar{x}_A$ and $\bar{x}_B$, derived from samples of sizes n_A and n_B drawn by random numbers singly and without stratification from two groups of patients A and B is

$$\text{Var}\,(\bar{x}_A - \bar{x}_B) = \sigma_A^2/n_A + \sigma_B^2/n_B$$

wherein σ_A^2 and σ_B^2 are the variances between the patients within the hospitals in the two groups.

The optimum allocation of resources in analytic studies is different from the optimum allocation in enumerative problems. For analytic studies, the optimum allocation of skill and effort is found by setting

$$\frac{n_A}{n_B} = \frac{\sigma_A}{\sigma_B}\sqrt{\frac{c_B}{c_A}}$$

wherein c_A and c_B are the costs per case. One may note that the sizes of the groups A and B do not enter into this formula.[1, p.240]

It so happens that in most studies σ_A and σ_B will not be greatly different, nor the costs c_A and c_B. Under such circumstances, one may write the useful approximation

$$n_A = n_B$$

This is a very simple equation. It tells us that if we wish to find the effect of two different treatments, we simply take equal numbers of patients from each group, regardless of how many patients are in each group.

Of course, if we already have on hand observations on 100 patients from one source and on 1000 patients from another source, we do not discard data to make the two groups equal in size. We take what data we have, as it is too late to plan samples that would have been economical.

The enumerative and analytic problems are competitive; that is, the allocations are different. In an enumerative study, the size of sample is proportionate to the size of the hospital. For an analytic study, the size of sample would be the same for one group as for another, even though one group is ten times as big as the other. In carrying out a study that is simultaneously enumerative and analytic, we are confronted with the fact that efficient sample design for enumerative purposes may not be the best allocation for analytic purposes. Therefore, some compromise is usually necessary in a study that serves both aims. It may happen, of course, that the two groups under comparison are, by good fortune, about the same size.

Application to an Analytic Problem

A further aim of the study of schizophrenics is analytic, to discover differences between different types of orientation, or to discover differences between communities, or differences between the two periods, 1934-36 and 1954-56, or between the upper and lower parts of New York State. One might ask, for example, whether the number of readmissions per patient has increased between the two periods, or whether the proportion of married schizophrenics has changed, or the average age of admission (including readmission), or the number of children ever born. One might ask whether these characteristics differ between groups of hospitals, or between the upper and metropolitan parts of New York State. Again, we may bear in mind that the statement of aims in any problem is not statistical. Here, they belong to medical genetics.

The decision in the present study was to give preference to the enumerative aims of the study in each period. The sample was accordingly distributed among the hospitals in proportion to their sizes. Fortunately, because the number of admissions in the upper and lower portions in the state are not greatly different, being in the ratio of about one-third in the upper part to two-thirds in the lower part, this allocation caused no serious loss for analytic use.

ALLOCATION OF THE SAMPLE IN THE STUDY OF SCHIZOPHRENICS

Thus, on the basis of the foregoing theory, we arrived at the following steps for the selection of the sample of schizophrenics:

1. The size of sample will be 8000 admissions in 1934-36, and the same number in 1954-56.

2. Distribute the sample proportionately among all the hospitals in the study.

3. Decide the number of subsamples (10 in this case).[2]

4. Compute the zoning interval.

5. Draw 10 random numbers in each zone for each hospital. Each random number is a hospital consecutive number.

Use of Subsamples

The random numbers in the table draw the sample, not as one big sample, but as ten independent smaller samples, called subsamples, or — according to Mahalanobis[2,pp.186-187] who introduced their use in 1936 — an interpenetrating network of samples. There is a great advantage in the use of independent subsamples, as they facilitate estimation of the standard errors, and detection of human errors. Many illustrations of the use of subsamples appear in the author's book on sample design.[2] I include for illustration a portion of one of the sampling tables.

SAMPLING TABLE FOR THE METROPOLITAN INSTITUTIONS 1954-1956

Zone	1	2	3	4	5	6	7	8	9	10
0001 - 0080	0032	0015	0050	0055	0058	0041	0021	0079	0011	0054
0081 - 0160	0139	0087	0130	0096	0159	0129	0148	0106	0086	0095
0161 - 0240	0211	0228	0192	0197	0189	0217	0202	0193	0214	0163
etc.										

The sample of hospital admissions was naturally bigger than the desired number of schizophrenic patients that we hope to investigate. Actually, it was by intention about four times as big. In the first place, some trial studies showed that only about half the admissions are schizophrenic, and in the second place, the prediction was that it would be possible to follow up on only about half the cases selected but not now in the hospital.

In relation to the task of thinning the sample for the fieldwork—both for patients not now in the hospital and for relatives — it may be mentioned in conclusion that there is a further contribution which statistical theory can make toward conservation of resources. Many cases in this study, possibly 70 per cent of them, have left the hospital before they ended their reproductive ages. They will require further investigation, beyond information obtainable from hospital records, to ascertain whether any more children were born to these patients. Such information will be fairly easy to obtain when records of the Department of Mental Hygiene indicate that a patient was readmitted to a state hospital after 1936 or after 1956, respectively.

However, investigation of some cases can proceed only by attempts to find the patient, or to find some relative or other possible informants. Letters addressed to informants or relatives named in the hospital records, or to the patient himself, will undoubtedly yield some valid addresses. On the other hand, some letters will come back marked "Unknown," or "Deceased." Social workers may in some cases be able to find a patient. As a last resort, actual scouting to the last-known address of a relative, or of an informant, or of the patient himself, may be necessary. This is expensive, and requires time and skill.

At the point where the cost of further information suddenly rises to a relatively high figure, statistical theory indicates that one may wisely reduce the work-load by retaining for investigation only a randomly selected portion of such patients. The proportion to retain is determinable by consideration of costs. The formula for the optimum thinning ratio is $1 : \sqrt{r}$, where r is the ratio of the two costs. For example, if the average cost of further information rises to nine times the cost of acquiring the same information from records in the hospital, or by mail, then the optimum thinning-ratio for patients that require scouting would be $1 : 3$.

The actual thinning would be done by random numbers. Thus, for a ratio of 1:3, random numbers would retain one patient from every three consecutive patients. Examples of balanced thinning are given in the book previously mentioned.[2,p.337]

One would of course not do any thinning if it were necessary to retain all cases in order to achieve a prescribed goal of precision. What the statistical plan of thinning does is to yield the maximum amount of information (greatest precision) for a total allowable expenditure of skills and of resources for the entire investigation.

REFERENCES

1. DEMING, W. E.: Some Theory of Sampling. New York, Wiley, 1950.
2. ———: Sample Design in Business Research. New York, Wiley, 1960.
3. SHEWHART, W. A.: Economic Control of Quality of Manufactured Product. New York, Van Nostrand, 1931.
4. TIPPETT, L. H. C.: Methods of Statistics. London, Williams & Norgate, 1931.

6

Mating and Fertility Trends in Schizophrenia

CHARLES GOLDFARB, M.D., AND L. ERLENMEYER-KIMLING, PH.D.

PREVIOUS STUDIES of mating and fertility patterns in schizophrenia, conducted in different countries and at different times, have shown schizophrenic populations to be characterized by low rates of marriage and reproduction in comparison with their general populations.[1,4,5,7-9,12,13-15] The relative fertility of given genotypes in a population is designated as their adaptive value. In this sense, schizophrenics have been found to have a relatively low adaptive value. That biological infertility, however, is not the principal factor in the diminished reproductive rate has been demonstrated by studies, in which fertility of schizophrenics within marriage was found to be comparable to the marital fertility of the general population.[1,14,15]

Until recently, life expectancies for schizophrenics were relatively low, and the incidence of "social atrophy" comparatively high, probably due, at least in part, to prolonged confinement in mental institutions. Moreover, the reduced reproductive rates found in schizophrenic populations suggested a high probability of the phenomenon referred to by Dobzhansky as "genetic death."[3]

Advances in medical science may now be changing the expectations of the schizophrenic individual. Improvements in medical techniques and public health programs enhance the prevention, early detection, and control of such diseases as tuberculosis and pneumonitis to which schizophrenics tend to show lowered resistance.[1,8,10] At the same time, modern somatic therapies in psychiatry may permit the schizophrenic individual to function within the community at a higher level of integration during longer periods of remission. Thus there has been a building up of buffers that may not only reinforce the schizophrenic's chance of survival, but may also revitalize his social role.

Hand-in-hand with these developments which have benefited the physical and possibly the social stability of the affected individual may go changes in the marriage and fertility patterns of the schizophrenic population. Analysis of these changes requires consideration of corresponding trends in the general population. During the past two decades, there has been a notable rise in marriage and fertility rates in the United States. Among special factors contributing to this changing fertility pattern we find a marked trend toward earlier marriages with childbearing at younger ages, a decrease in the number of childless and one-child marriages, and an increase in marriages with two, three or four children.[2,6,11,16]

In evaluating the reproductive fitness of schizophrenics, the reproductive trends in the general population serve as a frame of reference. Changing patterns in the general population may be reflected in the marital and re-

42

productive patterns of schizophrenics. With the concurrent and independently determined influence of new medical achievements, an increase in the schizophrenics' rate of reproduction might now not only parallel, but relatively exceed the general one. If the reproductive gain is comparatively greater in schizophrenics than in the general population, the adaptive value of schizophrenics will be higher than it was previously, and their proportional contribution to the gene pool of succeeding generations will be expanded.

From a genetic as well as a psychiatric point of view, the possibility that schizophrenics are increasing their relative contribution to the gene pool has far-reaching implications. For this reason, the present statewide study has been undertaken with a twofold goal: (a) to study possible changes in schizophrenic mating and fertility patterns, including the specific problems of assortative mating and of differential pre- and post-psychotic patterns; (b) to examine the relationship between trends in the schizophrenic and general populations.

PROCEDURAL ASPECTS OF THE STUDY

Under the design of the study, a random sample of schizophrenic patients admitted to New York State mental hospitals during the three-year period 1934-36 is compared with a like sample admitted in 1954-56. All cases in the sample are reviewed and diagnostically verified before being accepted as index cases. A minimum sample of about 2400 schizophrenic cases will be obtained for each survey period, of which about 1200 will be investigated through direct field contact. The sampling design for the study has been discussed by Dr. Deming in Chapter 5.

Detailed marital and reproductive histories are obtained for each index case, with attention to the pre- and post-psychotic patterns. In this context, the terms "pre-psychotic" and "before disease onset" refer to the period before the earliest occurrence of psychiatric symptoms as recorded in the patient's case history.

Additional data needed for an analysis of all marriage and fertility aspects include hospitalization and treatment histories as well as such personal data as religion, education and occupation. Wherever possible, the psychiatric histories of the parents, siblings, children and spouses of the index cases are also recorded, as is information on the reproduction of the siblings. Special attention is given to the problem of assortative mating, and a detailed study of the marriages between two schizophrenics is in progress.

The first year of this study was spent in collecting data from three upstate hospitals and from two hospitals in the downstate metropolitan area. At present, marriage and fertility data are available for 1552 cases (approximately one-third of the final sample) up to the time of their admission during the survey years 1934-36 or 1954-56.

Obviously, the figures reported here are preliminary data, intended mainly to point out trends discernible at this stage of the investigation. Corrections will be applied for age at onset and at first admission, for number of admissions and total length of hospitalization, for duration of marriage, etc., when more complete data are available for detailed statistical analyses. This first report compares some trends in the schizophrenic population with those in the general population of the United States.

The term "admission" as used here refers to the admission of an index case to a state hospital during the years 1934-36 or 1954-56, regardless of whether it was a first, second, or later admission. Use of data relevant to the admission during the survey years provides a standard time-period for all cases, which would not be true of first admissions. Only legitimate live births are considered in the present fertility data. In future reports examination of illegitimacy and stillbirth rates may be warranted.

DATA ON MARRIAGES AND FERTILITY

Figure 1 presents the *age distributions* of the two samples by sex, at onset and at admission. At onset, the age distributions for the two samples of like sex are quite similar. At admission, there is a slight skewing toward the older

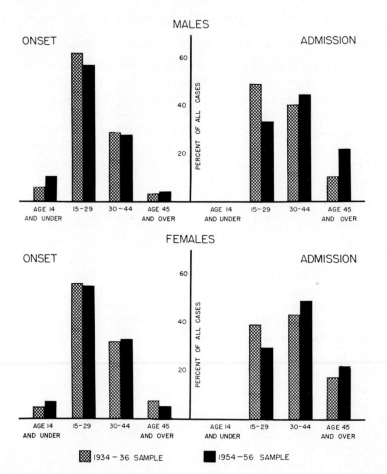

FIG. 1.   Age distribution of the two schizophrenic samples at onset and at admission.

age groups in the 1954-56 sample, compared with that of 1934-36. As seen in table 1, there is less than one year's difference between the samples in the mean age at onset, while the females of the 1954-56 sample were, on the

TABLE 1. AVERAGE AGE (MEAN AND STANDARD ERROR) AT DISEASE
ONSET AND AT SURVEY ADMISSION

Average	Males		Females	
	1934-36 (N = 380)	1954-56 (N = 319)	1934-36 (N = 491)	1954-56 (N = 362)
Age at onset	26.0 ± .45	25.1 ± .55	27.5 ± .46	27.0 ± .51
Age at admission	31.4 ± .54	36.0 ± .66	34.1 ± .52	36.7 ± .62
Onset-admission interval	5.4 ± .71	10.9 ± .86	6.6 ± .69	9.7 ± .81

average, admitted 2.5 years later than the 1934-36 cases, and the males 4.6 years later. Correspondingly, the average interval between onset and admission was longer for the 1954-56 sample.

Table 2 shows the per cent of schizophrenic index cases *ever-married* at onset and at admission to a hospital during the survey years. Several trends are indicated here. First, in agreement with previous studies [4, 8] the majority of all marriages occur before onset of the disease. Second, the proportion of married persons at onset appears to be higher in the 1954-56 sample than in the earlier sample. Among the 1954-56 females there were 5.4 per cent more married cases at onset than in the 1934-36 sample; among the males, 10.8 per cent more cases were married. The small dissimilarity in the age distributions at onset, shown in figure 1, is not sufficient to account for the increase in the marriage rate.

A third observation is that the 1954-56 sample shows a considerably increased frequency of marriages occurring in the interval between onset and admission (table 2). In fact, the percentage of post-onset marriages is approxi-

TABLE 2. MARRIAGE AND FERTILITY OF SCHIZOPHRENICS
AT DISEASE ONSET AND AT SURVEY ADMISSION
(ALL AGES, 15 AND OVER)

Survey period	Number of cases at admission	Per Cent Ever Married		Interval Between Onset and Admission			Total Children		Percent born between onset and admission
		At onset	At admission	Number marrying in interval	Per cent of marriages that occur in interval	Rate of marriage per year of interval	At onset	At admission	
			WOMEN						
1934-36	491*	51.3	54.2	27	10.1	4.1	405	539	24.9
1954-56	362*	56.7	66.3	49	20.4	5.0	276	441	37.4
			MEN						
1934-36	380†	22.1	24.7	15	15.9	2.8	146	183	20.2
1954-56	319‡	32.9	42.3	42	31.1	3.9	151	230	34.3

* 25 cases under age 15 at onset.
† 23 cases under age 15 at onset.
‡ 36 cases under age 15 at onset.

mately twice that of the earlier sample. Even with correction for the length of the interval between onset and admission, the rate of marriage per year of the interval indicates that the post-onset marriages of the 1954-56 sample exceed those of the 1934-36 sample.

Of the total number of children produced up to the time of admission, the majority were born before disease onset (table 2), as was found by earlier investigators.[4,7,8] However, just as more marriages were contracted between onset and admission in the 1954-56 sample, more children were also born in that interval than in the 1934-36 sample.

The nearest general census period for comparison with our 1934-36 sample was that of 1940. For the 1954-56 sample, the Current Population Reports of 1954 have been used as the best comparative source available.

Figure 2 presents graphically the per cent of schizophrenic cases in each age

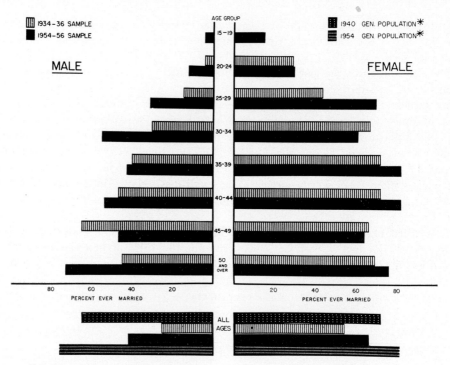

Fɪɢ. 2.　Marital status (per cent ever-married) of schizophrenics at admission compared with the general population.

group that were ever-married at admission. The per cent ever-married in the general population of the United States in 1940 and 1954 is also given for all ages combined. In both sexes, for almost every age group, there was a higher incidence of marriage among the 1954-56 schizophrenic cases than among the 1934-36 cases.

Although schizophrenics of both sexes continue to show a much lower frequency of marriage than the general population, the difference between the schizophrenic and general populations has narrowed in the later survey period for most of the age groups (table 3). For all ages combined, the proportion of married women in the 1934-36 sample was 18.2 per cent lower than in the general population, and 15.2 per cent lower in the 1954-56 sample; between the schizophrenic males and the general population males it was 40.5 per cent in 1934-36, and 34.2 per cent in 1954-56.

TABLE 3. MARITAL STATUS (PER CENT EVER MARRIED) OF
SCHIZOPHRENICS AT ADMISSION AND OF GENERAL POPULATION

Age	MEN				WOMEN			
	Schizophrenics		General population*		Schizophrenics		General population*	
	1934-36	1954-56	1940	1954	1934-36	1954-56	1940	1954
All ages, 15 and over	24.7	42.3	65.2	76.5	54.2	66.3	72.4	81.5
15 - 24	2.7	9.1	14.0	20.8	21.6	24.5	32.0	42.6
25 - 34	22.1	44.6	71.4	83.0	55.6	65.8	81.0	90.2
35 - 44	43.2	48.6	84.9	91.0	72.6	82.1	89.6	93.1
45 and over	55.0	62.0	89.3	92.2	68.2	71.6	91.1	92.7

*United States Bureau of Census, Current Population Reports,
Series P-20, No. 33 and No. 56.

While both the schizophrenic and the general populations disclose an increase in the frequency of *married persons,* the relative increase (i.e., the difference between the two periods taken as a percentage of the initial figure) was greater for the schizophrenics than for the general population. According to these preliminary data, schizophrenic women had a relative increment of 22.3 per cent in marriage, between the two survey periods, compared with a relative increase of 12.6 per cent in marriage for women in the general population between 1940 and 1954. The trend is even more striking for schizophrenic males. Their relative increase in marriage between the two survey periods was 71.2 per cent, while the percentage of married men in the general population showed an increase of only 17.3 per cent.

Two points may be noted in regard to the *average age at first marriage* given in table 4. Schizophrenics appear to marry somewhat later than individuals

TABLE 4. MEDIAN AGE AT FIRST MARRIAGE (IN YEARS)

Sex	Schizophrenics		General Population*	
	1934-36	1954-56	1940	1954
Men	25.4	26.1	24.3	23.0
Women	21.7	21.8	21.5	20.3

*United States Bureau of Census, Current Population Reports, Series P-20, No. 72.

of the same sex in the general population. This finding will warrant further analysis with special attention to the relationship between ages at onset and at marriage. Curiously, also, the trend toward earlier marriage, which is a part of the changing overall pattern, is not evidenced in the schizophrenic population.

Fertility trends may be considered in terms of the proportion of individuals who fail to reproduce, as well as in the number of children produced. Moreover, fertility figures may be based on only those individuals that marry and reproduce, or on all married persons, or on all persons, married and single. The latter measure of fertility estimates the total reproduction of a population.

Shown in table 5 are the number of married schizophrenics who remained childless, those who produced children, and the total number of children produced.

TABLE 5. CRUDE MARRIAGE AND FERTILITY DATA ON SCHIZOPHRENICS AT ADMISSION

Age	Survey Period	MEN				WOMEN			
		Total number of cases	Number ever married Without children	Number ever married With one or more children	Total children	Total number of cases	Number ever married Without children	Number ever married With one or more children	Total children
All ages, 15 and over	1934-36	380	22	72	183	491	60	206	539
	1954-56	319	29	106	230	362	53	187	441
15-24	1934-36	112	1	2	3	125	12	15	24
	1954-56	66	2	4	4	53	4	9	9
25-34	1934-36	140	7	24	51	135	19	56	116
	1954-56	92	10	31	74	111	13	60	136
35-44	1934-36	88	7	31	91	146	13	93	236
	1954-56	90	11	33	75	117	18	78	198
45 and over	1934-36	40	7	15	38	95	16	42	163
	1954-56	71	6	38	77	81	18	40	98

TABLE 7. REPRODUCTION OF SCHIZOPHRENICS AND OF WOMEN IN THE GENERAL POPULATION

Age	Characteristic	Schizophrenics				General Population Women*	
		Men 1934-36	Men 1954-56	Women 1934-36	Women 1954-56	1940	1954
15 to end of reproductive period	Total number	360	278	406	281	—	—
	Ever married (%)	23.6	37.8	51.2	64.7	65.0	76.3
	Childless (% of married persons)	23.5	26.7	22.5	19.2	26.5	18.1
	Childless (% of all persons)	81.9	72.3	60.1	47.7	52.2	37.5
	Total children	161	187	376	343	—	—
	Children per married person	1.9	1.8	1.8	1.9	1.9	2.0
	Children per reproducing person	2.5	2.3	2.3	2.3	2.5	2.5
	Children per person	0.4	0.7	0.9	1.2	1.2	1.5

* Source: Derived from U. S. Bureau of Census, Current Population Reports, Series P-20, No. 108, Table 1.

TABLE 6. PERCENTAGE DISTRIBUTION OF MARRIED WOMEN
(AGED 15-44) WITH SPECIFIED NUMBER OF CHILDREN

Number of Children	Schizophrenics		General Population*	
	1934-36	1954-56	1940	1954
0	22.5	19.2	26.5	18.1
1	27.3	27.5	25.4	23.8
2	23.4	25.3	20.3	27.2
3	14.8	16.5	11.4	15.8
4	4.3	4.9	6.5	7.2
5 and 6	5.3	5.5	6.1	5.6
7 or more	2.4	1.1	3.7	2.3

*United States Bureau of Census, Current Population Reports, Series P-20, No. 46 and No. 65; 1950 Census of Population, Vol. IV, Special Reports, Part 5, Chapter C, Fertility.

The patterns of *family-size* for schizophrenic women and for women in the general population are seen in table 6. In both populations, there was a decrease in families with no children, and an increase in families with two or three children. Schizophrenic women, however, did not exhibit the general population's decline in one-child families, nor were the increases in two- and three-child families as great as in the general population. Also, among schizophrenic women families of four or more children were less common.

FERTILITY TRENDS

Fertility data calculated in several ways are presented in table 7 for the schizophrenic samples, and for women generally. Since fertility figures are not available for men in the general population, comparisons for schizophrenics of both sexes are made with statistics for women in the general population. The fertility data in table 7 are for individuals within the reproductive period, i.e., ages 15 through 44 for women and ages 15 through 49 for men.

It is of interest that *childless marriages* do not seem to occur more frequently in the schizophrenic sample than in the general population. Indeed, a slightly smaller proportion of childless marriages is noted among schizophrenic women of the earlier period than among women in general. However, it is clear that in schizophrenics as a whole, both married and unmarried, there is a much higher frequency of individuals who produce no children than there is in the general population. The explanation lies in the relatively high proportion of *unmarried schizophrenics*. Accordingly, the proportion of childless individuals is highest among the males.

Examination of the various trends reveals that the decline in the percentage of childless women, both in schizophrenics and in the general population, stems from the simultaneous increase in marriages and the decline in childless marriages. The decrease in childless individuals is not as great among schizophrenic women as among women in the general population. Only the schizophrenic males show some increase in childlessness within marriage. Correspondingly, the proportion of the total group remaining childless does not decline to the extent which might otherwise be expected on the basis of the substantial rise in marriages.

By considering the rates of reproduction as shown in the bottom three rows of table 7, one obtains a picture of the *complete fertility pattern* within marriage. Not only do schizophrenics tend to have as few childless marriages as the general population, but they also have nearly as many children per marriage and per fertile marriage. As noted previously, the decrement in reproduction of the total group is caused primarily by the lowered marriage rate.

Based on our preliminary data, the absolute increase in the number of children per individual, 0.3 children per individual, is the same for schizophrenics of either sex as for women in the United States population. The relative increase, however, calculated as a per cent of the initial rate, projects a remarkable picture. This increase in the reproductive rate is 25 per cent for women in the general population, 33 per cent for schizophrenic women, and 75 per cent for schizophrenic men. Thus, although schizophrenics on the whole continue to fall below the general population in the production of children, they appear to be at least paralleling the general population's trend in the direction of *increased fertility,* and possibly surpassing it.

CONCLUSIONS

Although it would be premature to draw definite conclusions at this stage of the study, a few general points may be summarized here. In line with the findings of previous investigators, the present data show marriage and total reproductive rates for schizophrenics below those of the general population, with a larger decrement for male than female schizophrenics. As reported by Essen-Möller[4] and Kallmann,[8] the low pre-psychotic marriage and reproductive rates are even further curtailed after onset of the disease. In the present study as well as in the investigations of Böök[1] and Ødegaard,[14,15] the lowered reproduction of schizophrenics would seem to be attributable to the preponderance of unmarried persons, with no real reduction of fertility within marriage itself.

While some of the major trends in the general marriage and fertility patterns are followed by the schizophrenics, others are not. Both populations have experienced an increase in the frequency of marriage, but schizophrenics do not maintain the general trend toward earlier marriages. The decrease in childless marriages shown by women generally is reflected by schizophrenic women, but not by schizophrenic men.

Although changes in the fertility pattern of American women include a decrease in the number of families with one child and an increase in two- and three-child families, there is no evidence of a decline in one-child families among schizophrenic women. However, their increase in two- and three-child families follows the trend of the general population.

In general, it may be said that during the 20-year period covered by our survey,* both the pre- and post-psychotic frequencies of marriage and reproduction in schizophrenics increased. Probably our most significant preliminary finding is that of relatively greater increases in marriage and total reproduction among schizophrenics than in the general population. Should this trend con-

*The contributions of several members of our staff are gratefully acknowledged. We are especially indebted to Mrs. Joan Rudolph for her valuable assistance.

tinue to be borne out as the investigation proceeds, the implications for the health of future generations will require careful appraisal by both geneticists and psychiatrists.

REFERENCES

1. Böök, J. A.: A genetic and neuropsychiatric investigation of a North-Swedish population with special regard to schizophrenia and mental deficiency. Acta Genet. 4:1 and 345, 1953.
2. Coale, A. J.: Population growth. Science 134: 827, 1961.
3. Dobzhansky, T.: Man and natural selection. Am. Scientist 49: 285, 1961.
4. Essen-Möller, E.: Untersuchungen über die Fruchtbarkeit gewisser Gruppen von Geisteskranken. Acta Psychiat. Neur. Scand. (suppl. 8) 1935.
5. Gibbs, C. E.: Sex development and behaviour in female patients with dementia praecox. Arch. Neurol. & Psychiat. 11: 179, 1924.
6. Grabill, W. H., Kiser, C. V., and Whelpton, P. K.: The Fertility of American Women. New York; Wiley, 1958.
7. Kallmann, F. J.: The Genetics of Schizophrenia. New York, J. J. Augustin, 1938.
8. ——: Heredity, reproduction and eugenic procedure in the field of schizophrenia. Eugen. News 6: 105, 1938.
9. ——: The genetic theory of schizophrenia. An analysis of 691 schizophrenic twin index families. Am. J. Psychiat. 103: 309, 1946.
10. ——: Heredity in Health and Mental Disorder. New York. Norton, 1953.
11. Kiser, C. V.: Current mating and fertility patterns and their demographic significance. Eugen. Quart. 6: 65, 1959.
12. Norris, V.: A statistical study of the influence of marriage in the hospital care of the mentally sick. J. Ment. Sc. 102: 467, 1956.
13. Ødegaard, Ø.: Marriage and mental disease: A study in social psychopathology. J. Ment. Sc. 92: 35, 1946.
14. ——: Discussion on families with manic-depressive psychosis. Eugen. Quart. 6: 137, 1959.
15. ——: Marriage rate and fertility in psychotic patients before hospital admission and after discharge. Internat. J. Soc. Psychiat. 6: 25, 1960.
16. Whelpton, P. K.: A generation of demographic change. In Francis, R. G., Ed.: The Population Ahead. Minneapolis, Univ. Minnesota Press, 1958.

7

Deafness and Schizophrenia: Interrelation of Communication Stress, Maturation Lag and Schizophrenic Risk

KENNETH Z. ALTSHULER, M.D., AND BRUCE SARLIN, M.D.

IN A RECENT SYMPOSIUM entitled "Genetics and Behavior"[19] the well picked bones of the nature-nurture controversy were solemnly laid to rest with the verdict that the whole argument had been spurious and unfounded. Behavior was recognized by experts from the behavioral sciences as being inextricably rooted in biology. Patterns of disordered behavior were said to be structuralized by biological processes with an early "knick" representing a part of innate personality potentials.

While this harmony of view looks well on paper, the old ghost, in fact, still walks. In appraising the development of a schizophrenic process, a cursory nod may be given to constitutional factors, but the emphasis continues to be placed on disordered patterns of communication or disturbances in the mother-child relationship. [1, 5] More often than not, the evidence of genetic studies is simply ignored, out of frank personal preference for other theories.[15,16,21]

One method of assessing the relevance of such extrinsic determinants of schizophrenia is to compare the schizophrenia risk in the population at large with the risk in groups where external influences are particularly strong. In this way, cautious credence can be given to the implications of carefully documented genetic data, without neglecting the possible significance of various precipitating factors.

PSYCHOLOGICAL IMPLICATIONS OF EARLY TOTAL DEAFNESS

Persons with early total deafness constitute a group that lends itself well to this kind of scrutiny. Disordered communication and disruption of the early child-parent relationship typify the conditions under which the young deaf person develops. To make up for the lack of hearing by providing other tools for communicating, years of special schooling are necessary. In many instances, this training cannot be effective unless it takes place in residential schools and begins at a very early age, entailing long periods of separation from the parental home.

This report is the twenty-first in a series dealing with the Mental Health Project for the Deaf conducted by this department. The project has been aided by a grant from the Office of Vocational Rehabilitation of the U. S. Department of Health, Education and Welfare.

Another disturbing factor is that parents are rarely encouraged to learn the manual (sign) language. Instead, verbalization is practiced to induce the child to speak, thus adding another element to the power struggle between child and parent. The result is a mutually frustrating, bewildering and tension-producing situation in which both sides seek to convey and gratify personal needs. Where parents are unable to control feelings of guilt, resentment or disappointment over the child's defect, emotional communication is further distorted.

Speech development in normal children, according to Spitz,[20] acts as an "organizer of the psyche" and is necessary for both personality expansion and the formation of "relationships in the human pattern." Hampered by his handicap, the deaf child remains relatively fixed and isolated so that unbalanced development results. While his physical maturation may proceed normally, the emotional and intellectual aspects of his growth lag behind, limiting the expression and codification of evolving age-specific interests.

Many psychological studies of the deaf have shown such pronounced residual limitations in abstract conceptual ability that it is not certain that this developmental imbalance can ever be fully righted.[4,13] Rorschach tests confirm that normal deaf persons are distinguished by ego rigidity and deficient emotional adaptability, descriptions usually applying to personalities that tend to be vulnerable to breaks in adaptation.[12]

In short, the net effect of early hearing loss and its sequelae is extremely stressful, and is likely to disrupt and distort normal personality development. Nevertheless, all other things being equal, the consequences of this disordering stress can hardly be equated with a schizophrenia-like process.

SCHIZOPHRENIA IN THE DEAF

The clinical features of a *real schizophrenic psychosis in the deaf* were described in a previous report.[3] Despite various modifications in symptomatology, the basic personality disorder was shown to be clearly discernible. Interestingly enough, the paranoid form of the disease was not found to be more common in the deaf than in the hearing.

The schizophrenia rate for the deaf computed at that time was 2.5 per cent. Derived from a survey of hospitalized patients, this estimate, if generally applicable, would represent an increase over the one per cent rate for comparable hearing populations. Calculations for both groups were made by means of the abridged Weinberg method.[11,22] A further correction, adding one extramural schizophrenic for every two institutionalized,[8] was used to bring the rate obtained for a hearing (control) group of hospitalized patients into agreement with the one per cent general population rate. The same procedure was employed in the deaf group.

Acceptance of the 2.5 per cent schizophrenia risk figure for the deaf would presuppose that the basic numbers of deaf and hearing schizophrenics were truly comparable. Differentials in rates of hospital admission or discharge, differences in the ratio of hospitalized to nonhospitalized cases, or gradients in diagnostic standards would so alter the basic figures as to preclude valid comparisons.

That such differentials exist is shown in table 1. Comparable census figures

TABLE 1. DISTRIBUTION OF SCHIZOPHRENIC HOSPITAL PATIENTS IN
NEW YORK STATE ACCORDING TO LENGTH OF HOSPITALIZATION

Hospitalized Schizophrenics in New York State		Percentage of Schizophrenics Hospitalized		
Hearing status	Total	Less than 5 years	5 years and over	20 years and over
Hearing*	52,225	24.2	75.8	35.4
Deaf	120	10.8	89.2	47.5

*State of New York, Department of Mental Hygiene, annual report, 1957.

for deaf and hearing patients reveal a significantly greater proportion of deaf schizophrenics to have been hospitalized for more than five years, or even more than 20 years. Having observed no variation in age of onset, severity of illness or the like, we have to ascribe these differences mainly to an accrual of institutionalized deaf patients in the wake of social factors unrelated to the psychiatric condition. Existing difficulties in clinical evaluation and convalescent sheltered placement of destitute patients with limited communication skills lend weight to this interpretation.

On the whole, hospitalized schizophrenics represent 1.16 per cent of the total deaf population of New York State, as compared with .43 per cent in the hearing. Taking into account the increment among undischarged deaf patients, the ratio of hospitalized to nonhospitalized cases would not be the same for the two groups. In other words, the assumption of one extramural patient for every two in a hospital, necessary to bring the figures for hospitalized hearing schizophrenics into accord with the expectancy rate for the general population, is not applicable to data on the deaf.

As to the comparability of diagnostic classifications, it was found in the earlier survey that nearly 25 per cent of all deaf patients carried a hospital diagnosis of "psychosis with mental deficiency."[3,18] Comprehensive clinical evaluation, using all avenues of communication, especially the short cut to understanding afforded by manual language, reduced this unusual figure considerably. While many of these cases were reclassified as schizophrenic, some in the schizophrenic group were also placed into other diagnostic categories (personality disorder, psychoneurosis). Despite the lack of a similar diagnostic survey in hearing patients, there was little doubt that the criteria for classifying psychiatric hospital patients tend to vary between the two groups, the communication barrier making diagnosis less precise among the deaf.

Certainly, no comparison of schizophrenia rates for deaf and hearing populations would be valid without taking into account the effect of certain genetic constellations. With heredity playing an important role in deafness, it is not surprising that the parental consanguinity rate in deaf families has been found to vary between 6 and 10 per cent.[14] In our own survey, the observed consanguinity rate approximates 8 per cent for the parents of all deaf persons in New York State, and 5 per cent for the parents of deaf schizophrenics.[17] Cousin marriages in the general population are probably fewer than one per cent. [7]

An increased frequency of parental consanguinity would influence schizophrenia rates for the deaf only if vulnerability to a schizophrenic process were more likely to be found under conditions favoring the manifestation of recessive traits. In line with the statistical considerations of Dahlberg,[18] the actual increase found in consanguinity would not be expected to significantly alter the actual schizophrenia risk in this special group.

Generally speaking, therefore, the following considerations apply to our analysis of families affected by both deafness and schizophrenia. The schizophrenia rate of 2.5 per cent estimated for the deaf is not fully acceptable, nor is it an accurate index of a change in schizophrenia risk because of disrupted personal relationships, disordered communication or lack of harmony between the elements of psychological development and biological maturation. Special care is required in appraising this problem through hospitalized cases alone, and the need for some other technique of investigation is evident.

Through the years, genetic studies have been made of the risk for various psychiatric disorders in relatives of affected patients (index cases) in virtually all kinship categories.[2] Despite differences in diagnostic standards, statistical procedures, availability of relatives and special demographic conditions affecting the manifestation of gene-specific disorders, there has been a remarkable unanimity of findings. The results of these well controlled studies are summarized in table 2 which shows the consistently observed graded increase in schizo-

TABLE 2. FREQUENCY OF SCHIZOPHRENIA IN THE GENERAL POPULATION AND IN RELATIVES OF SCHIZOPHRENICS

Source	Frequency of Schizophrenia in General Population	Step-sibs	Half-sibs	Frequency of Schizophrenia in the Relatives of One Schizophrenic			
				Full sibs	Dizygotic co-twins	Monozygotic co-twins	Parents
Various Investigations (1916 to 1953)	0.3-2.4	—	7.6	4.5-12.0	12.5-14.9	68.3-81-7	7.1-12.0
Kallmann 1946 (twin index cases)	0.85	1.8	7.0	14.3	14.7	85.8	9.2

phrenia rates with the increase in degree of genetic similarity to a schizophrenic index case. Representing an American (New York State) population which was ascertained and diagnosed according to conservative contemporary standards, Kallmann's 1946 study[9] warrants special note.*

If the stress effect of deafness alone were to increase appreciably the manifestation of schizophrenia without gene-borne vulnerability, the schizophrenia risk for sibs and parents of deaf index cases should fall below the rates found for relatives of hearing probands. That is, persons with deafness would be more likely to develop schizophrenia, regardless of genetic predisposition. Hence, relatives of deaf schizophrenics, with neither the perceptual defect nor the

---

*Despite the choice of twin rather than single-born index cases, the schizophrenia rates obtained for sibs and parents approximated those reported by others. Since Kallmann's study was similar to the current one in many respects, e.g., New York State population, comparable diagnostic standards, and personal investigation, it would seem to offer the best base for comparison. Nonetheless, the longitudinal nature of his investigation (5 years) and the selection of twin index cases are variables which serve to emphasize the lack of perfectly comparable data between investigations. In the absence of such data, gross deviations from the whole range of findings are required to regard observed differences as really meaningful.

genetic potential for schizophrenia, should be roughly similar to the general population. The morbidity risk among them should then approximate 1 per cent, rather than show the increase reflecting shared genetic vulnerability as postulated in other family studies. Also, there should be a marked difference between hearing and deaf relatives of deaf index cases, since in the presence of similar genetic endowments, deafness as such should cause a significant increase in the frequency of schizophrenia. By studying the families of deaf schizophrenics along these lines, we can assess the influence of stresses exerted by total hearing loss on the risk of schizophrenia.

STATISTICAL DATA ON THE FAMILIES OF DEAF SCHIZOPHRENICS

Toward this end, our departmental survey of the deaf population of New York State was organized in such a way as to include all deaf persons admitted to mental hospitals. Of the 286 patients seen during this 6-year period, 138 met our stringent diagnostic criteria for both deafness and schizophrenia. *Deafness* was defined as a "stress producing hearing loss at an early age, making effective auditory contact with the world impossible and necessitating special educative efforts."[10] The diagnosis of *schizophrenia* was established in each case by a committee of three clinical psychiatrists trained in working with the deaf. No psychotic case was accepted without unanimity of opinion, nor was any undue pressure exerted to achieve uniformity of classification.

The diagnostic criteria employed were on the conservative side, and for purposes of comparison may be equated with those used in our previous investigations. Essentially, these criteria were focused on a clearly discernible personality change with repudiation of reality relationships, disintegration of personality and impaired concept formation or loosened conceptual frame of associations, coupled with blunting, apathy or other incongruities between thought and feeling. Disordered behavior and impaired judgment were always present, but delusions, hallucinations or deteriorating tendencies, while commonly found, were not prerequisite for the diagnosis.

In classifying the sibs and parents of deaf index cases, no relative, regardless of history, was labeled schizophrenic, unless there were adequate hospital records or extensive personal interviews to substantiate the diagnosis. Shiftless individuals with suspicious histories remained unclassified or were placed in the category of "probable schizophrenia." On the other hand, fairly positive life performance reports by other relatives, even where possibly biased, led to the classification of a missing hearing person as nonschizophrenic. Since the communication problem of the hearing-impaired may mask an underlying personality disorder, no deaf person was given any mental status classification whatsoever, unless historical records were supplemented by personal psychiatric interview. In this way, any difference between the two groups, hearing and deaf, would be maximized, keeping to a minimum the ascertainment of schizophrenia cases among hearing relatives, and increasing the proportion of schizophrenics found among the hearing-impaired.

The general data on the *siblings* of our sample of deaf schizophrenics are tabulated in tables 3 and 4. Of the total of 349 sibs, 18 died before they entered the age of risk for schizophrenia, which was assumed to extend from

TABLE 3.   AGE DISTRIBUTION OF THE SIBLINGS
OF DEAF SCHIZOPHRENICS

Age	Living		Deceased		Total
	Male	Female	Male	Female	
0-14	0	0	12	6	18
15-24	0	7	6	3	16
25-34	14	18	2	2	36
35-44	38	43	3	1	85
45-54	52	37	6	2	97
55-64	30	26	6	1	63
65 and over	7	11	8	8	34
Total	141	142	43	23	349

TABLE 4.   HEARING STATUS OF THE SIBLINGS OF DEAF SCHIZOPHRENICS

Age	Deaf	Hard of Hearing	Hearing	Undetermined	Total
0-14	1	0	11	6	18
15-24	1	1	14	0	16
25-34	0	1	35	0	36
35-44	11	0	74	0	85
45-54	5	3	89	0	97
55-64	2	1	60	0	63
65 and over	2	1	31	0	34
Total	22	7	314	6	349

the ages of 15 to 45 years. The other 48 deceased relatives survived all or part of this period and were recorded as of the age at death.

No significant early impairment of hearing was present in 314 sibs, although a few did develop some degree of hearing loss late in life. Six others died in infancy with hearing status undetermined. Of the remaining 29 sibs, 22 (including one who had died at the age of 3) met our criteria for deafness. The other seven were classified as hard of hearing. Except for degree of deafness or age of onset, their developmental histories were substantially the same as those of the deaf.

Comparable information about the *parents* of 138 index cases is presented in tables 5 and 6. All but 21 of them lived through the age of risk for schizophrenia. In 38 couples, the only information obtained was the fact that they had died. With more than 70 per cent of the parents deceased, hearing status

TABLE 5.   AGE DISTRIBUTION OF THE PARENTS
OF DEAF SCHIZOPHRENICS

Age	Living		Deceased		Total
	Male	Female	Male	Female	
15-24	0	0	0	1	1
25-34	0	0	3	1	4
35-44	1	1	8	6	16
45-54	5	8	14	9	36
55-64	3	10	17	19	49
65 and over	28	25	59	58	170
Total	37	44	101	94	276

TABLE 6. HEARING STATUS OF THE PARENTS
OF DEAF SCHIZOPHRENICS

Age	Deaf	Hard of Hearing	Hearing	Undetermined	Total
15-24	0	0	1	0	1
25-34	0	0	4	0	4
35-44	0	0	16	0	16
45-54	0	0	28	8	36
55-64	0	1	37	11	49
65 and over	4	0	109	57	170
Total	4	1	195	76	276

could be determined only in 200 of them, including 4 cases of deafness and
one of marked hearing impairment. Since the mode of transmission in deafness
is generally assumed to be recessive, the limited number of deaf parents in this
sample comes as no surprise.

Psychiatric classification as to the presence or absence of schizophrenia has
been possible in 310 of the 331 siblings known to have survived at least part
of the age of risk (table 7). The remaining 21 cases consist of 19 hearing and

TABLE 7. PSYCHIATRIC CLASSIFICATION OF THOSE 331 SIBLINGS OF
DEAF SCHIZOPHRENICS WHO LIVED BEYOND THE AGE OF 14 YEARS

Age	Schizophrenia Definite*		Probable		Without Schizophrenia		Undetermined		Total
	Male	Female	Male	Female	Male	Female	Male	Female	
15-24	1	0	0	0	5	9	0	1	16
25-34	3	3	0	1	13	16	0	0	36
35-44	4	5	1	1	35	38	1	0	85
45-54	4	2	2	1	48	34	4	2	97
55-64	1	5	0	0	31	16	4	6	63
65 and over	0	0	0	0	14	17	1	2	34
Total	13	15	3	3	146	130	10	11	331

*Includes 15 cases who were not hospitalized.

2 deaf siblings who could not be satisfactorily diagnosed. Eighteen siblings
died before age 15.

An unequivocal diagnosis of schizophrenia was made in 28 sibs, while another 6 were classified as probably schizophrenic because of our inability to
confirm the classification through hospital records or personal interview. Typical
of the latter group was an extremely suspicious woman who for several years
had remained in self-imposed house confinement. She entered only very briefly
into bizarre bits of conversation with our visiting team, all the while refusing
to unbolt her door.

If only fully verified cases are considered, the corrected schizophrenia risk
figure for all sibs is 11.6 per cent. It increases to 14.1 per cent if the 6 doubtful cases are included (table 9). These and subsequent computations relate
the number of schizophrenics to an age-corrected frame of reference based on
all psychiatrically classified cases. In the comparisons to follow, only the minimum rate will be used.

TABLE 8. PSYCHIATRIC CLASSIFICATION OF THE PARENTS
OF DEAF SCHIZOPHRENICS

Age	Schizophrenia Definite*		Probable		Without Schizophrenia		Undetermined		Total
	Male	Female	Male	Female	Male	Female	Male	Female	
15-24	0	0	0	0	0	1	0	0	1
25-34	0	0	0	0	2	1	1	0	4
35-44	1	1	0	0	7	6	1	0	16
45-54	1	1	2	0	11	12	5	4	36
55-64	2	2	1	0	12	21	5	6	49
65 and over	3	2	5	3	45	47	34	31	170
Total	7	6	8	3	77	88	46	41	276

*Includes 4 cases who were not hospitalized.

TABLE 9. SCHIZOPHRENIA RISK IN THE SIBLINGS
AND PARENTS OF DEAF SCHIZOPHRENICS

Relatives of Deaf Schizophrenics	Surviving age 15	Psychiatrically classified	Definitely schizophrenic	Corrected frame of reference*	Crude risk (%)	Corrected risk (%)
Hearing sibs	303	284	25	223	8.8	11.2
Deaf sibs†	28	26	3	19	11.5	15.8
Total	331	310	28	242	9.0	11.6‡
Parents of deaf index cases	276	189	13	179	6.9	7.3

*The sum of all cases over 45 and one-half the cases between 15 and 45, for whom
information was available.
†Includes seven cases with marked hearing loss.
‡14.1% if probable cases are included.

The most interesting finding is the absence of a statistically significant difference between the schizophrenia risks for hearing and deaf sibs. With 25 cases of schizophrenia among the 284 hearing sibs, their corrected expectancy rate is 11.2 per cent. The corresponding rate for the 26 siblings with impaired hearing who were available for classification is 15.8 per cent. This rate is reduced to 14.3 per cent if the 3 cases of schizophrenia are related to a total of 28 hearing-impaired sibs, including those two who were reported to have been emotionally well adjusted but could not be interviewed. Because of the smallness of the sample, removal of the 7 hard of hearing sibs raises this figure to 23 per cent without letting it reach the level of a statistically significant difference.

Of similar importance is the finding that all groups of siblings, the hearing as well as the deaf and the combined total, have significantly greater risks for schizophrenia than the general population (1 to 2 per cent). Compared with the general population, the risks for these groups are roughly of the same order of magnitude as those computed in other family studies. In particular, they closely approximate the rate of 14.3 per cent reported by Kallmann (1946) for the siblings of schizophrenic index cases without a hearing loss.[9]

As previously mentioned, our rates were obtained under selective conditions which tended to maximize differences between the findings for hearing and deaf siblings. An even larger difference is observed if the number of schizo-phrenics is related to the *total* number of siblings in each group, whether psychiatrically classified or not. This method requires the additional assump-tion that there were no schizophrenics among the siblings who could not be classified. In this uncertain case, the divergence between rates for hearing and deaf sibs comes closer to, but still does not reach, the level of statistical sig-nificance (10.4 per cent for hearing and 14.3 per cent for deaf sibs).* At the same time, our rate for hearing sibs, while lower than the one reported by Kall-mann for the sibs of schizophrenic twins, comes closer to those observed by some other investigators.

In any case, we cannot say that there are statistically significant differences in schizophrenia risk between deaf and hearing siblings of deaf schizophrenics. On the whole, all groups of siblings of our deaf index cases show a definite in-crease in morbidity risk over the general population, similar to the one that has been so consistently reported in earlier studies. Although the findings do not preclude the possibility of some role played by stressful factors in the simul-taneous occurrence of deafness and schizophrenia, the weight of evidence indi-cates that early total deafness, with all its deprivations and distortions in the normal development patterns, has little bearing on the statistically demonstrable risk of schizophrenia.

Although less precise because of the large number of deceased, our data on the parents of deaf schizophrenics point in the same direction (tables 8 and 9). In many instances, classifications had to be based on descriptions provided by their children, and thus may have been subject to victimization or eulogy.

In a total of 189 members of the parental generation, the information obtained was considered sufficient to warrant classification. For this group, 13 persons, none of whom were deaf, were diagnosed as schizophrenic through psychiatric interview or hospital records, yielding a minimum schizophrenia rate of 7.3 per cent for the parents of deaf schizophrenics. This figure is only slightly below the rate observed by other investigators in parents of schizo-phrenics without perceptual defect (approximately 9 per cent). Again, if in-completely studied parents are counted as normal, the schizophrenia risk varies from 5.1 to 9.5 per cent, depending on whether "probable" cases of schizo-phrenia are included or excluded.

CONCLUSIONS

With the nature of the genetic vulnerability factor in the etiology of schizo-phrenia still uncertain, various current theories attempt to explain the total range of schizophrenic phenomena on developmental grounds alone. While the importance of nongenetic influences in the molding of life processes is recog-nized in modern genetics as well as in psychiatry, disagreement remains over the more or less central role assigned to them in the causation of specific forms of psychopathology.

The present study approaches this problem through a statewide census of

---

*Although the absolute difference in percentages actually decreases with this method of calculation, the difference comes close to significant levels by virtue of narrowing the range of "chance" results when a larger denominator is used.

deaf schizophrenics, combined with a computation of schizophrenia risk figures for their siblings and parents. Early total deafness was chosen as an additional criterion for the ascertainment of schizophrenic index cases, because it imposes unusually stressful and disruptive conditions on childhood development and later life. These stresses include disturbed and distorted communication, developmental imbalances and marked disorder of parent-child relationships.

In view of these extreme hardships, a significantly increased frequency of schizophrenia might be expected to be typical of the deaf. Another working hypothesis would be to ascribe an anticipated reduction in schizophrenia rates to the presumably "sheltered" home milieu or the lifelong "emotional immaturity" postulated for the deaf. In either case, significant differences in schizophrenia risk should emerge not only between the sibships of deaf and non-deaf schizophrenics, but especially between the hearing and non-hearing sibs of deaf schizophrenics.

If adequately trained, psychiatrists can recognize the clinical symptoms of schizophrenia in the deaf as readily as in the hearing. Considered as a separate population, the deaf of New York State show a slightly increased schizophrenia rate (2.5 per cent) over that of the general population 1 to 2 per cent. However, since our sample of deaf schizophrenics has been ascertained from hospitalized cases, with a standard correction for those living on the outside, this slight excess seems largely attributable to a combination of extrinsic factors, especially the prolonged duration of time which deaf patients spend in mental hospitals. A more valid schizophrenia rate for the deaf is virtually unobtainable.

It is more important that no significant difference in schizophrenia risk has been found either between the hearing and deaf sibs of our index cases, or between either group of siblings and comparable sibships of non-deaf schizophrenics, even under conditions which are apt to maximize expected variations. On the other hand, all groups of siblings yield significantly higher schizophrenia rates than the general population. The observed rates for the parents of deaf and hearing schizophrenics are in line with these findings.

We may therefore conclude that sibship consanguinity to a schizophrenic person results in the expected marked increase in morbidity risk whether or not there is a perceptual defect in the index case or the relative. In other words, the severe and varied stresses associated with early total deafness apparently do little to increase the chance of developing clinical symptoms of schizophrenia.

REFERENCES

1. ALANEN, Y. O.: The Mothers of Schizophrenic Patients. Copenhagen, Munksgaard, 1958.
2. ALTSHULER, K. Z.: Genetic elements in schizophrenia: A review. Eugenics Quart. 4: 92, 1957.
3. ———, AND RAINER, J. D.: Patterns and course of schizophrenia in the deaf. J. Nerv. & Ment. Dis. 127: 77, 1958.
4. BARKER, R. G., et al.: Adjustment to Physical Handicap and Illness: A Survey of the Social Psychology of Physique and Disability. New York, Soc. Sci. Res. Council, 1953.
5. BATESON, G., et al.: Toward a theory of schizophrenia. Behav. Sc. 1: 251, 1956.
6. DAHLBERG, G.: Mathematical Methods for Population Genetics. Basel, Karger, 1948.
7. FREIRE-MAIA, N.: Inbreeding levels in different countries. Eugenics Quart. 4: 127, 1957.

8. GOLDHAMER, H., AND MARSHALL, A. W.: Psychosis and Civilization. Glencoe, Ill., Free Press, 1953.
9. KALLMANN, F. J.: The genetic theory of schizophrenia. Am. J. Psychiat. 103: 309, 1946.
10. ———: Objectives of the mental health project for the deaf. Proc. 37th Conv. Am. Instructors of the Deaf. Washington, D. C., U. S. Govt. Printing Office, 1956.
11. ———, AND RAINER, J. D.: Genetics and demography. In Hauser, P. M., and Duncan, O.D., Eds.: The Study of Population. Chicago, Univ. Chicago Press, 1959.
12. LEVINE, E. S.: Youth in a Soundless World. New York, N.Y. Univ. Press, 1956.
13. ———: The Psychology of Deafness. New York, Columbia Univ. Press, 1960.
14. LINDENOV, H.: The Etiology of Deaf-Mutism with Special Reference to Heredity. Copenhagen, Munksgaard, 1945.
15. MURPHY, B. W.: Genesis of schizoid personality: Study of two cases developing schizophrenia. Psychiat. Quart. 26:450, 1952.
16. PERRY, J. W.: A Jungian formulation of schizophrenia. Am. J. Psychotherapy 10: 54, 1956.
17. RAINER, J. D.: Marriage patterns and family composition in early total deafness. Second Internat. Conf. Hum. Genet. (Rome, 1961). Amsterdam, Excerpta Medica, 1961.
18. ———, AND KALLMANN, F. J.: Genetic and demographic aspects of disordered behavior patterns in a deaf population. In Pasamanick, B., Ed.: Epidemiology of Mental Disorder. Washington, D. C., Publication No. 60 of A. A. A. S., 1959.
19. SCOTT, J. P.: Genetics and the development of social behavior. (With discussions by J. HIRSCH AND J. D. RAINER.) Am. J. Orthopsychiat., in press.
20. SPITZ, R. A.: A Genetic Field Theory of Ego Formation. New York, Internat. Univ. Press, 1959.
21. SZALITÁ-PEMOW, A.: Remarks on the pathogenesis and treatment of schizophrenia. Psychiatry 14: 295, 1951.
22. WEINBERG, W.: Zur Probandenmethode und zu ihrem Ersatz. Ztschr. Neurol. 123: 809, 1930.

8

Discussion

Dr. Robie

I was greatly impressed by Dr. Rainer's emphasis on the psychotherapeutic aspects of genetic family counseling, especially in relation to mate selection and parenthood problems. It is a notable sign of progress that a realistic appraisal of possible genetic health deterrents no longer implies a hopeless outlook. Actually, coupled with the judicious use of psychopharmacological drugs in combating the psychotic symptoms of our patients, the recognition of serious health hazards which may arise from an unwanted pregnancy in a poorly stabilized setting, can be converted into a valuable psychotherapeutic tool for promoting in clinically improved patients an understanding of the important principles of self acceptance, self reliance and social responsibility.

Dr. Furst

As a practicing psychiatrist, I have also gained the impression in the last few years that the marital fertility of schizophrenics, studied so thoroughly by the team of Dr. Goldfarb and Dr. Erlenmeyer-Kimling, seems to have increased with the use of phenothyazines. Obviously, indifference or contemptuousness would be the least desirable attitudes toward this problematic side-effect of modern treatment methods. A particularly difficult problem is posed by the tendency of the narcissistic schizophrenic to regard his own reproductivity as the most important thing in the world. I am wondering how these conflicting results of active psychiatric treatment procedures can be satisfactorily reconciled with each other: the maintenance of clinical remissions and the trend toward increased marital fertility with its consequent stresses on unstable family situations.

Dr. Bender

The results of a recent investigation by Dr. Kris and Dr. Carmichael (Psychiatric Quar. 31: 690, 1957) may be of some interest here. In this study, the children of schizophrenic patients, who became pregnant while placed on convalescent care and receiving chlorpromazine, have been followed. At birth, no signs of abnormality were detectable in these infants. It will be important to see whether all the children in this series develop normally as they grow older.

Dr. Rainer

We appreciate the factual statements made by Dr. Robie, Dr. Furst and Dr. Lauretta Bender. A better understanding of family problems, combined with more effective treatment methods, is certain to be encouraging to both patients and their psychiatrists.

Dr. Holt

According to the data presented by Dr. Altshuler and Dr. Sarlin, the schizophrenia risk for the deaf siblings of deaf schizophrenics is 23 per cent, and that for the hearing sibs, 11.2 per cent. It has been emphasized that the former group is very small, and that the difference between the corrected expectancy rates for the two groups of siblings is not statistically significant. Nevertheless, there seems to be a definite trend toward a higher schizophrenia risk among the deaf members of the given sibships, and it may not be warranted to discount this trend altogether.

Dr. Altshuler

The schizophrenia rates for the nonhearing sibling of deaf schizophrenics have been calculated in two different ways: (1) by combining the hearing-impaired with the deaf siblings and (2) in order to maximize the difference between deaf and hearing members of the given families, by omitting the hard of hearing. The latter series included only 7 persons and was numerically too small to be treated as a separate group. It may also be stressed that the schizophrenia risk figure for deaf siblings is based only on three cases of schizophrenia. Although the difference between the schizophrenia risks of hearing and deaf siblings (11.2 and 23 per cent, respectively) appears to be large, it may be noted that our sample of deaf siblings of deaf schizophrenics is too small to lend itself to reliable predictions. The only statement that can be made with confidence is that although we attempted to maximize the observed difference between the two groups of siblings, a level of statistical significance was not reached.

Dr. Alexander

May I say that Dr. Altshuler's method of studying the expectancy of schizophrenia in the presence or absence of deafness impresses me as a particularly elegant one. In looking for a similar quantifying approach, I have thought at times that the genetic mechanism resulting in homosexual behavior might also be investigated profitably by comparing groups of homosexuals with and without color blindness. As far as the etiology of schizophrenia is concerned, I cannot resist the temptation to play the role of a devil's advocate for a while, although I personally favor the genetic theory of this disorder.

It seems to me that the mode of communication between mother and child, stressed by psychodynamically oriented schools, is largely of the nonverbal variety. This type of communication may be enhanced rather than impaired in the upbringing of deaf children, but it has not been taken into consideration in Dr. Altshuler's study. In line with my own observations, deaf children are sometimes smothered by the extraordinary love of their mothers. This factor of an excessive degree of "primary communication patterns" may play a significant part in the psychopathology of deaf schizophrenics.

Dr. Altshuler

Although Dr. Alexander's arguments appear to be well founded, may I reiterate that the schizophrenia rates for deaf and hearing persons have not been found to differ significantly in either direction, that is, in the direction of considerably higher or considerably lower frequency levels.

SECTION II: PROGRESS IN BASIC GENETICS

9

Introduction

H. BENTLEY GLASS, PH.D.

FOR 25 YEARS, psychiatric genetics was to us a field of specialization, where we could rely on the research data emanating from Dr. Kallmann's department. By the same token, these studies always showed a healthy reliance on, and a close relation to, the basic biological sciences. This affinity was particularly strong to the discipline of *basic genetics* as is evidenced by the manner in which the program of this symposium was arranged. With an entire section devoted to basic human genetics, the present volume provides indisputable proof of the remarkable technical progress which has taken place in this sector in recent years.

The field of *microgenetics,* that successfully developed the techniques for the experimental manipulation of chromosomes, is brilliantly represented by Prof. Kopac of New York University. At that noted institution of learning, he occupies the rooms which long ago housed one of the great pioneers in this experimental discipline, Robert Chambers. What is more, he works there with the same endurance and ingenious spirit to carry on the worthy tradition of this well equipped laboratory. In fact, the instruments available today are so highly refined that he has far surpassed the achievements of those older biologists who began micromanipulation, microdissection and microradiation studies with chromosomes many years ago.

While Prof. Kopac is showing us how much the invention of new tools for experimental work has contributed to recent advances in basic genetics, one of the younger workers in *cytogenetics* is demonstrating conclusively how much has been accomplished with these improved techniques within a very short time. Dr. Malcolm Ferguson-Smith is now Lecturer in Medical Genetics at the University of Glasgow, but we had the good fortune in Baltimore to be closely associated with him and his work during the past two years. For a while, he even left with us his wife and a young "coacervate" composed of DNA, RNA, protein and lipids when he returned to Scotland to carry on his investigations into the cytogenetics of sexual development.

These studies have convincingly substantiated not only the association between chromosomes and sex anomalies, but also that between chromosomes and behavioral (psychiatric) problems. Although a word of caution seems justified regarding the finding of so many Klinefelter and Turner cases among the patients of mental institutions (no comparable data are as yet available on the frequency of these syndromes in the general population), recent developments in our knowledge of chromosomal disarrangements have been at an amazing pace. Actually, it is hard to believe that it was no more than five years ago that the correct chromosome number in human cells was established by the work of Tjio and Levan as being 46 and not 48.

Similar progress has been made in the area of *biochemical genetics,* represented here by a first rate biochemist who by force of his own experimental interests, has also become a very good geneticist. Presently serving as visiting professor of biochemistry at the American University in Beirut, Eugene Knox happens to be the man to whom I write a letter whenever we have a real problem regarding some aspects of "biochemical genetics and human metabolism," the subject of his contribution to this symposium. He always has the right answer to our questions, and my only regret is that when he has a difficult genetic problem — as we all do have occasionally — he is perfectly capable of supplying his own answer and has no need to apply to me or my fellow geneticists.

Special cytochemical phenomena connected with the biological function of DNA are to be reviewed by another old friend of mine, Prof. Carl Lindegren of Southern Illinois University, whose ideas are always extremely interesting even though criticized by many of us. With Richard Goldschmidt dead and sorely missed by all of us, our present generation of geneticists is fortunate, indeed, to have in Carl Lindegren another skeptic and iconoclast, another man who is given to breaking or building conceptual models.

It happens sometimes that the use of a new scientific tool becomes such a profound part of an investigator's work that it hinders rather than helps further discovery. Instead of using the tool to explore an intricate problem, he is preoccupied with thinking of new things which he may do with the tool. The history of genetics from the time of Gregor Mendel serves to demonstrate dramatically that the development of a new conceptual model — be it that of a gene, a functional chromosome, or some other aspect in the structure of the hereditary system — is likely at first to lead to a great surge of experimental activity. Much investigative work must be done to unravel the details of an imaginative discovery. However, these methodological inquiries are often followed by a period of mental stagnation. With newly developed concepts becoming firmly fixed in the investigators' minds, original discoveries tend to grow into scientific dogmas.

Therefore, every era needs its model breakers as well as its model builders, its skeptics as well as its enthusiasts. The previous generation of biologists owed a great deal to Richard Goldschmidt, who was one of these courageous men. Often laughed at and not infrequently wrong, he nevertheless proved to be profoundly right in many instances, pointing out the ways in which geneticists had become absorbed in their models. Time and only time will tell, perhaps, whether and to what extent Carl Lindegren may have been as profoundly right in the present generation as Richard Goldschmidt often was in the preceding one.

The final report in this section of the symposium was also concerned with *the relation between genes and enzymes,* tying together the various biochemical concepts of the basic processes of gene action and mutation which continue to be of focal interest to our present generation of geneticists. Paradoxically, at least from the standpoint of classic genetics, the report of Prof. K. C. Atwood of the University of Illinois was along relatively conservative lines of conceptualization, although it could by no means be regarded as that of an "old-timer."

In actuality, this brilliant scientist is a fast traveler who has accomplished a great deal, moving at a rapid pace from Columbia University, where he did his graduate studies, via Oak Ridge and the University of Chicago to his present position which entails all the responsibilities connected with a professorship in microbiology. Of even greater significance may be the fact that although Prof. Atwood started out with microbes and then worked with slightly larger organisms, his most recent interest has been the heredity of human red cells. As you may imagine, this is quite a feat since erythrocytes have no nucleus, no DNA, and not even any chromosomes.

Unfortunately, the recording of Kimball Atwood's valuable contribution to this symposium proved to be technically so imperfect that only a very brief abstract can be included here. If the memory of a plain human recorder can be trusted as much as the tape of an ingenious but delicate recording machine, the fragmented statements summarized in Chapter 14 were the highlights of his interesting report.

10

Structure and Microsurgery of Chromosomes

M. J. KOPAC, Ph.D., Sc.D.

CHROMOSOMES are fantastically dynamic structures. Not only are the chromosomes structurally different from time to time within the same cell, but quite frequently major structural differences in chromosomes can be demonstrated in the differentiated cells of the same organism. In all probability the dynamic structural aspects of chromosomes are a reflection of their functional activities which, on one hand, can be replication in preparation for the next generation or, on the other hand, the transfer of genetic information. Other changes occur especially during mitosis.

CHANGES IN CHROMOSOMAL STRUCTURES DURING MITOSIS

The dynamic features of typical somatic chromosomes are best shown during mitosis. In figure 1, six stages in the life cycle of a cell in mitosis have been more or less arbitrarily designated. The interphase is characterized primarily by the diffuse condition of the chromosomes and, among other properties, there is usually at least one prominent nucleolar body. Chromosomes at this time are in their best architectural configuration for the purpose of replicating or for transmitting genetic information (fig. 2). However, when the cell is committed to replicate, some striking changes occur in the chromosomal structures. For example, during prophase the chromosomes become linearly condensed after replication. There are also cyclic changes in the nucleolar material, and it is usually at early prophase that the association between the nucleolus and one or more paired chromosomes becomes most clearly apparent.

During prometaphase the chromosomes have not only replicated, but have just about become fully condensed. In addition, the nucleolar body has disappeared and the nuclear membranes become disorganized. Apparently, the centromeric region is the last to replicate so that the two new chromosomes (derived from one) remain attached at this region, clearly represented by the primary constriction. The replicated chromosomes, now the chromatids, have a "bow tie" configuration. The primary constriction designates the site of the centromere from which spindle fibrils are generated. Those chromosomes associated with nucleoli possess a secondary constriction.

At metaphase, the primary constrictions of the chromatids line up at the equator. Each pair of chromatids has apparent fibrillar components leading to each of the two polar regions represented by the centriolar apparatus. At this time, the mitotic spindle may be disrupted by colchicine or other mitostatic drugs to such an extent that mitosis is interrupted.

The subsequent events in mitosis are well known and include (a) the separation or disjunction of the chromatids at anaphase; (b) the migration of the separated chromosomes to the respective poles; and (c) the reorganization

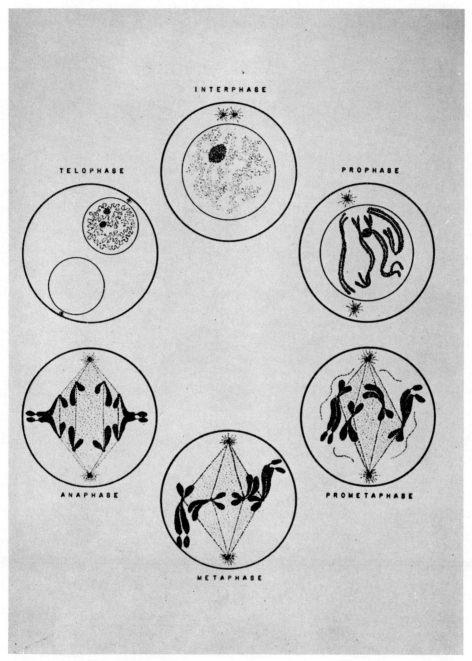

Fig. 1. Principal stages in mitosis. Six arbitrarily selected stages in mitosis in a prometaphase to anaphase.
hypothetical cell containing two nucleolar chromosomes and two non-nucleolar chromosomes. Note: the secondary constrictions and satellites in nucleolar chromosomes from

of the two daughter nuclei during telophase. During this phase, the chromosomes become less distinct by decondensing, and the nucleoli reappear. If the nucleolar organizers of the chromosomes are close together, the emerging nucleolar bodies may fuse to form a larger body.

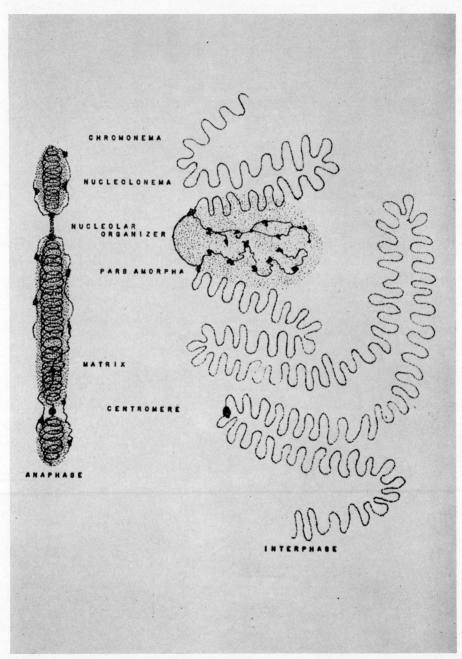

FIG. 2. Diagrammatic representation of the nucleolar chromosome at anaphase and interphase. Nucleolus in interphase shows nucleolonema and pars amorpha.

NUCLEOLAR CHROMOSOMES

The nucleolar chromosome is shown in two stages in figure 2. At interphase, the chromosome is in maximal linear extension, together with the maximal development of the nucleolar body. Moreover, the chromosome has the optimal configuration for replication and also for transferring genetic information. At anaphase, the chromosome shows the maximal linear condensation with the nucleolar organizer region limited to the secondary constriction. The metamorphosis from the fully extended interphasic chromosome to the condensed anaphasic chromosome is accomplished primarily by a spiralization of the fundamental structure of the chromosome, the *chromonema*. The primary constriction of the chromosome designates the position of the centromere from which spindle fibrils are generated during prometaphase.

The nature of the *nucleolar organizer* has not been fully solved. Depending on the species, considerable variations are found in the fine structures within the nucleolus. Frequently, extensions of the nucleolar organizer which is a part of the chromosome may establish continuity with the *nucleolonema* as fibrils or a reticulum. The persistence of the *nucleolonema* on the mitotic chromosomes has been reported by Estable and Sotelo,[8] who are also responsible for the terms, *nucleolonema* and *pars amorpha*. The main bulk of the nucleolar body, which disappears in late prophase, is the *pars amorpha*. It is probably this material that provides some or all the material in the matrix that coats the chromosomes during mitosis. The nucleolar organizer and the *nucleolonema,* regardless of their structure, persist and replicate for the next generation. This replication presumably occurs at the time the chromonema is replicated.

HUMAN NUCLEOLAR CHROMOSOMES

Since human cells possess one or more nucleoli, it would be of interest to establish which of the chromosomes may be associated with nucleoli. In this connection, the acrocentric chromosomes — groups D and G (according to the Patau classification) or 13, 14, 15, 21 and 22 (according to the Denver classification) — may be satellited.[3,18] Satellites are frequently a characteristic of nucleolar chromosomes, especially if the nucleolar organizer is near the terminal portion of the chromosome. Inasmuch as altogether 5 pairs of chromosomes may be satellited, this possibility might mean that human karyotypes could have as many as ten nucleolar chromosomes and, accordingly, as many as 10 nucleoli if fusion did not occur.

Some of these difficulties have been cleared up convincingly by Ohno et al.[17] Although chromosomes 13, 14, 15, 21 and 22 may carry satellites, not all carry satellites in the same karyotype. Moreover, not all satellited chromosomes, at any one time, necessarily generate a nucleolus.

It has been pointed out that chromosomes 13 and 21 may occasionally be associated with the same nucleolus.[17] The nucleolar organizer region (frequently long and attenuated), and the satellite as well as the nucleolus, can be seen clearly in early prophase. At prophase, breaks may occur in the chromosomes and give rise to reconstitution of various types. For example, when a break occurs in the nucleolar organizers of both 13 and 21, a translocation may follow in which the large satellite that originally belonged to 13 now becomes a part of chromosome 21. The result is an exchange of satellites with a partial exchange of nucleolar organizers. There are other possibilities which may lead to translocations in satellited chromosomes.

LAMPBRUSH CHROMOSOMES

The lampbrush chromosome is an architectural variant that occurs in certain vertebrate oöcytes prior to maturation. The loops which provide the lampbrush configuration are lateral extensions of the principal linear configuration of the chromosome.[9] These lampbrush loops tend to be rich in RNA and are presumably concerned with the synthesis of RNA or possibly even ribonucleoprotein (RNP). Only certain sites on the chromosome appear to be active at any one time.[5]

There are other sites that are nonfunctional. Such sites appear merely as chromomeres with no lateral loops. It is the loop that is the apparent functional component. The lampbrush chromosome seems to be primarily suited for the purpose of generating what appear to be copious amounts of RNA-rich substances. It may be assumed, therefore, that the active sites of the chromosomes are transmitting or transferring genetic information.

The physiology of lampbrush chromosomes has been studied by Duryee,[7] who described numerous microsurgical explorations on these chromosomes. In addition to stretching experiments, Duryee applied reagents with a micropipette to individual loops in order to determine their differential solubilities. It was thus established that chromosomes, immersed in calcium-free media, could be stretched to 4.5 times their original length; while chromosomes in 0.001 M CaC1$_2$ solutions could be stretched only about twice their length before breaking. In general, loop segments could not be stretched as much as the structures existing between the loops, namely, the principal chromosomal axis.

POLYTENE CHROMOSOMES

Another type of chromosome found in the salivary glands, intestinal cells, and malpighian tubules of larval Diptera is the *polytene,* so-called giant, chromosome. These chromosomes are several hundred times larger than conventional somatic chromosomes. They are characterized by prominent basophilic transverse bands. The giant salivary gland chromosomes of *Drosophila* are composites of several hundred, or indeed thousands, of individual chromosomal strands of *chromonemata* cabled together. Somatic synapsis also occurs.

Microsurgery on these chromosomes has been performed by several investigators.[14] One of them, D'Angelo,[6] may be singled out. A band in *Chironomus* chromosomes could be resolved, by transverse stretching, into a series of dots which represent chromomeres of the individual chromonemata. Furthermore, by delicate teasing with a microneedle, a single strand could be pulled out. This information, together with other studies, clearly demonstrates that these chromosomes are a composite cable of hundreds or thousands of individual *chromonemata*. The band is the concerted effect of the chromomeres which, depending on their size and shape, will form bands of various sizes, patterns, and staining intensities.

As in lampbrush chromosomes, the giant polytene chromosomes also show signs of localized intense activity.[2] In *Drosophila,* such activity is manifested by the formation of puffs or swellings, which appear to be centers of intense synthetic activity and produce RNA as well as proteins. In other Diptera, in addition to puffs, the Balbiani ring configurations are formed.

Both the puffs and Balbiani rings are specialized regions of activity within chromosomes. It is possible that the products elaborated from these sites may be subsequently involved in some particular biochemical activity which the cell is destined to enter at a precise time. Indeed, in *Drosophila melanogaster,* Becker[1] catalogued some 70 puffs, perhaps indicating that during development, ranging from the second instar to the pupa, at least 70 gene sites become unusually active. The polytene chromosomes might, therefore, represent a self-amplified system in which local gene action can be seen clearly. Local gene site activity in conventional somatic chromosomes cannot be so clearly demonstrated.

MICROSURGERY ON SOMATIC CHROMOSOMES

Another microsurgical operation on chromosomes is illustrated in figure 3.

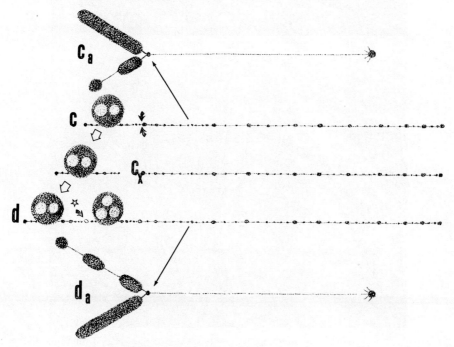

FIG. 3. Microsurgical translocation of nucleolar organizer. Chromosomes c and d are homologous at leptotene. Nucleolar organizer is cut off chromosome c at point indicated by arrows and is brought to chromosome d at point indicated by arrow and star. Chromosome c_a is the appearance of chromosome c prior to removal of nucleolar organizer at anaphase, while d_a is the anticipated appearance of chromosome d, also at anaphase. Chromosomes c_a and d_a show positions of centromere with spindle-attaching fibril, as well as secondary constrictions, indicating positions of the nucleolar organizers (from Kopac, Tr. New York Acad. Sc. 23: 200, 1961).

This is an attempt to produce an experimental chromosome with two nucleolar organizers, instead of the one that it normally has by a synthetic translocation.

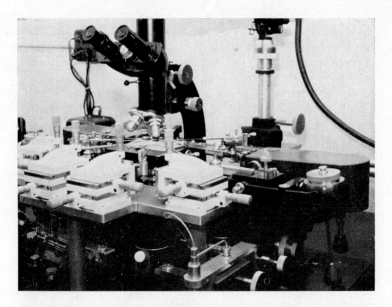

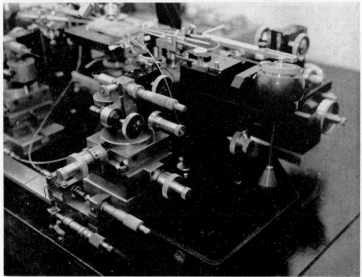

FIG. 4. Multi-unit micromanipulator assemblies. *(Top)* Right side of micromanipulator unit consisting of two volumetric submicromanipulators, two Leitz 1959 micromanipulators and two precision micromanipulators, with facilities for accommodating ten microneedles and micropipettes. *(Bottom)* Eight micromanipulators grouped around a microscope. Four micropositioners mounted on elevated subbase in front of microscope are used for holding recipient cells, for nucleolar transplantation. Leitz 1959 and 1961 micromanipulators, two on each side of microscope, are used for transplanting nucleoli. This unit is equipped with eight microinjectors, including two of the differential piston microinjectors (from Kopac and Harris, Ann. New York Acad. Sc. 97: 331, 1962).

Some progress is being made in this direction.[14] The main obstacle to the goal in this type of microsurgery is to get consistent anastomosis between the cut end of the chromosome and the end of the chromosome to which the fragment should become attached.

The instrumentation needed to accomplish such operations is much more sophisticated than the instrument with which Robert Chambers originally started. One of the newer instruments, shown in figure 4 *(top)*, was designed to accommodate ten microneedles or micropipettes.[15] There are six micropositioners in this instrument, two of them being volumetric submicromanipulators designed to handle and measure volumes of liquid of the order of one micro-microliter.

TRANSPLANTATION OF NUCLEOLI

Another useful and informative microsurgical procedure involves the transplantation of a *nucleolus*. Nucleoli have been successfully transplanted into the

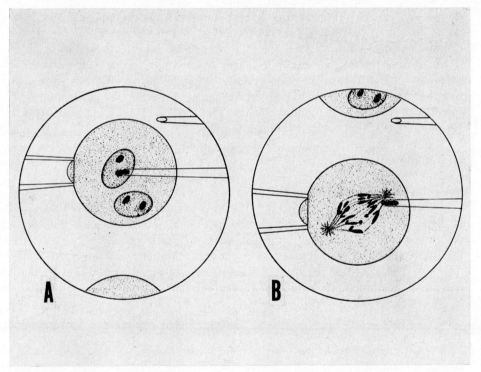

FIG. 5. Procedure for transplanting nucleolus into nucleus. (A) Donor cell is held by the microelastimeter which consists of a larger micropipette connected to the microinjector (see Kopac, 13). Part of the host cell is in view. One small micropipette is inserted into nucleus of donor cell showing partial extraction of nucleolus. The other small micropipette is in standby position. (B) Nucleolus inserted into host cell, in midanaphase, behind one set of chromosomes. This cell is also held by microelastimetry. Donor cell moved out of position. Diagram shows preferred orientation of mitotic spindle and the best position for inserting nucleolus to avoid damaging the spindle or deranging the chromosomes (from Kopac, Tr. New York Acad. Sc. 23: 200, 1961).

cytoplasm.[12,13] The transplantation of a nucleolus into an intact nucleus is much more difficult and requires a special procedure.* From a technical point of view, it would be easier to insert a nucleolus with a micropipette into the nucleus than it is to take out the nucleolus. The difficulty is that, probably 80 times out of a hundred, as soon as a nuclear membrane is punctured, especially with a larger micropipette, a series of events is initiated that eventually leads to the complete disintegration of that nucleus.

If the nuclear membrane does not exist as in anaphase, then there is nothing to puncture (fig. 5). The placement of a nucleolus behind one of the anaphase sets of chromosomes can be done without interrupting mitosis. During telophase, when the reconstitution of nuclei occurs, the nucleolus that was implanted becomes a part of the new nucleus. In all nucleolar transplants, there is the possibility that nucleolar chromosomes may be transplanted along with the nucleolus. It is not known how much chromosomal material is transplanted, because of the extreme difficulty in seeing conventional chromosomes during the interphase.

Examples of nucleoli successfully transplanted into the nucleus of a cell are shown in figure 6. These are cells of the renal adenocarcinoma of the frog grown in cell cultures. In figure 6A it can be seen that the nucleolus was accidentally fragmented during transplantation with the fragments held by delicate strands. Nevertheless, the nucleolus was "adopted" by the nucleus. The large nucleolus (fig. 6B) was also successfully "adopted" by the nucleus. Not only was this nucleolus fully incorporated by the nucleus, but the *in situ* nucleoli fused with the transplanted nucleolus. The fusion of nucleolar bodies is a common event if they are close enough together.

A system has been devised to solve the problem of timing. When a cell is undergoing mitosis, there is little that can be done to slow down the process without stopping it completely. In order to allow for the possibility that a nucleolus could not be extracted from a nucleus at the right time, instrumentation is now available to handle the problem.[15] This instrument is illustrated in figure 4 *(bottom)*. With the given instrument, four cells each held by a separate micropositioner can be lined up at various stages of mitosis. At the instant a nucleolus is taken out of a nucleus, the cells are inspected to see which one is ready to receive a nucleolus. There are four additional micromanipulators for removing nucleoli from the donor cells and implanting them into recipient cells.

TRANSPLANTATION OF NUCLEI

In recent years, *nuclei* have been successfully transplanted in a number of instances, including the *Amoeba,* various *Amphibia*[4] and *Acetabularia.*[10] Of particular interest were Kroeger's experiments on nuclear transplantation which also gave information on chromosomal changes. [16] The nuclei were explanted from prepuparium stages of *Drosophila busckii* into the preblastoderm

*The microsurgery of somatic chromosomes, nucleolar transplantation, and special instrumentation were supported in part by Grant C-2018 from the National Cancer Institute, National Institutes of Health, Public Health Service, and Grant DRG-271 from the Damon Runyon Memorial Fund for Cancer Research, Inc., New York, N. Y.

or blastoderm egg contents of *Drosophila melanogaster* extruded into a fluoro-carbon oil (Kel-F-I). After three hours in the preblastoderm or blastoderm egg contents, the nuclei were stained and squashed in order to reveal the banding and puffing patterns of the chromosomes.

Several interesting features were noted. Some of the puffs persisted through-out, as they normally did through to the puparium stage (achieved approxi-mately three hours after onset of the prepuparium). Other puffs disappeared in the preblastoderm or blastoderm egg content environment. In one instance, a huge puff, not heretofore seen, appeared on the second chromosome in nuclei explanted into preblastoderm egg contents, but did not appear in nuclei ex-planted into the blastoderm egg contents. Thus, the altered nuclear environ-

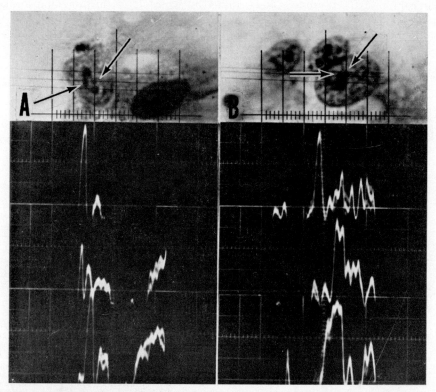

Fig. 6. Nucleoli transplanted into nucleus of renal adenocarcinoma of frog. Photo-graphs were taken from the video monitor screen with a standard polaroid camera by triple exposure to show each line selected for analysis on the oscilloscope. These selected lines appear as black horizontal lines on the video images (using Kin Tel closed circuit television) and correspond to the oscilloscope traces in sequence, top line and top trace, and so on. Positioning of traces and vertical adjustment of sweep time permits registry of pulses, with the structure shown in corresponding vertical segments in the video images. One vertical division on video image equals 7.6 microns. Cells fixed 30 hours after trans-plantation and stained with hematoxylin and eosin. (A) Nucleolus, fragmented during transplantation, consists of principal mass with two smaller satellites (indicated by arrows) attached to it by strands. (B) Large transplanted nucleolar mass with two smaller nucleoli (indicated by arrows) apparently attached to it (from Kopac, Tr. New York Acad. Sc. 23: 200, 1961).

ment had dramatically changed some of the structures of chromosomes, thereby illustrating the effects of ecology on chromosomal configurations.

ROLE OF CHROMOSOMES AND NUCLEOLUS IN CELLULAR DIFFERENTIATION

One of the major problems in biology is *cellular differentiation.* It is always a remarkable event that following fertilization, every stage in the development of a zygote proceeds on schedule. If the embryology is known, one can predict precisely when the various stages will appear. Along with the complex structural changes, there are also biochemical differentiating systems. For example, islet cells of the pancreas produce the protein, insulin. Muscle cells, among other substances, produce the protein, myoglobin.

A hypothetical situation in reference to these two cell types and the characteristic proteins they produce is illustrated in figure 7. In this diagram, a small

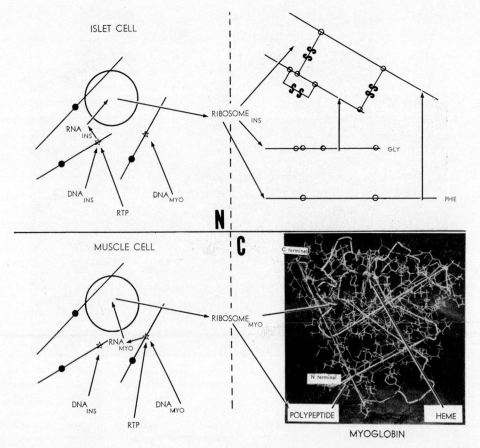

FIG. 7. Diagram illustrating hypothetical transfer of genetic information in islet cell and muscle cell. Nucleus (N) is to left of broken line (nuclear membrane); cytoplasm (C) is to the right. Only three chromosomes, one with a nucleolus, are shown. Islet cell shows hypothetical site of DNA with coded information needed to synthesize insulin. In muscle cell, a similar site is shown for producing coded RNA that will enable the cell to synthesize myoglobin. Figure of myoglobin is after Kendrew. [11]

fraction of the cell's genetic mechanism is shown, including one nucleolar chromosome with its nucleolus. The pancreatic islet cell obviously has the genetic information needed to synthesize insulin. Reasons have been established for believing that this information is stored on a specific chromosomal locus as coded DNA. There are also reasons for believing that this DNA does not directly participate in protein synthesis, but rather another nucleic acid, RNA, which must first be produced. For example, it is presumed that from a given region of DNA, specific RNA is copied off that carries the same code as represented by DNA.

The nucleolus probably plays a part in the next step. This RNA, the so-called messenger RNA, as it comes off of a particular gene locus, gets into the nucleolus where it is then integrated with other proteins, and also presumably with certain specific polymerizing enzymes. The resulting particles are probably the ribosomes which are generally found in the cytoplasm. The ribosome apparently passes through the nuclear membranes into the cytoplasm where, along with cytoplasmic membranes, it can then produce insulin. In the cytoplasm, the ribosome, which is coded specifically for insulin, must assemble the various adapted and activated amino acids to produce the 21-amino acid glycine chain and the 30-amino acid phenylalanine chain. Then, the ribosome must link these two chains together with three properly positioned disulfide bridges.

The muscle cell, on the other hand, produces myoglobin which has more amino acids than insulin and is also integrated with heme. Furthermore, there is considerably more structural complexity in the folding of the polymerized amino acids as has been suggested by Kendrew's[11] x-ray diffraction studies. The problem which arises is that of assembling some 150 amino acids in precise sequence as well as the folding of the long chain of amino acids into the intricate pattern which, when coupled with heme, constitutes the myoglobin molecule.

It may be presumed that in the chromosomes of muscle cells there is a gene locus, distinct from the insulin locus, with the information required for myoglobin synthesis. Here again, messenger RNA must be copied off the DNA template, and integrated with proteins and enzymes in the nucleolus, where a ribosome designed specifically for myoglobin synthesis is produced.

An interesting problem is the following: Do islet cells and muscle cells carry at the same time the genetic information needed for both insulin and myoglobin synthesis? If it is true that these cells still bear both kinds of genetic information, then another question arises: Why does the islet cell produce insulin and not myoglobin, and the muscle cell produce myoglobin and not insulin? Are the nucleoli in islet cells different from those in muscle cells? These are major problems in differentiation.

SUMMARY

There are three fundamental types of chromosomes: the somatic chromosomes, generally with a single chromonema; the lampbrush chromosome, whose lateral loop structures reflect localized hyperactivity in the synthesis of RNA or RNP; and the giant polytene chromosomes where repeated replication of chromonemata has occured without separation. Localized hyperactivity in the polytene chromosomes is shown through the development of puffs or Balbiani rings. Quite frequently, the environment may modify the chromosomal structures as has been revealed in the Kroeger experiments. In addition, the chromosomes may undergo changes in structure by spontaneous deletions or translocations.

A continued study of chromosomes and nucleoli, augmented with experiments which may alter their structures directly as by microsurgery or, indirectly by changes in ecology as produced by subcellular transplantations, may help us in unravelling the mysteries of *cellular differentiation,* probably one of our foremost biological problems.

REFERENCES

1. BECKER, H. J.: Die Puffs der Speicheldrüsenchromosomen von Drosophila melanogaster. I. Beobachtungen zum Verhalten des Puffmusters im Normalstamm und bei zwei Mutanten, Giant und Lethal-Giant-Larvae. Chromosoma 10: 654, 1959.
2. BEERMANN, W.: Chromosomal differentiation in insects. In Rudnick, D., Ed.: Developmental Cytology. New York, Ronald Press, 1959.
3. BÖÖK, J. A., et al.: Proposed chromosome nomenclature. Am. Inst. Biol. Sci. Bull. 10: 27, 1960; J. Hered. 51: 214, 1960.
4. BRIGGS, R., and KING, T. J.: Nucleo-cytoplasmic interactions in eggs and embryos. In Brachet, J., and Mirsky, A. E., Eds.: The Cell. New York, Academic Press, 1959, Vol. 1.
5. CALLAN, H. G., and LLOYD, L.: Lampbrush chromosomes of crested newts Triturus cristatus (Laurenti). Phil. Trans. Roy. Soc. Lond., B. Biol. Sci. 243: 135, 1960.
6. D'ANGELO, E. G.: Salivary gland chromosomes. Ann. N. Y. Acad. Sc. 50: 910, 1950.
7. DURYEE, W. R.: Chromosomal physiology in relation to nuclear structure. Ann. New York Acad. Sc. 50: 920, 1950.
8. ESTABLE, C., AND SOTELO, J. R.: Una nueva estructura celular: el nucleolonema. Publ. Inst. Invest. Ciencias Biol. 1: 105, 1951.
9. GALL, J. G.: Chromosomal differentiation. In McElroy, W. D., and Glass, B. Eds.: The Chemical Basis of Development. Baltimore, Johns Hopkins Press, 1958.
10. HAMMERLING, J., et al.: Growth and protein synthesis in nucleated and enucleated cells. Exp. Cell Res. (suppl.) 6: 210, 1958.
11. KENDREW, J. C.: The three-dimensional structure of a protein molecule. Scientific Am. 205: (Dec.) 96, 1961.
12. KOPAC, M. J.: Micrurgical studies on living cells. In Brachet, J., and Mirsky, A. E., Eds.: The Cell, New York; Academic Press, 1959, Vol. 1.
13. ———; Experimental studies on malignant nucleoli. In Proc. Symp. Fundamental Cancer Research, Vol. XIV (Cell Physiology and Neoplasia). Austin, Univ. Texas Press, 1960.
14. ———: Exploring living cells by microsurgery. Tr. New York. Acad. Sc. 23: 200, 1961.
15. ———, and HARRIS, J.: Microsurgery and visible light television. Ann. New York Acad. Sc. 97: 331, 1962.
16. KROEGER, H.: The induction of new puffing patterns by transplantation of salivary gland nuclei into egg cytoplasma of Drosophila. Chromosoma 11: 129, 1960.
17. OHNO, S., et al.: Nucleolus-organizers in the causation of chromosomal anomalies in man. Lancet 2: 123, 1961.
18. PATAU, K.: The identification of individual chromosomes, especially in man. Am. J. Human Genet. 12: 250, 1960.

11

Human Cytogenetics and Sex Determination

MALCOLM A. FERGUSON-SMITH, M.B., Ch.B.

IN HUMAN CYTOGENETICS the sex chromosomes are at present unique in that they are the only chromosomes to which specific genetic functions can be ascribed. Among these functions is included their role in sex determination and in the formation of sex chromatin, in addition to the more obvious and well known sex-linked traits such as color blindness and hemophilia.

In the past 3 years, the cytological demonstration of human sex chromosome aberrations has shed considerable new light on the mechanism of normal sex determination in man. It is the purpose of this paper to discuss these developments and, in addition, describe more recent information concerning the genetic role of the X chromosomes as shown by studies in patients who have gross structural anomalies of the X chromosomes.

It is well known that, in man, the sex of the individual is determined at the time of fertilization by the type of sex chromosome contributed by the paternal gamete. If the fertilizing sperm carries a Y chromosome, the resulting zygote has an XY sex chromosome constitution and will become a male. On the other hand, if the sperm is X-bearing, the zygote has an XX constitution and will become a female. A similar mechanism operates in a large number of species including *Drosophila,* from which very precise information about the exact genetics of sex determination has been obtained.

The actual way by which the sex chromosome constitution determines sex in Drosophila was shown by Bridges[4] and others over 40 years ago. They found that there was a delicate balance between male-determining genes carried on the autosomes and female-determining genes carried by the X chromosomes. This conclusion was derived partly from observations made by Bridges on the inheritance of sex-linked characters in Drosophila. He noted that in certain strains of Drosophila, exceptional females appeared which resembled the mother in all sex-linked characters and apparently carried no sex-linked characters from the father. These experiments suggested that such exceptional females inherited both X chromosomes from the mother.

Bridges was able to confirm this hypothesis by demonstrating cytologically that these flies had an XXY constitution. He also showed that exceptional males bearing sex-lined characters, inherited from the father, had an XO sex chromosome constitution; these males were sterile. Breeding the exceptional female with a normal male produced two further exceptional flies, the XXX or "super-female," and the XYY, a fertile male. Moreover, breeding the XYY male with the XXY female resulted in another viable female with an XXYY sex chromosome constitution.

On the basis of these experiments it was assumed that two X's in the presence of a normal diploid complement of autosomes produced a female, whereas the presence of only one X led to male differentiation. The Y chromosome apparently made no contribution to sex determination, although it was necessary for fertility.

In 1921, Bridges[5] described certain types of intersex in triploid flies, which were the result of imbalance produced by the increased dose of male-determining genes carried by the autosomes. The situation in Drosophila may be summarized by the following scheme, with A representing the haploid complement of autosomes:

2A + XX   = normal female
2A + XY   = normal male
2A + XXY = exceptional female (fertile)
2A + XO   = exceptional male (sterile)
2A + XXX = superfemale (usually nonviable)
2A + XYY = exceptional male (fertile)
2A + XXYY = exceptional female (fertile)
3A + XX   = intersex

Through these classic investigations it was possible for Bridges to provide an explanation for numerical abnormalities of the sex chromosomes in his exceptional flies. His hypothesis was that an abnormal cell division occurred during gametogenesis in the mother. At the first meiotic division of oogenesis, the XX chromosome bivalent fails to disjoin at anaphase so that both remain in the egg or pass out into the polar body. The fertilization of the resulting XX or O eggs by X or Y sperm from a normal male fly will produce the first three exceptions; namely XXY, XO and XXX individuals. Another type, YO, was assumed to be inviable and was never found.

The given defect in cell division, referred to as *nondisjunction,* apparently occurred during the first meiotic (reductional) division rather than the second (equational) division, because according to Bridges, females which were heterozygous for recessive characters and bred to normal males, produced only heterozygous-dominant characters and no homozygous-recessive characters. With nondisjunction taking place at the second meiotic division, the ensuing exceptional daughters would have been expected to show recessive traits.

Before the recent discoveries in human cytogenetics were made, it was widely held that sex determination in man followed the same type of balance mechanism as in Drosophila. However, the new developments have furnished evidence for the operation in man of a different mechanism, in which the Y chromosome plays a very important part. Nonetheless, Bridges' work remains the foundation of knowledge in this area, and nondisjunction is the most probable explanation for almost all the numerical abnormalities of human chromosomes which have meanwhile been described. It seems appropriate at this point to make a brief mention of the discovery of the sex chromosome aberrations on which our knowledge of sex determination in man is based.

HUMAN SEX CHROMOSOME ABNORMALITIES

The first indication of sex chromosome anomalies being not only viable but also not uncommon came from the results of nuclear sexing studies in the

Klinefelter and Turner syndromes. These studies were made before the techniques for human chromosome analysis were available.

In common with all mammalian cells, [29] human interphase nuclei show visible sex dimorphism in the form of a characteristic sex chromatin mass (fig. 1). This mass is present in 30 to 60 per cent of female nuclei, but is entirely absent in male nuclei (fig. 2). By means of the simple buccal smear technique, [22] normal individuals may invariably be assigned their correct *genetic sex* by microscopic determination of their nuclear sex. In 1954, it was discovered by Polani et al. [27] and Wilkins et al. [31] that certain females with short stature, primary amenorrhoea, ovarian agenesis and other stigmata of Turner's syndrome, had a male-type (or chromatin-negative) nuclear sex. Similarly in 1956, certain males with primary testicular atrophy and a variety of other features of Klinefelter's syndrome were found by Plunkett and Barr [26]

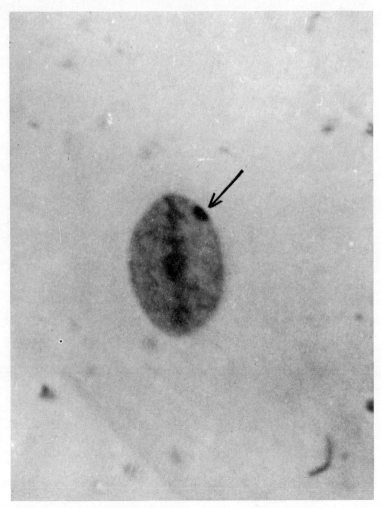

FIG. 1. Nucleus of an oral mucosal cell from a normal female showing sex-chromatin lying close to nuclear membrane. Cresyl echt violet x 4,000

and Bradbury et al.[3] to have a female-type (or chromatin-positive) nuclear sex.

Interest in these two syndromes was soon aroused, especially when it became clear that both conditions were much more common than had previously been supposed. In fact, the chromatin-positive Klinefelter's syndrome was found to account for three per cent of all subfertility at a male infertility clinic[11] and for about one per cent of male patients in an institution for the mentally retarded.[7] The latter frequency has been confirmed by various investigators. [8,23,28] In the general population, Klinefelter's syndrome occurs in approximately one in 400 male births,[21] whereas chromatin-negative Turner's syndrome is much rarer, with an estimated frequency of one in 1,000.

In searching for the basic etiology of these two disorders it became particularly important to know what the discrepancy between nuclear sex and

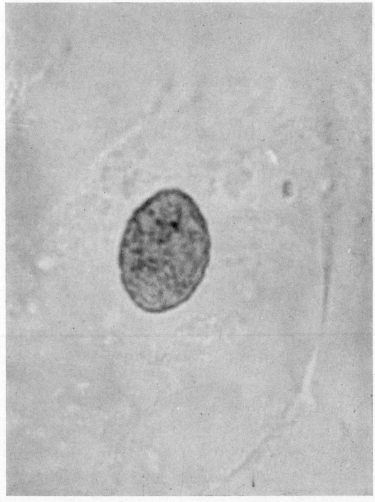

Fig. 2. Nucleus of an oral mucosal cell from a normal male. Chromatin-negative. Cresyl echt violet x 4,000

somatic appearance could mean. The obvious line of approach was to study the chromosomes and, if possible, determine the sex chromosome constitution of patients with anomalous nuclear sex. The elucidation of this problem has led to the discovery of an unexpectedly large group of sex chromosome aberrations in man.

As a result of the technical improvements which enabled Tjio and Levan[50] in 1956 to establish 46 as the correct somatic chromosome number in man, a reasonably accurate analysis of the human chromosome complement was possible by 1959. In that year, Ford et al.[12] reported that in chromatin-negative Turner's syndrome the somatic chromosome number was 45, and the sex chromosome constitution, XO. From the chromosomal point of view, these patients were similar to the exceptional XO individuals in Bridges' Drosophila experiments, the only discrepancy being that their phenotype is female instead of male. Almost simultaneously, chromosomal studies by Jacobs and Strong [16] in chromatin-positive Klinefelter's syndrome revealed that these patients had 47 chromosomes with an XXY sex chromosome constitution. Chromosomally, they had the identical anomaly of the XXY exceptional female fly, but their phenotype was male. These findings have since been confirmed by many investigators including our own group[9] and are illustrated in figures 3 and 4, which show the typical karyotype analyses in chromatin-negative Turner's syndrome and chromatin-positive Klinefelter's syndrome respectively.

Extension of surveys of nuclear sex among the mentally defective population has revealed two more types of "exceptional" individual. Analogous to the superfemale in Drosophila is the triple-X individual (fig. 5), who is usually fertile[9,14,17] and shows no characteristic syndrome recognizable on clinical grounds and attributable to the additional X chromosome.[19] The triple-X/Y individual (fig. 6) is male and presents the features of chromatin-positive

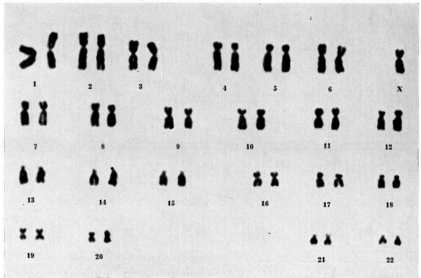

Fig. 3.   Karyotype of a somatic cell in a patient with chromatin-negative gonadal aplasia (Turner's syndrome). $2n - 1 = 45$ (XO).

Klinefelter's syndrome.[10] Both XXYY[24] and the XXXXY[13] individuals also resemble males with Klinefelter's syndrome, while the tetra-X individual is female and apparently not distinguished by a specific clinical syndrome.

All of these exceptional individuals can be recognized by their nuclear sex, as the maximum number of sex chromatin bodies per diploid nucleus is always one less than the number of X chromosomes (table 1). For example, in both

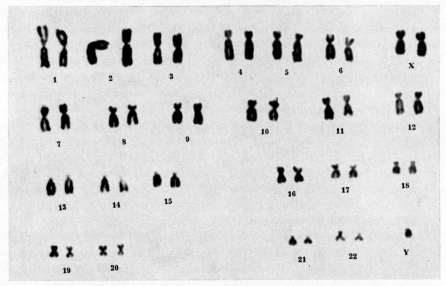

FIG. 4.   Karyotype in chromatin-positive Klinefelter's syndrome. 2n + 1 = 47 (XXY).

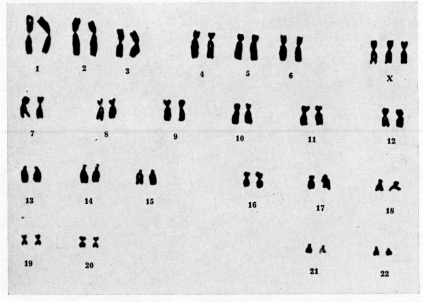

FIG. 5.   Karyotype in the triple-X syndrome. 2n + 1 = 47 (XXX).

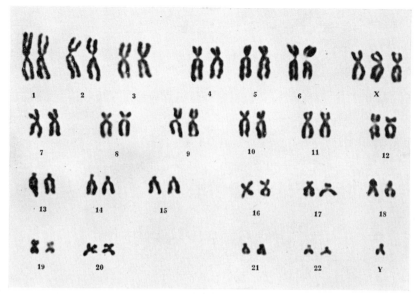

FIG. 6. Karyotype in the triple-X/Y syndrome. 2n + 2 = 48 (XXXY).

TABLE 1. EXCEPTIONAL SEX CHROMOSOME COMPLEMENTS IN MAN

	Sex Chromosome Constitution	Nuclear Sex	Phenotype
Chromatin-negative Turner's syndrome	XO	negative	sterile female
Chromatin-positive Klinefelter's syndrome	XXY	positive	
	XXXY	double positive	
	XXYY	positive	sterile male
	XXXXY	triple positive	
The extra-X syndromes	XXX	double positive	
	XXXX	triple positive	fertile female

the triple-X and the triple-X/Y syndromes the nuclear sex is double-positive (fig. 7), each sex chromatin body being of the same size as the single sex chromatin present in normal female nuclei. These various findings are summarized in table 1.

It may be concluded, therefore, that sex determination in man depends on one factor: the presence or absence of a Y chromosome. Irrespective of the number of X chromosomes present, one Y chromosome seems to carry sufficient male determiners for male sex determination. Similarly, additional X chromosomes over the normal XX female sex chromosome complement apparently have no effect on sex differentiation. The only exception to the rule of female sex differentiation, in the absence of a Y chromosome, is the rare situation encountered in true hermaphroditism. Here a testis that is defective may differentiate unilaterally despite an XX sex chromosome constitution.[10,15] These findings suggest that *normally* the Y chromosome carries strongly male-determining genes.

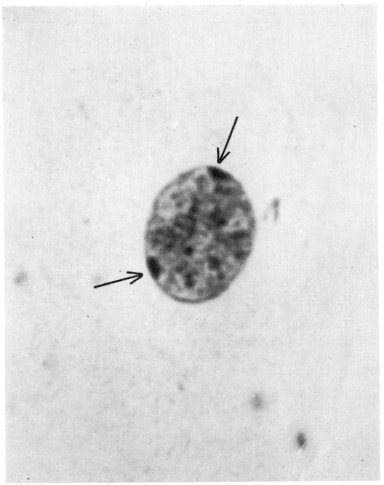

Fig. 7. Nucleus of an oral mucosal cell from a patient with the triple-X-Y syndrome. Double chromatin-positive. Cresyl echt violet x 4,000

THE ROLE OF THE X CHROMOSOME

What specific role does the X chromosome play in human sex determination? Apparently it plays an insignificant part, although, like the Y in Drosophila, it probably is necessary for fertility. Some indication of its importance in this regard has been derived from findings in patients with variants of Turner's syndrome, who are *chromatin-positive* in their nuclear sex. It is shown in table 2 that we have studied 19 patients with primary amenorrhoea, short stature, and associated anomalies of Turner's syndrome, who had various types of chromatin-positive nuclear sex (report is in preparation). In 17 patients, a definite chromosome abnormality has been demonstrated. Although seven different types of sex chromosome constitution have been identified in this group, the basic defect common to all of them is loss or deletion of the short arm of one X chromosome in at least a significant proportion of cells.

In 10 cases, there is evidence of sex chromosome mosaicism. In other words, each individual is composed of cells from two or more stem lines, with each

TABLE 2. SEX CHROMOSOME ANOMALIES IN TURNER'S SYNDROME

Sex Chromosome Constitution*	Number of Cases	Nuclear Sex	
		Proportion of positive cells	Size of sex chromatin
XO	7	none	—
XO/XX	9	low count	normal
XO/XX/XXX	1	low count, single and double	normal
Xχ	1	high count	large
XO/Xχ	2	normal count	large
XO/Xχ/XXX	1	low count, single and double	some large
XO/Xx	2	very low count	small
Xx	1	low count	small
XX	2	normal count	normal

* In this column, the symbol X denotes a normal X chromosome; χ, a presumed isochromosome for the long arm of X and x, a partially deleted X chromosome.

stem line having a different sex chromosome constitution. In another case (figs. 8 A and B), an abnormally large X chromosome has been found, indistinguishable from chromosome No. 3, and interpreted as an isochromosome for the long arm of the X chromosome. Such an isochromosome may be produced during cell division by transverse instead of longitudinal fracture of the centromere. This abnormal division results in the formation of two metacentric chromosomes which may be of unequal length. The arms of each individual daughter chromosome are genetically identical so that the abnormality may be considered a very gross type of duplication-deficiency.

Two other cases show a similar isochromosome in addition to mosaicism, while a third case is distinguished by an abnormally small X chromosome

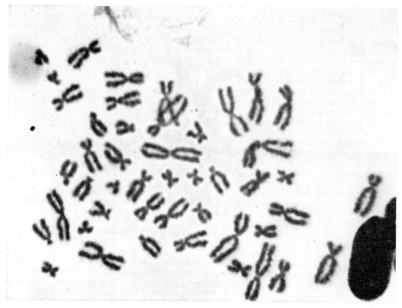

FIG. 8. (A) Squash preparation of a bone marrow cell in a case of chromatin-positive Turner's syndrome. Aceto-orcein x 4,000

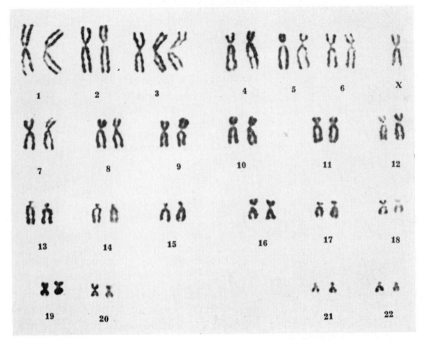

Fig. 8.   (B) Karyotype of above cell showing an abnormally large X chromosome indistinguishable from chromosome 3.

comparable in size but distinguishable from chromosome No. 18 (fig. 9). The karyotype of the last case may be interpreted as the result of deletion of one X chromosome, because examination of the nuclear sex reveals a very low count of small sex chromatin bodies (fig. 11 and table 2).

Only very recently Jacobs et al.[18] have described 3 cases of chromatin-positive Turner's syndrome, who have structural abnormalities of one X chromosome. While one is an isochromosome for the long arm of an X chromosome, the second has been interpreted as a partial deletion of the long arm of one X, and the third appears to be an almost complete deletion of the short arm of one X. Laparotomy, with examination of the internal genitalia, has been performed in the second case of Jacobs et al.[18] and in 8 of the 17 chromatin-positive cases in table 2. The findings in all cases have been identical, and indistinguishable from the chromatin-negative group. In the usual ovarian site, there are "streak" gonads in place of the ovaries. These structures are composed of dense fibrous tissue resembling ovarian stroma, but they contain no germinal cells.

These observations suggest that the genetic material of both X chromosomes is necessary for initiation of normal differentiation of the ovary, but is not essential for female differentiation of the genital ducts and external genitalia. This conclusion is in perfect accord with certain findings in experimental embryology. According to Jost's work,[20] the fetus will differentiate along female lines, irrespective of genetic sex, if the gonad is destroyed at a critical period of development.

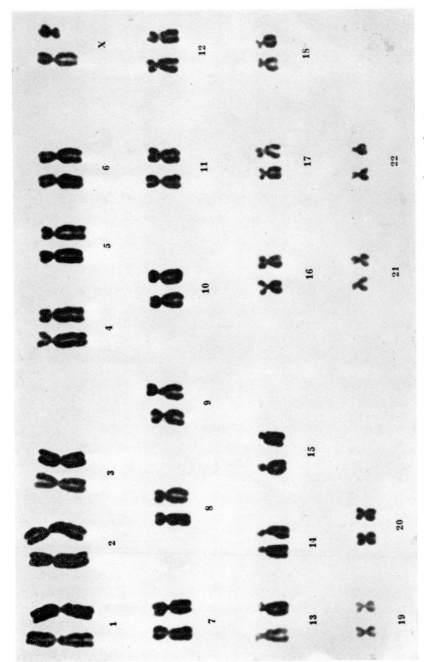

FIG. 9. Karyotype in a patient with chromatin-positive Turner's syndrome showing one abnormally small X chromosome.

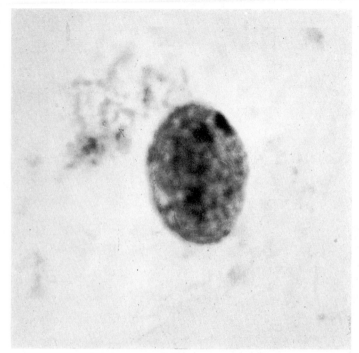

Fig. 10.   Nucleus of an oral mucosal cell in a patient who has an isochromosome for the long arm of one X chromosome (same case as fig. 8). Cresyl echt violet x 4,000

THE ORIGIN OF SEX CHROMATIN

Chromosome analyses in the group of chromatin-positive variants of the Turner syndrome have provided very strong evidence relating the sex chromatin body directly to the X chromosome.

According to an earlier hypothesis,[2] the sex chromatin body represents heteropyknotic portions of the two X chromosomes which are visible in the resting nucleus due to somatic pairing. By and large, this hypothesis was based on circumstantial evidence. The sex chromatin was observed only in individuals with two X chromosomes, and it sometimes appeared as though formed by two distinct bodies. Its absence in the male was interpreted as indicating that the equivalent portion of a single X chromosome was either not large enough to be distinguished from the other nuclear chromocenters, or was not heteropyknotic.

A more likely alternative hypothesis, proposed recently, implicates only one of the X chromosomes and thus does not require somatic pairing. Supporting evidence comes from observations on nuclear sex dimorphism in lower species. In birds, butterflies and moths, the female also shows a nuclear sex chromatin mass. However, as the female and not the male is the heterogametic sex, this sex chromatin is associated with only one X chromosome.

Investigations of Ohno et al.[25] have given support to the hypothesis that the sex chromatin in mammals is derived from heteropyknotic portions of one X chromosome. These studies have demonstrated that in the prophase stage of mitosis in the female one of the X chromosomes is heteropyknotic and is

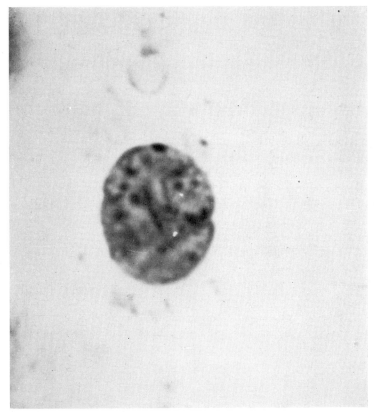

FIG. 11. Nucleus of an oral mucosal cell in a patient who has an abnormally small X chromosome (same case as fig. 9). Cresyl echt violet x 4,000

thus distinguishable from the other chromosomes. In the rat, this X chromosome is bent acutely at its center and resembles the shape of the sex chromatin at interphase. The male reveals no differential heteropyknosis of any of the prophase chromosomes and, of course, shows no sex chromatin. Corroborative evidence is furnished by the nuclear sex findings in the triple-X and triple-X/Y syndromes. In line with the earlier hypothesis of sex chromatin being formed by the combined effects of two X chromosomes, the observation of double sex chromatin bodies in these two syndromes should indicate the presence of 4 and not of 3 X chromosomes.

Finally, in our patients with structural anomalies of the X chromosomes, variation in size of the sex chromatin body can be closely related to the size and composition of the abnormal X chromosome. For example, the patient with the isochromosome of the long arm of the X chromosome (fig. 8 A) has a very large, single sex chromatin body (fig. 10), while the case with the presumed deletion of one X chromosome (fig. 9) has a very small, single sex chromatin body (fig. 11). Of course, a much larger series is needed to determine what parts of the X chromosome contribute to the formation of sex chromatin. Nevertheless, observations of this kind have definitely established that it is not an autosomal product.

One major implication of recent studies on the origin of the sex chromatin still defies adequate explanation; namely, that in female somatic cells the two X chromosomes are different, at least to the extent that one forms sex chromatin and the other does not. We can only speculate how such differentiation may occur. Two possible opportunities for the differentiation of the two X chromosomes are during gametogenesis and at the time of fertilization.

DISCREPANCIES IN NUCLEAR SEX

The previously described correlations between nuclear sex anomalies and sex chromosome constitutions seem to provide an answer to two further questions which have been a source of confusion in the past. The first concerns discrepancies in nuclear sex diagnosis made in different tissues in the same individual. There have been several reports on Turner and Klinefelter cases with a different nuclear sex in skin or buccal smear, as well as in white blood cells. Hence, some investigators[1] questioned whether the polymorphonuclear "drumstick," first described by Davidson and Smith,[6] is the same structure as the sex chromatin body. However, in our mosaic XO/XX and XO/XX/XXX cases it is not unusual to find some tissues in which sex chromatin is absent, while other tissues have low counts of sex chromatin, and yet other tissues have nuclei with two sex chromatin bodies. With this degree of variation being consistently observed in sex chromosome mosaics, the diagnosis of mosaicism may be predicted before chromosome analysis.

The view that the polymorphonuclear "drumstick" is the sex chromatin body is firmly substantiated by studies of two of our cases with structural anomalies

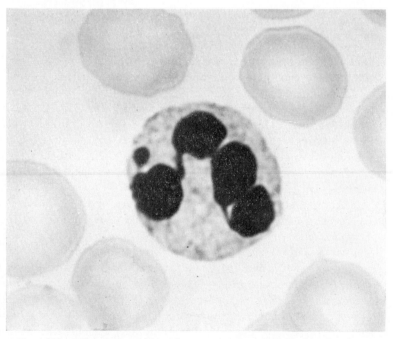

Fig. 12. (A) Polymorphonuclear leucocyte in a normal female showing typical "drumstick." x 4,000

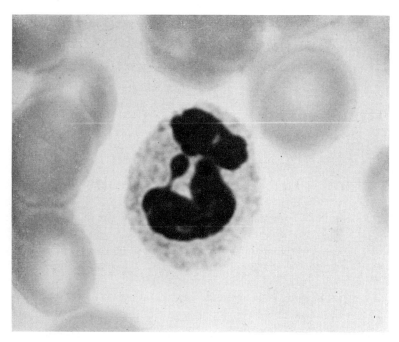

Fig. 12 (B) Large polymorphonuclear "drumstick" in a patient with an isochromosome for the long arm of an X chromosome (same case as fig. 8 A). x 4,000

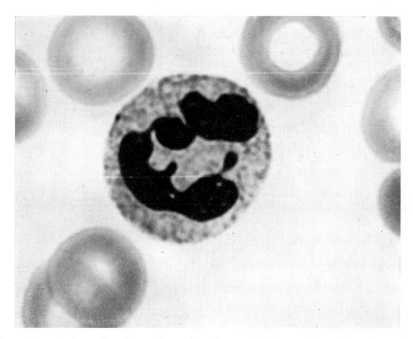

Fig. 12. (C) Small polymorphonuclear drumstick in a patient with a large deletion of an X chromosome. x 4,000

of the X chromosome. Figure 12 A shows a typical "drumstick" in a preparation from a normal XX individual. In fig. 12 B, the drumstick is recognizably larger than normal in the case with the isochromosome of the long arm of the X, while in an individual with deletion of the large part of the long arm of the X the drumstick is much smaller than normal (fig. 12 C). The size of the drumstick is, in fact, dependent on the size and composition of the X chromosome in entirely the same way as the sex chromatin mass.

SUMMARY

The discovery of various human sex chromosome abnormalities in the past three years has led to a revision in current views on the mechanisms of sex determination in man. In line with the accumulated evidence, the Y chromosome carries strongly male-determining genes, while the X chromosome plays no significant part in sex determination although it is essential for fertility.

Study of 17 patients with chromatin-positive gonadal aplasia (Turner's syndrome) indicates that the genetic material in two X chromosomes is necessary for the initiation of normal differentiation of the ovary. The nuclear sex and chromosomal findings in these patients and in other types of sex chromosome anomaly provide strong support for the hypothesis that the sex chromatin body is derived from a single X chromosome. These observations also give proof to the hypothesis that the polymorphonuclear "drumstick" is the sex chromatin body, and lend support to the view that discrepancies in nuclear sex diagnosis from different tissues in the same individual may be attributable to sex chromosome mosaicism.

REFERENCES

1. ASHLEY, D. J. B.: Occurrence of sex chromatin in the cells of the blood and bone marrow in man. Nature 179: 969, 1957.
2. BARR, M. L.: Sex chromatin and phenotype in man. Science 130: 679, 1959.
3. BRADBURY, J. T., BUNGE, R. G., AND BOCCABELLA, R. A.: Chromatin test in Klinefelter's syndrome. J. Clin. Endocrinol. 16: 689, 1956.
4. BRIDGES, C. B.: Non-disjunction as proof of the chromosome theory of heredity. Genetics 1: 107, 1916.
5. ———: Triploid intersexes in Drosophila melanogaster. Science 54: 252, 1921.
6. DAVIDSON, W. M., AND SMITH, D. R.: A morphological sex difference in the polymorphonuclear neutrophil leucocytes. Brit. M. J. 2: 6, 1954.
7. FERGUSON-SMITH, M. A.: Chromatin positive Klinefelter's syndrome (primary micro-orchidism) in a mental deficiency hospital. Lancet 1: 928, 1958.
8. ———: The prepubertal testicular lesion in chromatin positive Klinefelter's syndrome (primary micro-orchidism) as seen in mentally handicapped children. Lancet 1: 219, 1959.
9. ———, AND JOHNSTON, A. W.: The human chromosomes in disorders of sex differentiation. Tr. A. Am. Physicians 73: 60, 1960.
10. ———, ———, AND WEINBERG, A.: The chromosome complement in true hermaphroditism. Lancet 2: 126, 1960.
11. ———, et al.: Klinefelter's syndrome: Frequency and testicular morphology in relation to nuclear sex. Lancet 2: 167, 1957.
12. FORD, C. E., et al.: A sex chromosome anomaly in a case of gonadal dysgenesis. Lancet 2: 711, 1959.
13. FRACCARO, M., KAIJSER, K., AND LINDSTEN, J.: A child with 49 chromosomes. Lancet 2: 899, 1960.

14. FRASER, J. H., et al.: The XXX syndrome: Frequency among mental defectives and fertility. Lancet 2: 626, 1960.

15. HUNGERFORD, D. A., et al.: The chromosome constitution of a human phenotypic intersex. Am. J. Human Genet. 11: 215, 1959.

16. JACOBS, P. A., AND STRONG, J. A.: A case of human intersexuality having a possible XXY sex determining mechanism. Nature 183: 302, 1959.

17. ———, et al.: Evidence for the existence of the human "superfemale." Lancet 2: 423, 1959.

18. ———, et al.: Cytogenetic studies in primary amenorrhoea. Lancet 1: 1183, 1961.

19. JOHNSTON, A. W., et al.: The triple-x syndrome: Clinical pathological and chromosomal studies in three mentally retarded cases. Brit. M. J. 2: 1046, 1961.

20. JOST, A.: Réchérches sus la differenciation sexuelle de l'embryon de lapin. III. Rôle des gonads foetales dans la differenciation sexuelle somatique. Arch. Anat. Micr. Morphol. Exp. 36: 271, 1947.

21. MOORE, K. L.: Sex reversal in newborn babies. Lancet 1: 217, 1959.

22. ———, AND BARR, M. L.: Smears from the oral mucosa in the detection of chromosomal sex. Lancet 2: 57, 1955.

23. MOSIER, H. D., SCOTT, L. W., AND COTTER, L. H.: The frequency of the positive sex chromatin pattern in males with mental deficiency. Pediatrics 25: 291, 1960.

24. MULDAL, S., AND OCKEY, C. H.: The "double male": A new chromosome constitution in Klinefelter's syndrome. Lancet 2: 493, 1960.

25. OHNO, S., KAPLAN, W. D., AND KINOSITA, R.: Formation of the sex chromotin by a single X-chromosome in liver cells of Rattus norvegius. Exp. Cell Res. 18: 415, 1959.

26. PLUNKETT, E. R., AND BARR, M. L.: Congenital testicular hyperplasia. Lancet 2: 853, 1956.

27. POLANI, P. E., HUNTER, W. F., AND LENNOX, B.: Chromosomal sex in Turner's syndrome with co-arctation of the aorta. Lancet 2: 120, 1954.

28. PRADER, A., et al.: Die Häufigkeit des echten, chromatin-positiven Klinefelter Syndroms und seine Beziehungen zum Schwachsinn. Schweiz. med. Wchnschr. 88: 917, 1958.

29. SMITH, D. R., AND DAVIDSON, W. M. (Eds.): Symposium on Nuclear Sex. London, Heinemann, 1958.

30. TJIO, J. H., AND LEVAN, A.: The chromosome number of man. Hereditas 42: 1, 1956.

31. WILKINS, L., GRUMBACH, M. M., AND VAN WYK, J. J.: Chromosomal sex in "Ovarian Agenesis." J. Clin. Endocrinol. 14: 1270, 1954.

12

Biochemical Genetics and Human Metabolism

W. EUGENE KNOX, M.D.

THE RECENT ADVANCES in biochemistry and genetics have significantly changed the way we must think about hereditary mechanisms. In order to review the new principles, we may apply them to the explanation of one hereditary disease of the mind, phenylketonuria. But if these principles have the general validity we think they do, analogous explanations must hold for all other diseases.

A disease, or any hereditary character, is not inherited as such. It is a consequence of a long series of interactions in the individual, some of which were initiated by gene actions and some by environmental actions. Therefore, the following three main parameters are to be considered: (1) the effects of heredity, (2) the effects of environment, and (3) the interactions of "pathogenetic mechanisms." They will be considered in that order.

All too commonly, emphasis is placed on heredity or environment in discussing the etiology of disease. This dichotomizing attitude holds especially true for diseases of the mind. Yet, it is really incorrect to consider each disease to be poised somewhere between the extremes of nature and nurture, dependent more upon the nearer pole and less upon the farther pole. Heredity *and* environment necessarily cooperate to produce every case of clinical disease. This truism now has substance in the detailed knowledge of the chemical mechanisms, by which heredity and environment can determine the nature of the individual.

For the sake of convenience, that which determines the physiological nature of an individual may be referred to as *information*. For example, the information of the hereditary gene is intrinsic in its chemical properties. This information is, in fact, chemically inscribed instructions about *some* of the activities that can occur.

The stimulus of the environment also contains information. One of the great unifying principles of our time is the realization that information, embodied in any kind of signal, is thermodynamically the same as free energy. Disorder of the signals, or noise, is the same as entropy. The orderly arrangement of atoms in a molecule, and even the concentration of a chemical substance, as we shall see, is associated with certain information just as it is associated with a certain free energy. The immediate problem is to see how much information makes an individual what he is.

The notions of information and noise are easier to use than the energetic concepts of $-\Delta F$ and $T\Delta S$, especially for certain applications. Nothing would seem to prevent the extension of these ideas beyond the biochemical level into the realm of behavior and learning, thus amplifying the already familiar use of the word information in these fields with its powerful thermodynamic connotations. However, in this report we shall not go so far. Here it would seem preferable to explicitly exclude that kind of information which determines adaptive behavior and learning.

HEREDITARY INFORMATION

It is first necessary to appreciate the singularly limited nature of the hereditary information. It has been common knowledge for a century that a store of information in each germ cell told it whether to develop into a mollusk or a man. Cytology localized this information store in the nuclear chromosomes. Genetic research on the various inherited peculiarities or "characters" was able to recognize in this total informational content of a species some more or less hypothetical but independently acting units called genes. Although much has been imputed to it, the *genetic gene* represented only a modicum of information concerned ideally with one thing or one character, like a paragraph in a book.

More recently, it was possible to identify DNA (deoxyribonucleic acid) as the *chemical carrier* of the hereditary information. Once the essential chemical structure of DNA was discovered, the kind of information inscribed on the chemical gene was definable in structural (molecular) terms. This advance marked the fusion of genetics with chemistry: the informational gene, previously a theoretical construct, has finally been placed on a material basis.

In the rush of this remarkable progress toward such new concepts as the gene's subdivision into recons, cystrons and mutons, the image of what the gene really is has become somewhat blurred, simply because its structure can now be studied in its *minute details* — its sentences, words, and even letters. We can work with the "molecular graininess" of the hereditary material, instead of only with whole paragraphs of genetic information. Curiously, however, the extreme simplicity of this information seems to have taken many biologists by surprise.

Chemically, the DNA substrate of the gene consists of very long double threads which are formed by monotonously repeating sugar molecules joined one after another by phosphate bonds. These backbones carry little information. To each sugar thread is attached a sequence of the four bases: adenine, thymidine, cytosine, or guanine. Their initial letters, A, T, C and G, make up the alphabet of the new hereditary language. The two threads with their projecting bases are opposed in a ladder-like structure, which tends to be wound into a helix. There is little in this chemical picture of DNA to resemble the infinitely complex and modulating germ plasm expected by some biologists. Yet chemists believe that the structure described is admirably suited to the limited functions the gene is supposed to perform:

1. It has to replicate exactly in order to supply the next generation with precisely the same information. While replication for the next generation of individuals does not concern us here, replication from the egg to all the body cells is similar to the former phenomenon and central to our present problem. According to current theory, the latter form of replication is facilitated by the double helical nature of DNA. The two strands with projecting bases are exact

complements of one another, like a die and its pressing. This is an admirable basis for any replication.

2.   The gene has to be remarkably stable to chemical change throughout countless generations. The cumulative strength of the hydrogen bondings between the bases stacked flat one upon the next within the double helix can confer unusual chemical stability, equal to that required of the hereditary substance. Barring the effects of the intense energy of ionizing radiation, and some chemical mutagens, the given structure is almost immutable. It cannot, for example, be modified during the life of an individual, although modifications of this kind would help us explain the modulations and chronologies of some apparently hereditary traits.

3.   Finally, the gene must carry a good deal of unambiguous information. The amount poses no problem. With the DNA strands being very long, they are coiled into helices and folded, gene after gene, into a large number of chromosomes. The crux of the problem is how precisely and completely the limited kind of information carried by the gene can specify the type of organ structure or function that is to be created.

The information held by the DNA can only be coded into the varying sequences of the four bases along its length. There is no other possibility. The most efficient use of the four bases, taken three at a time, would give exactly 20 triplet sets, or words, like ATC and ATG. These 20 words do not need punctuation to show where one leaves off and the next one begins. Forty other possible words like TCA and CAT have been omitted in this particular vocabulary, because they would occur within a repetition of the word ATC (— ATCATC—), and so cause ambiguity.   Fortunately, only twenty different words are necessary to express the kinds of hereditary messages which have been deciphered.

TRANSCRIPTION FROM GENE TO OPERATOR

The information on the gene must be materialized into something to affect the individual. The transduction is mediated through the equation of the twenty different words of DNA with the twenty different amino acids which make up all proteins. This equivalence provides striking confirmation for the gradual emergence, over the past fifty years, of the view that *proteins* are often the operative products of genes. In fact, the ability of the information on DNA to display extreme specialization in mapping protein structure and, conversely, the apparent dependence of genetic information on being expressed through some proteins would seem to indicate that all genes may form patterns for structuring proteins and that all proteins are likely to have equivalent genic patterns. This, at least, is the well supported current hypothesis.

The first clues that the hereditary instructions transducted through the gene were materialized in proteins were derived from that class of functional proteins called enzymes. In 1908, Sir Archibald Garrod [1] recognized that a defective enzyme caused a specific abnormality in metabolism which resulted from a stoppage at the metabolic step controlled by the enzyme, "just as when the film of a biograph is brought to a standstill, the moving figures are left foot in air." Then "the intermediate product in being at the point of arrest will escape further change," and by accumulating will give rise to the discernible symptoms of disease. Since several such enzyme deficiency diseases were found to be inherited, Garrod named them the *inborn errors of metabolism.* Modern genetic theories simply extend the concept of the inheritance of defects in enzyme proteins to all proteins, including some which have not yet been recognized.

It was another class of proteins, the hemoglobins, which provided the first direct proof of the gene-protein relationship. In effect, they served as the Rosetta stone in revealing the hereditary language. The essential structure of hemoglobin, like that of DNA, is a linear string. The strings of the hemoglobin protein are made up of the twenty different amino acids and are about 150 amino acids long. A string, called a polypeptide chain, is made by a particular gene. Two chains of each kind controlled by different genes (α and β) are coiled together in a worm-like manner to form the globular protein molecule of adult hemoglobin. Therefore, hemoglobin has the structure $\alpha_2 \beta_2$ and is produced by two analogous genes, α and β, which are located on different chromosomes.

The secret of the hereditary control of protein function lies in the linear correspondence between each of the twenty different three-letter words on the DNA chain and each of the twenty different amino acids on the polypeptide chain. The study of the hemoglobins has disclosed that the hereditary information is marked by the purine and pyrimidine bases along something like ticker tape. It is transcribed by the machinery of the cell onto a similar tape marked with amino acids. The analogy is very close to the way instructions for modern computers are handled on punched tapes.

The sequence of discoveries began with Ingram's finding that the genetic mutation producing sickle-cell anemia could not have changed more than just one word on the DNA, because there was a precise alteration of just one amino acid on one of the polypeptide chains of hemoglobin from patients with sickle-cell anemia. [2] The alteration was the substitution of valine for the usual glutamic acid in the sixth position from the amino end of the β-polypeptide chain of adult hemoglobin. No alterations were found at any of the other 150 sites on the β-chain, and none on the α-chain.

Actually, it was possible to carry the demonstration of the exactness of the relation between one gene and one polypeptide chain one step further. Only a homozygous individual with both genes for the β-chain abnormality was shown to be abnormal in all his hemoglobin and to have sickle-cell anemia. The heterozygous individual with both a normal and an abnormal gene had both normal and abnormal kinds of hemoglobin. There was no blending of inheritance at the molecular level. At the clinical level, however, although the red cells of the heterozygous individual can be made to sickle under extreme conditions, the complement of normal hemoglobin so dilutes the effect of the abnormal that no serious pathological consequences result.

There is good reason to believe that the mutations, which cause the defective enzymes in the inborn errors of metabolism, produce their effect in the same way. Through a change in a single amino acid, the ability of the whole enzyme molecule to catalyze its reaction is apt to be impaired or completely lost. It is already well established that specific enzyme activities are missing in a number of these diseases, with such losses being sufficient to account for the major clinical findings. There is even the analogy between the effects of one and two abnormal genes. In several diseases of this kind, the homozygous individual has no active enzyme, while the heterozygous individual has active enzyme but in less than the normal amount.

Similar alterations of proteins with some as yet unrecognized functions may well be the primary causes of *all* the hereditary diseases. The principle is not in question. What is holding us up is our current ignorance of the physiological roles of a great number of proteins and of the subtle dysfunctions which can result from the interaction of altered proteins and their environment.

For the causation of disease in an individual, an error in the hereditary information may be necessary, but it may not suffice in itself. Sufficient environmental "information" or stimulus tending to evoke the disease may occur so haphazardly that even the hereditary basis of the disease will remain uncertain. The chemical principles underlying these environmental stimuli will now be described.

ENVIRONMENTAL INFORMATION

It is commonly implied in specialized discussions of genetics that the store of hereditary information completely determines the important elements of an individual. All biology, then, would simply depend on the ordering of a few amino acids in particular sequences. Thereafter, life would run its course like a wound-up clock.

It is now known, however, that the environment inside and outside the cell supplies additional information in such a way that it can control the nature of an individual almost as fully as can his heredity. It does so in precise chemical ways that are complementary with the workings of the hereditary information. This objective is achieved through the supply of a different kind of information than is furnished by heredity. The limited nature of the hereditary information is able to determine only the *qualitative* patterns of the proteins. Information for the *quantitative* control of gene product formation must come from the chemical environment of the gene and cell. The actions of these two kinds of information are diagramed in figure 1, one controlling through the gene structure the *structure* of the enzyme, and the other through the gene action the *amount* of the enzyme.

Reflection will impel us to realize that gene action cannot be automatic. All genes cannot possibly be forming products all the time, and those in action cannot be working at constant and equal rates. Unless some genes were quiescent until turned on, the liver would not have a different enzymatic machinery than has the brain. Indeed, if all genes were continuously active, all hereditary abnormalities would appear in the embryo and never, like Huntington's chorea, during middle age. Unless some gene actions could be speeded up or slowed down, tissue repair would not be possible. Even the phenomena of growth and maturation would not occur. Some aspects of sickle-cell anemia and phenylketonuria will also serve to illustrate the workings of this quantitative control of gene action by the environment.

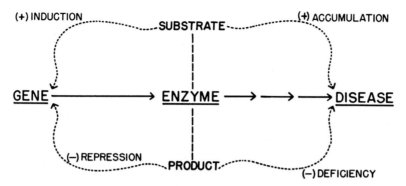

FIG. 1. Hereditary and environmental controls of enzyme action and disease production. The qualitative nature of the enzyme is determined by the gene structure, and the quantity of the enzyme by components of the chemical milieu, which induce or repress gene action. For an individual the consequence of a blocked metabolic step is the same whether the enzyme is inactive because imperfectly structured or because it is not formed.

An individual who is homozygous for the gene which predisposes to sickle-cell anemia does not have the disease as an infant. The explanation is that the human fetus makes and uses a different hemoglobin until after birth. The fetal hemoglobin (Hgb F) contains a γ-polypeptide chain which is replaced by the chemically distinct β-polypeptide chain of adult hemoglobin (Hgb A). The genes α and γ determine the structure of the α- and γ-chains of fetal hemoglobin. After birth the γ-gene ceases to act and the β-gene becomes active, producing the adult hemoglobin. In sickle-cell anemia the normal β-gene is replaced by a mutant β^s which produces the abnormal β^s-polypeptide found in the hemoglobin of patients with sickle-cell anemia (Hgb S). Only after birth,

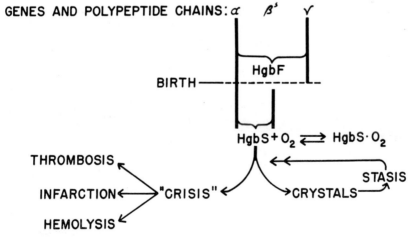

FIG. 2. Pathogenesis of sickle-cell anemia. Environmental information acting at the time of birth suppresses γ-gene action and initiates β-gene action with formation of the abnormal hemoglobin. This molecule's low solubility when deoxygenated can initiate the vicious cycle shown to precipitate a clinical crisis.

when the β-gene becomes active will an affected child begin to accumulate abnormal hemoglobin and to show symptoms of sickle-cell anemia (fig. 2). However, the γ-gene persists in the cell, becoming active in conditions like thalassemia when all the body's resources for hemoglobin synthesis must be exploited. Obviously, some kind of information is signaled at the time of birth to stop the operation in the γ-genes and to start the β-genes, thereby switching over production from the fetal to the adult type of hemoglobin. In the absence of this information, the individual would not develop sickle-cell anemia!

A similar situation occurs in phenylketonuria. None of us reading this have mental deficiency of the kind caused by a lack of phenylalanine hydroxylase, yet all of us lacked this enzyme until some time after birth! The gene with the information to make this enzyme was inoperative until, fortunately for us, something turned on its function during early childhood. It would be fair to say that we escaped mental deficiency because we were exposed to the essential effect of this postnatal stimulus.

THE ACTION OF THE ENVIRONMENTAL INFORMATION

If the first appearance of phenylalanine hydroxylase in the liver after birth is induced by the excess of phenylalanine in the food we eat, this causal relation would accord with what we know about the quantitative control of gene action. We do not yet have such detailed knowledge for phenylalanine hydroxylase. But other enzymes, including tryptophan pyrrolase, a similar amino acid metabolizing liver enzyme, have been studied intensively. Administration of an excess of the substrate tryptophan to an animal will induce a several-fold increase in the enzyme within five hours. When the extra tryptophan has been metabolized, the level of the enzyme in the liver cells returns to normal. Similar phenomena have been thoroughly investigated in microorganisms. There is much uncertainty about the detailed chemical mechanism of this effect, but the information for a cell to make more of an enzyme can surely be embodied in the concentration of the substrate of the enzyme.

Information for a cell to make less of an enzyme can be incorporated in the concentration of the product of the enzyme reaction. Such a relationship can constantly regulate the amount of product formed. In informational terms, the control represents a negative feedback loop like the one by which a thermostat controls the temperature of a room, with more enzyme forming when the product is too low, and with less when it is too high.

Animals have evolved still more complex regulations than are seen in unicellular organisms. In these regulating mechanisms, the actions of chemicals from distant tissues, such as the hormones, may be superimposed upon the primitive controls exerted at the cellular level by local substrates and products. Yet, in at least one known instance, the action of the hormones follows essentially the same primitive design. Hydrocortisone has been found to induce an increase in the activity of tryptophan pyrrolase in much the same way as tryptophan. Recent experiments in our laboratory by Dr. Goldstein have demonstrated this hydrocortisone-induced increase of tryptophan pyrrolase in the isolated perfused liver. These findings add materially to the theory that the action of a hormone is independent of the similar action exerted by the substrate. There is also reason to believe that this is a bona fide mode of action of a hormone.

Extensive data on the quantitative controls of cellular enzymes by the body's chemical components are being rapidly accumulated. It would appear that it rarely is the concentration of only a single component which governs the amount of an enzyme. Instead, the effect of one compound is modified by the entire aggregate of components which at the cell's particular metabolic state are present at the time. In other words, the effective information acting on any one gene is the result of the concentrations of many substrates, products and hormones. These concentrations are in turn controlled by the products of other genes or are introduced from the exterior environment of the organism.

There is a similarity between the information embodied in the concentrations of the many cellular metabolites and the information handled as quantities by an analog computer. If the many information stores of an analog machine were set to drive a digital computer, which handles its many kinds of information qualitatively, as position, the result would be a fair model for the determination of the biochemical nature of an individual from the interaction of these given kinds of information on metabolites and genes (fig. 3).

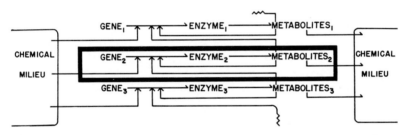

Fig. 3. Control of kind and amount of enzymes. The interdependencies of gene, gene action, enzyme action and chemical milieu in each gene-enzyme set, and among the many such sets which make up any individual, produce consequences which are not necessarily predictable from the nature of the initial disturbance.

The single sets of interdependencies among gene, gene product and environment are easily comprehended. Yet, the individual who has a disease is the resultant of very many such sets and their myriad interactions. Pathogenesis is the study of these interactions.

PATHOGENETIC MECHANISMS

Sickle-cell anemia again provides an example of how completely a pathogenesis can be worked out. Pauling [3] called sickle-cell anemia a molecular disease, because its signs and symptoms could be properly referred to the hereditarily altered chemical structure of the hemoglobin molecule. We have seen, however, that there is also the role of chemical environment which must signal the timing and probably the amount of the abnormal hemoglobin synthesis. Only when given both the altered gene and the stimulus that results in the synthesis of the abnormal protein can the clinical consequences be explained almost completely. Functional disturbances in the individual result from structural alterations within the hemoglobin molecule, because structure and function are one at the molecular level.

The abnormal hemoglobin, Hgb S, is chemically different from the usual Hgb A, and behaves differently. It carries oxygen quite well, but its dysfunction lies in another property. This is the diminished solubility of the deoxygenated form, which causes it to crystallize within the red cell when too much oxygen has been lost. Since red cells tend to be distorted by the projecting crystals, they lose their usual smooth oblateness and take on the jagged sickle shapes. The flow of these irregular cells in the blood stream is impeded and the circulation slows. Still more extensive deoxygenation results from the stasis, so that a vicious cycle ensues of crystallization, stasis, deoxygenation and more crystallization, with the explosive clinical result called a crisis (fig. 2). Blood flow to the part stops, infarction occurs, and there is hemolysis of the cells enmeshed in the thrombus. The accumulated damage from repeated crises causes death by middle age.

Hence, such a mechanistically simple disease as sickle-cell anemia does not develop from the necessary hereditary information like a wound-up clock. Even if given sufficient environmental information to make the abnormal protein, there is still no dysfunctional crisis. The full-blown disease picture depends on some chance restriction of the blood circulation or some trivial deoxygenation of a tissue. Only then is dysfunction superimposed upon the biochemical abnormality to produce disease. Even more subtle interactions can be expected in the pathogenesis of diseases affecting tissues whose functions are more complex than those of red blood cells.

A pathogenetic mechanism for the observed mental deficiency in phenylketonuria, constructed on similar principles, may be posed as a working hypothesis. Stated baldly, what has been said implies that the phenylketonuric actually "acquires" his mental deficiency. He inherits only the pattern for an ineffective phenylalanine hydroxylase, and this state itself is quite innocuous. Lack of this enzyme in fetal life and in infancy failed to hurt any of us. An ineffective enzyme *per se* did not innately handicap the intellectual development of those many patients who have been successfully treated for this disease by dietary means.

It is true that without the enzyme an individual accumulates excess phenylalanine from his diet to some thirty times its usual level in the body fluids, but this accumulation appears to be nearly innocuous throughout *most* of a person's life. Certainly, the accumulation of phenylalanine is not "toxic" in any usual sense. The relatively rare phenylketonurics with near-normal intelligence go through their lives with high phenylalanine levels. Similarly, high levels have produced no retrogression in the half-dozen successfully treated patients, who have been returned to a normal diet after five years of age. Since neither the lack of the enzyme nor the accumulation of phenylalanine is harmful as such, the mental deficiency may be said to be acquired by some unique interaction. This critical interaction appears to occur late in the first year of life. Before this period, institution of a low phenylalanine diet will prevent mental deficiency. After this period, mental deficiency develops and cannot be cured by any diet.

It may be postulated that human brains go through a period of chemical development or maturation at roughly the period of myelination. During that time they are susceptible to an irreversible change in function without producing any cytological evidence of damage. Very high phenylalanine accumulation is one of the factors that can induce such a change during the sensitive period.

Phenylketonurics happen to be the only known individuals who can accumulate sufficiently high levels of phenylalanine to reveal this susceptibility of human brains. Given such phenylalanine levels from any cause at the critical time, however, everybody among us would have "acquired" a state of mental deficiency similar to that of untreated phenylketonurics. According to this view, a high concentration of phenylalanine must carry information which can affect the nature and function of the developing brain. Information embodied in the concentrations of compounds has been shown to activate or suppress particular genes. What the phenylalanine does amounts to an alteration of the actions of the genes forming the brain. The result is that the organ is chemically imperfect and functionally defective.

CONCLUSIONS

Living things appear to act like the sort of self-regulating system to be expected from an hereditary repertory of enzymes making different metabolites, the sum of which can in turn determine the enzymes to be made from the repertory. The major biological problem of tissue differentiation, for example, can be understood in this way.

Although all of an individual's cells possess in common one pool of genetic information, they have been subjected to different chemical environments. In consequence, they have different enzyme concentrations and have developed along different lines. Such a differentiation of the brain may be subtly deranged by the altered chemical environment in phenylketonuria. If all brains, including those of animals, are indeed susceptible at a critical period to such an "acquirable" derangement, mentally defective brains can be produced in quantity for a chemical analysis of the derangement. Since structure and function blend at the molecular level, it is axiomatic that defective brains are chemically abnormal in some way.

In more general terms, it may be said that each disease results necessarily from an interplay of hereditary *and* environmental actions. The chemical mechanisms of these actions can now be seen in broad outline. Particular interest attaches to the pathogenetic interactions, because they are subject to some control in the individual. Even though the individual's hereditary information is fixed, its consequences can be altered.

REFERENCES

1. GARROD, A. E.: Inborn errors of metabolism (Croonian Lectures). Lancet 2: 73, 142, 214, 1908.
2. INGRAM, V. M.: A specific difference between the globins of normal human and sickle cell anaemia haemoglobin. Nature 178: 792, 1956.
3. PAULING, L., et al.: Sickle cell anemia, a molecular disease. Science 110: 543, 1949.

13

The Biological Function of DNA:
A Speculative View

CARL C. LINDEGREN, Ph.D.

Cytoplasm is to the biological universe what space is to the physical universe. It is the all-pervading, essential background against which all activities are manifested. It is so universally present that many biologists have ignored it, just as many physicists ignored space before Einstein.

CYTOPLASMIC CONSTITUENTS OF THE CELL

The *cytoplasm* is a clear, limpid fluid which in addition to the nucleus, contains a variety of other cell organs, or organelles, such as mitochondria, chloroplasts and microsomes. Without cytoplasm, however, none of these bodies is capable of biological activity, although some theorists favor the view that genes or nucleic acids are the prime movers in biological processes. Hence, since neither genes nor nucleic acids can simulate life in the absence of cytoplasm, it may be said in strictly speculative terms that the cytoplasm is the *sine qua non* of life. It may be added, however, that the composition of the cytoplasmic fluid is still more or less unknown.

The inheritance of cytoplasmic characters has been studied mainly by German geneticists, especially by Correns, Renner, Harder, Michaelis, von Wettstein, and Oehlkers. Distinguishing between *the genome* (the totality of the genes in an organism) and *the plasmon* (the totality of the cytoplasmic components of an organism), they performed many experiments which seemed to demonstrate both the autonomy and continuous interaction of these two major components of the protoplast.

According to Michaelis,[4] it may be said that "the cell is the unit of life, in which nucleus and cytoplasm form a self-perpetuating reaction system." As to the interactions between nucleus and cytoplasm, he suggested that the behavior of the nuclear genes can only be contrasted with that of the sum of all cytoplasmic constituents (plasmon). Actually, by contrasting "the autonomous genome with the autonomous plasmon," he gave each unit an equivalent self sufficiency and thus was able to define life in terms of "the interaction between these two different reaction-systems."

More specifically, the working hypothesis of Michaelis was the following:

a. In normal genome-plasmon combinations, the multiplying of plasmagenes and plasma organelles is correlated with the multiplying of nuclear genes and

This work has been supported by research grant C-4682 from the U. S. Public Health Service.

cell division, while "the distribution of cytoplasmic units during cell division proceeds in an orderly fashion."

b. In other genome-plasmon combinations, this coordination "is apparently broken and a segregation of plasma units is possible by irregular uncoordinated multiplication by an irregular distribution."

With respect to the notion of some biologists that "life originated with the gene," it may be emphasized that despite the present interdependence of nucleus and cytoplasm, there can be no question that the chromosomes and their genes are essential components of contemporary living things. Nevertheless, it does not follow that genes are "the primary components" of living material.

By analogy, one may say that electrical devices are essential components of the organism which we call Chicago. Without electrical devices, Chicago would undoubtedly perish and yield its place to some competing metropolis not similarly handicapped. It is equally clear, however, that such devices are not primary components of Chicago. Obviously, Chicago existed as an organism for a long time without them, although they now play a vital part in the city's life.

In fact, even proteins may represent fairly recent aspects of life, although it cannot be denied that they now appear to be inseparable from it.

THE THEORY OF THE COACERVATE

Hypothetically, it may be suggested that *the coacervate* of Bungenburg de Jong[2] deserves a central position in biological theory.

Originally described as an organized complex of different kinds of molecules held together in a specific pattern by mutual attractions, a coacervate is formed, as distinguished from coagulation, when solutions of hydrophilic colloids are left standing and separate into two layers: one rich in colloidal substances (coacervate) and the other almost free of colloids (the equilibrium liquid). If the coacervate does not separate out as a continuous layer, it appears in the form of very small droplets floating in the equilibrium liquid. Readily seen under the microscope, the droplets in Bungenburg de Jong's experiments with protein coacervates were found to vary from 2 to 670 microns in diameter. The stable association of different kinds of molecules in a coacervate is effected by forces at a level considerably below chemical bonds.

In the formation of a coacervate, electrostatic forces have been assumed by Bungenburg de Jong to act in the opposite sense to those of hydration. Apparently, the effect of hydration tends to stabilize the solution, while the electrostatic forces are acting to draw together the colloidal particles bearing opposite charges. "When the mutual attraction of the oppositely charged particles reaches a certain intensity, it can overcome the effect of hydration, and the particles combine to form a complex coacervate. Thus such a coacervate is always under the influence of two opposing forces, the electrostatic ones which keep it together and those of hydration which tend to drive the colloid back into solution."[2]

In Oparin's opinion,[5] life begins with the *first functional cytoplasm,* with the apparently limpid cytoplasm (coacervate) being the primeval biological material and with all other organelles—including mitochondria and nuclei which are also regarded as coacervates—having been superimposed upon the primeval cytoplasm. According to this view, living material is "a society" resulting from the association of a variety of coacervates into one organized structure, while the action of genes is assumed to be limited to the control of the synthesis of certain enzymes and the participation in the synthesis of the particular chromosomal coacervate of which they are a component part. Such distinctions are necessarily vague, but they imply that genes could "influence" but not "control" the synthesis of the other coacervates.

In line with this hypothesis, *structure* may be achieved in the coacervate by the association of molecules in a specific orientation due to their mutual attractions for each other. The idea that *"a hereditary particle,"* which is capable of being maintained and duplicated (without requiring enzyme action for its synthesis), could originate by the spontaneous association of molecules, might provide an explanation of the origin of the basic structures of living matter.

The pattern of such an existing structure has been assumed by Alexander and Bridges[1] to be capable of determining the continuity of the pattern. In other words, the orientation of the molecules already present in the living coacervate might guide and orient the molecules which are added to the coacervate. With the molecules in living coacervates arriving in this manner at their proper positions in the structures, it may be hypothesized that the pattern of the living coacervate would essentially be autonomous and self-directed. As a self-reproducing structure, the coacervate would have the characteristic of a hereditary particle.

THE NUCLEIC ACIDS AS MOLECULES CARRYING GENETIC INFORMATION

One of the important recent discoveries has been that an essential constituent of the nucleus, *the deoxyribonucleic acid* (DNA), is composed of nucleotides which are oriented in the molecules in a specific manner.[6] Another component which is also present in the nucleus is the cytoplasmic *ribonucleic acid* (RNA).

DNA is a long, fibrillar, duplex molecule, the two halves of which are complements of each other. The union of the fibrous molecule along the center line is fragile so that the molecule can be split along this center line. The splitting provides two nonidentical patterns, upon which two double strands identical with the original double strands can be reconstituted. The component nucleotides of each half can attract a set of complementary nucleotides from the milieu to reconstitute two new double-stranded nucleic acid molecules. Each of the complementary single strands thus provides a pattern for the reassembly of a complete new double strand. However, the difference between the assembly of a specific nucleic acid and that of a cytoplasmic coacervate is that although the attraction of the nucleotides may suffice to bring them into contact, only an *enzyme action* can make the union stable.

More specifically, it may be said that in DNA the different components are associated into what is unmistakably a molecule. In the coacervates, they are associated into complexes in which they retain integrity as molecules to a much greater extent. Hence, the *basic similarity* between DNA and the coacervate is that both depend upon the millieu in which they find themselves for their component parts. The *principal difference* is that with DNA being dependent upon enzymes to achieve the final state of a single structure, the components which are built into DNA must be activated by enzymatic reactions. Since the coacervate can be assembled without the mediation of the enzymatic activity, it could, and probably did, precede the accumulation of large quantities of DNA. This difference may be regarded as supporting the view that cytoplasm preceded the gene in the origin of life.

If the assumption is correct that each cell is *a society of autonomous organelles* which have become incorporated into a single system, the cell may be thought of as comprising a symbiotic association of a diversity of individual structures, each of which in some special manner serves to maintain the total society of the components which make up the cell. It is conceivable that one member after another may have been added to the membership of the society during the many millennia of precellular life, when life was manifested only as a slimy growth without boundaries. Each of the very ancient components of the society may have become a permanent component by selective synchronization of its growth rate or by direct attachment (coacervation) to some other component.

In other words, each component may have had its origin as a separate coacervate. It may have begun its association with the total society as an infectious agent, first preying upon the society and finally becoming adapted to it and, thus, *"essential."* In many instances, of course, both the host and the infectious parasite may have succumbed.

If contemporary living organisms are considered to be societies in which different kinds of aggregates have been integrated into a single whole, then the total integrated organism is the result of the interaction of a large variety of autonomous components, each of which controls its own growth and pattern (heredity). At present, our hypothetical list of *autonomous organelles* would include the limpid cytoplasm, the chloroplasts, the mitochondria, the cell membrane, the nuclear membrane, the centriole, the ribosomes, the solid spindle as well as the chromosomes with their genes and kinetochores. Most of these organelles may be assumed to have the principal features of a coacervate, with true chemical bonds in addition to the intermolecular coacervate bonds. Also, they would be autonomous in the sense that they can only be reproduced if a pattern is available. The different organelles in a living organism seem to be cross-linked to each other by the production of enzymes or nutrilites essential for the synthesis of each other. In the given circumstances, no individual organelle would be completely independent of the total organism.

THE THEORY OF THE CHROMOSOMAL COACERVATE (GENE SYSTEM)

In view of the fact that the phenomena associated with the action of a given gene occur in various places throughout the cell, it is possible to think of the mechanism controlling gene action in terms of a system which may be referred to as the *gene-system*. This hypothetical system may be postulated to comprise at least three separable entities: (a) the *receptor* which is located on the chromosomes at the place usually spoken of as the locus of the gene and which is assumed by the writer to be a globulin-like folded protein; (b) the *trans-*

mittor; and (c) the *effector.*[3] It is the contact of an inductor (entering the cell from the external milieu) with the receptor that apparently induces the synthesis of the specific enzyme controlled by the gene.

It is implied by the *one-gene-one-enzyme concept* that the production of each specific enzyme in the living organism is controlled by a separate specific gene. However, there is no compelling reason for the belief that all enzymes are produced by genes or that genes are the only source from which enzymes arise. If there are autonomous structures in the cytoplasm, they may produce enzymes independently of genes. However, since genetic analysis reveals only differences, it could not detect such a mechanism provided that the latter is universally distributed.

It is possible, for instance, that *mitochondria* produce enzymes independently of genes. The mitochondrion appears to be an autonomous structure from which certain oxidative enzymes may disappear without any noticeable effect having been produced on the genome. The *chloroplasts* may also be autonomous enzyme producers. It is conceivable that the cell wall and various other structures—apparently autonomous in the sense that they are not regenerated once they have been lost—may be able to generate endogenous enzymes which function in their respective constructions.

It may be assumed that the *nuclear nucleic acid* serves to orient the other components of the chromosome in a linear manner, maintaining a linear structure of a precisely limited "coded" length. The "code" of DNA provides a very effective device for achieving this end. It insures not only that the chromosomes will synapse at meiosis in a precisely homologous manner, but also that unequal crossing-over which occurs occasionally, even in the "coded" region, will be reduced to a minimum. It may be that the other components of the chromosome are associated *by coacervation* to the nucleic acid backbone, since coacervation is the most economical device for preserving the association of complex patterned structures.

One of the principal components of the chromosome is a basic protein, *histone.* With the nucleic acids being acidic, it seems reasonable to suppose that the basic histone and the acidic acid form a coacervate. A tentative hypothesis of gene action and gene structure may be based on the assumption that the gene at its locus on the chromosome is a coacervate of RNA (cytoplasmic nucleic acid), DNA (nuclear nucleic acid), and a folded protein-like globulin, all three members coacervated together with histone.

In line with the previously described gene-system theory (fig. 1), the given locus is a protein folded to form the *receptor,* while the ribonucleic acid template is a crucial component of the *transmittor* of the system.[3] Hence, enzymes are synthesized in the cytoplasm by the alignment of a series of activated amino acids on a ribonucleic acid template assembling the amino acids into a protein which is the enzyme.

With the RNA *template* being assumed to arise from the locus of the gene on the chromosome, there are some exposed nucleotides of single-stranded DNA available at the locus, which bind RNA and receptor-protein in the locus. Double helices of DNA bound to the histone foundation-protein may also be present to give the chromosome structural integrity. However, it is single-

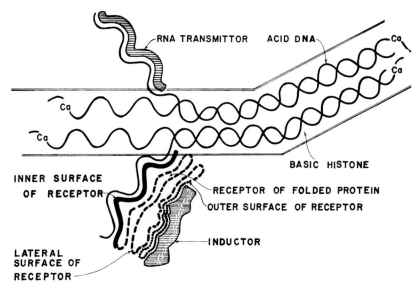

Fɪɢ. 1.   Theoretical gene system.

stranded DNA that is associated with the RNA and the receptor. At each locus, the structural DNA is held in its place in the linear continuum of the chromosome by a calcium bond at each end. The locus is also occupied by an RNA nucleotide, corresponding in length and in the distribution of similar or complementary nucleotides with those of the DNA chain.

While the RNA chain is not bound into the long axis of the chromosome by calcium bonds, the DNA-RNA-protein-receptor complex becomes unstable when the inductor unites with the receptor-protein. The RNA template is released from the complex, because it is not calcium-bonded and thus is free to leave the locus.

According to this theory, one element of the transmittor of each gene-system is the moiety of RNA (template) which passes from the nucleus into the cytoplasm to effect the synthesis of the enzyme in the cytoplasm. The nucleolus is a temporary organelle possibly containing transfer RNA appearing in a restricted region of a chromosome during the interphase between nuclear divisions, while the effector of the gene-system comprises the mechanism synthesizing the enzyme in the cytoplasm.

THE THEORY OF ADAPTIVE ENZYMES

As pointed out previously, the evidence that each single gene controls the synthesis of a single specific enzyme is very convincing, although not all the enzymes produced by an organism can simply be assumed to be under the control of genes. An alternative hypothesis might be that genes control only a very specific kind of enzyme, the *adaptive enzyme*. It may also be suggested that the chromosomal mechanism may not be the region in which gene-controlled enzymes are synthesized, but merely the place from which the impulse originates that evokes the synthesis.

The importance of adaptive enzymes to a multicellular organism which is constantly undergoing developmental changes cannot possibly be questioned. Obviously, an enzyme vitally important in one phase of development may be useless or detrimental in another. Thus, the organism, or rather each cell of the organism, should be prepared to synthesize a specific enzyme under a certain condition, but it should not fail to discontinue the synthesis of that particular enzyme when the conditions change. Only then would it be possible for cells descended from a single fertilized zygote to become *differentiated* into liver, brain or kidney cells and to synthesize the particular enzymes required by kidney cells in the one condition, and by liver or brain cells in the other. This process of differentiation takes place, although all cells are derived from the same original cell and therefore have the same basic heredity.

With a series of genes, each of which could act as a specific trigger for the synthesis of a *specific enzyme* upon stimulation by the proper molecule, the cell would be able in each new environment created by cell division or migration (where it would presumably be surrounded by different kinds of molecules, being in a different place) to produce new and different kinds of enzymes. Hence, the cell would develop into a different kind of cell because of its response to the new and different kinds of molecules in the new environment.

The advantage of the linear distribution of the genes along a chromosome which splits precisely in two at each cell division is obvious. By this procedure, the unused parts of the chromosome carrying genes (that would not be called forth to function until many generations later) could, nevertheless, be maintained. Distributed equally to every cell, they would be available when the time came. In other words, the differentiation achieved during development of a plant or an animal would occur, because division (or migration) placed each cell in an environment in which it was stimulated by specific local substances. The given stimulus induced the production of specific enzymes, precipitating either the synthesis of a component not present or the destruction of one already present. In this manner, gene action would be a factor in *differentiation*.

The merits of adaptive enzymes may be seen in the fact that the cell is not engaged in the manufacture of the enzyme until the moment for its use arrives. As to their origin in the early stages of the development of life, probably in living organisms not yet differentiated into tissues and organs, it may be assumed that the fluid, coacervated cytoplasm somehow achieved the ability to manufacture *proteinaceous enzymes*. This assumption is based on the observation that protein enzymes are folded to fit their substrates, and it would imply that the substrate served as a pattern for the origin of the first enzymes. Presumably, a single set of enzymes and an adequate amount of the organic substances, which had already accumulated, may have sufficed for continuous growth. When the supply was exhausted, growth ceased and had to wait upon the syntheses (abiotically) of more components.

Under these conditions, no repository in which the potential for producing adaptive enzymes could be stored would be required. At present, the nucleus is not so much an organ of synthesis as it is an *organ of storage,* in which the capacities for evoking a variety of syntheses are sequestered. If the actual synthesis of enzymes occurs in the cytoplasm, one may look upon the nucleus as a place in which the synthesis is initiated without being itself the factory in which the synthesis takes place. Hence, the gene is only the trigger, the activation of which initiates the production of the enzyme. The trigger may be activated by contact with a specific molecule. For example, the enzyme melibiase is brought forth when a molecule of melibiose (a disaccharide composed of glucose and galactose) comes in contact with the gene controlling the synthesis of melibiase. An interesting aspect of this adaptation may be seen in the fact that a molecule of galactose serves even better than a molecule of melibiose to induce the enzyme.

THE RECEPTOR THEORY OF THE GENE

As a corollary, it may be hypothesized that the receptor on the surface of the gene contains a *folded protein* which is different from the histone present in the body of the chromosome. In their outer aspect, the folds apparently conform to the shape of the substrate; for example, melibiose or a molecule of similar shape, like galactose, which also actuates this gene-system. A protein folded in such a mannner that a molecule of melibiose or galactose can fit its surface comprises the melibiose gene (or the receptor of the melibiase gene-system). Contact of a molecule of melibiose with the outer surface of the gene suffices to initiate the synthesis of the enzyme. The protein receptor is held in place on the chromosome by the specific configuration of the nucleotides at the locus.

The given hypothesis calls for distinguishing the following three aspects of the folded protein: (a) the *outer surface* which fits a specific molecule inducing the enzyme; (b) the *inner surface* which fits the conformation of the nucleotides at the locus; and (c) the *lateral surface* of folded protein which is the major factor in controlling the folding of the new gene reproduced at the reproduction of the locus. With the folded protein fitting on the DNA of the chromosome, it may be inferred that the specific sequence of the nucleotides is responsible for the folded protein being located at a specific position along the chromosome.

The specific nature of nucleic acid thus insures not only that the chromosome will not grow longer or shorter during the period of replication, but also that the genes will be maintained in the same relative linear position, especially during synapsis at meiosis and during crossing-over. It is also conceivable that at any locus such as that of the melibiose gene, many identical receptors are arranged around the periphery of the mitotic chromosome. With the DNA being present in both double and single strands, the chromosome may be thought of as being composed of thousands of multiple strands of DNA together with RNA, proteins and other substances in a complex coacervate. Each time the chromosomal coacervate grows to a specific limiting size, a longitudinal split occurs, which divides it into two new chromosomes. The receptors located around the periphery of the chromosome also multiply so that each new daughter chromosome has a sufficient complement of receptors at each locus. Thus, every daughter nucleus is apt to obtain a complete set of all the different kinds of genes.

Similarly, the sequence of the nucleotides making up the DNA of the chromosome acts at the reduction division to control homologous synapsis of the euchromatic regions carrying genes in order to insure that the reunions in crossing-over are precisely reciprocal; the chromosomes are neither shortened nor lengthened by the exchanges between partners in crossing-over. It is through the linear arrangement of coded DNA that the critical control of the over-all chromosome length is accomplished (unattainable through the multiplication of a coacervate without a DNA component). An enormous number of different genes may be located along this linear structure, since the folds in a protein molecule big enough to accommodate a single molecule (such as melibiose) would suffice to house the receptor for that particular gene. The size of an individual receptor might not differ by a large factor from the size of the molecule which acts as inductor of the enzyme. However, since the pattern is reproduced by a protein, the receptor might be considerably longer than the inductor molecule.

In addition to DNA and protein, the locus of a gene carries a short, free segment of RNA, held in place by RNA-to-DNA association of homologous, complementary nucleotides. Each gene locus is separated from each adjacent locus by calcium bonds which maintain the DNA in a single continuum, except for the calcium bonds. The contact of the inductor molecule with the receptor-protein at the locus renders the DNA-RNA association unstable, with some free fragments of RNA being released. These are the templates of the enzyme which travel to the cytoplasm. There they initiate the synthesis of an enzyme which is also a folded protein like the receptor. Following duplication of the folding of the receptor-protein, both the receptor and the enzyme would have a surface complementary to the substrate (or the inductor). Hence, the substrate (or inductor) will fit the protein surface. Fitting the substrate (imperfectly) to the protein would result in its splitting (or in the synthesis of two components into a single molecule).

THE THEORY OF ADAPTIVE ENZYME POTENTIALS STORED IN THE NUCLEUS

If the genome is a recent development which occurred after the evolution of the basic pattern of the cytoplasmic coacervate (with the capacity for enzyme synthesis), the storage of *enzyme potential* in morphologically undifferentiated "living slime" would evidently represent an extremely important function. In fact, any organism with the capacity for storing its cytoplasmic RNA-enzyme-producing mechanism in a repository where it would not be lost during non-functional periods would have a considerable advantage.

The storage organ may be assumed to have gradually developed into a structure which could be reproduced intact in a nonrandom manner without getting longer or shorter. Eventually, the chromosomes may have been stored inside a membrane separating them from the active cytoplasm, while the division of all the different chromosomes of one complex may have been organized under the control of a single central apparatus. It is this structure (called the nucleus) that was apparently transmitted to contemporary living organisms. Despite their great diversity, the stability of this structure, or rather the uniformity of its reconstruction, proved to be almost beyond belief. On this hypothesis, the genes controlling the differentiation of tissues and organs in complex plants and animals may be conceived as having had their origin in the storage of the enzymatic potential of the living cytoplasm.

GENES VERSUS CYTOPLASMIC COMPONENTS

It has already been stated that the cell may be regarded as a society composed of an enormous variety of different kinds of autonomous organelles which are embedded in autonomous cytoplasm and tend to be associated with an autonomous nucleus. On this basis, the interpretation of heredity, development and evolution differs considerably from the usual concepts of a cell unit, in which a nucleus is the only autonomous structure and controls all activity. For if the nucleus is the only autonomous member of the cell's society, then problems of evolution become problems of mutation, addition, subtraction or rearrangement of genes.

It is difficult for the writer to believe that the nucleus is the only autonomous member of the cell society. Instead, evolution would seem to involve much more than the addition or subtraction or mutation or rearrangement of genes. With evolution extending to the reproportioning of all the autonomous members of the cell society as well as to components of the nucleus, the effect of reproportioning would be to change the interrelations between different components of the society comprising the cell. Hence, the mechanism of evolution may be postulated to be different in complex and in simple organisms.

It may also be assumed that the different members of the cell society are not particularly dissimilar and that most of the differences are mainly due to changes in their *proportions* (interactions and balances between the members of the cell society) rather than to changes in the *kinds* of organelles. In this case it would be conceivable that environmental factors may, by a process of "epigenetic feed back" to the gonads, modify the course and direction of evolution.

In line with this theory, all the different kinds of original members of the society of animal cells may be supposed to have been developed to a specific balance in the early stages of each phylum. Also, many of the differences in evolution may have resulted from environmental influences which led to adaptations effected by changes in balance under the control of the epigenetic action. With an intensified effect in succeeding generations (feedback to the sex cells), many major changes may have been achieved with a cell society to which *no new kinds of members* were added, but in which *various new kinds of balances* were established by shifting the proportions of the materials present both in the genome and in the plasmon.

It would be possible to test this hypothesis by transplanting material from the cytoplasms of related organisms. In view of the highly stratified eggs of some of the amphibians, one might remove material from different strata and replace it with similar material from a different but relatively closely related form. In this manner, one might be able to observe the changes which occur in development.

CONCLUSIONS

In concluding this speculative view of the function of DNA, the writer would like to emphasize that biologists should set the *highest possible goals* as their objectives. There seems to be a tendency now to search for solutions to the problems of life in the analysis of the mechanism controlling the production of an enzyme by a gene. Although this is an endeavor worthy of the greatest effort, we should not lose sight of further goals. In particular, it would be quite dangerous to assume that the molecular biologist could achieve even a modicum of success without the help of the anatomist, the ecologist, the physiologist, the taxonomist, the cytologist, the immunologist, the psychologist, and above all *the philosopher*.

REFERENCES

1. ALEXANDER, J., AND BRIDGES, C. B.: Some physico-chemical aspects of life, mutation and evolution. In Alexander, J., Ed.: Colloidal Chemistry, Theoretical and Applied. New York, Chemical Catalog, 1928, vol. 2.
2. BUNGENBURG DE JONG, H. G.: La Coacervation et Son Importance en Biologie. Paris, Hermann & Cie, 1936, vols. 1 and 2.
3. LINDEGREN, C. C.: An hypothesis concerning the mechanism of gene action. Nature 189: 959, 1961.
4. MICHAELIS, P.: The genetical interactions between nucleus and cytoplasm in epilobium. Exp. Cell Res. (suppl.) 6: 236, 1958.
5. OPARIN, A. I.: Origin of Life, ed. 2. New York, Dover Publications, 1953.
6. WATSON, J. D., AND CRICK, F. H. C.: Genetical implications of the structure of deoxyribonucleic acid. Nature 171: 964, 1953.

14

Mutation and Gene Action

(Summary of Transcript)

K. C. ATWOOD, M.D.

RECENT ADVANCES TO BE CONSIDERED in the framework of the structure of DNA have taken place in relation to four aspects of basic genetics: replication, recombination, mutation and gene action.

The first basic experiment described was done by Meselson and Stahl in 1958[2] and was related to *replication*. By dissolving a given kind of DNA in a solution of cesium chloride, it is possible by very high speed centrifugation to observe a band representing the density of the DNA. This density tends to vary with the proportion of guanine-cytosine pairs in the given sample of DNA.

In the experiment in question, the investigators grew *E. coli* in a medium containing N_{15}. The DNA thus produced was more dense due to the heavy isotope and formed a density band that occupied a position in the linear density gradient somewhat different from the one it would normally occupy. When transferred to an ordinary N_{14} medium, these bacteria began to manufacture DNA of lesser density. The striking finding was that in one generation the density band of the DNA moves completely from its initial position to one exactly intermediate between pure N_{15} DNA and pure N_{14} DNA. In succeeding generations, the intensity of this band gradually decreases, while the band corresponding to N_{14} DNA appears, taking over the population.

These observations corroborate the mode of replication expected according to Watson and Crick's model of the double helix structure of DNA. In the first generation, the two strands of the helix are separated and the intact helix is replicated as each of the original strands manufactures a complementary strand from the nutrient medium. Therefore, the resulting DNA is made up of exactly half the original material and half the new (unlabeled) material.

The second experiment, cited to demonstrate the mechanism of *recombination,* was carried out by Meselson and Weigle in 1961. [3] They measured the density of the DNA that results from the recombination process in bacteriophage virus T2, and found the density of the recombinant DNA to be initially in the intermediate range. This observation reveals that recombinants must be formed, at least in part, by actual incorporation of segments of the parental strands following mechanical breakage of both parent strands, rather than by merely shifting the copying process from one parental strand to the other during replication. The given finding indicates that the phage chromosome does not need to be replicating in order for recombination to occur.

The next series of experiments presented dealt with the question of *muta-*

tion and served to illustrate the following three types of change in the DNA sequence:

1. Substitution of single nucleotide pairs by chemical analogs of the purine and pyrimidine bases (e. g., by 2-aminopurine and 5-bromo-deoxyuridine). Such mutagenic analogs are incorporated into the DNA, the frequency of mutation being directly proportional to the amount incorporated. The given type of mutation is reversible by the same type of analog.

2. Spontaneous mutations or proflavin-induced mutations. They are very rarely reversible and presumably involve changed sequences rather than substitution of single nucleotide pairs.

3. Substitution of one nucleotide pair for another in the nucleotide sequence through the action of an alkylating agent, such as ethylethane sulfonate.

The final group of experiments described provided clues to the nature of *gene action* and one of its most important aspects, namely, *its regulation*. To start with, we note that in the transformation of microorganisms incorporation of DNA from one to the other takes place only if they have sequences of purine and pyrimidine bases in common.[1] Other studies involve the sexual exchange of genetic material (chromosome strands) among microorganisms of different strains or species. Using this technique in a strain of *E. coli,* Pardee, Jacob and Monod [4] mapped the locus responsible for the formation of the enzyme β-galactosidase in the presence of inducer or substrate β-galactoside or lactose, respectively. They found one portion which determines the structure of the enzyme, and another which produces a "permease" that determines whether the substrate is pumped into the cell. But a third part was most interesting. A mutation in this region changes the capacity of the cell to make enzyme only whenever the inducer or substrate is present into one where enzyme is made all the time regardless of the presence or absence of the inducer or substrate. The experiment shows that the normal gene at this site actually represses the formation of the enzyme. It is a true "switch" or "operator" that regulates the activity of a particular gene-enzyme system. This experiment promises to be of classical importance in understanding how gene action can be turned on and off.

The following *general conclusions* were drawn:

1. The genetic material consists of DNA (or sometimes, as in the case of certain viruses, of RNA).

2. The information is carried in the form of certain nucleotide sequences, while mutations can be understood as changes in these specific sequences.

3. The recombination of linked sequences takes place, at least in part, by direct breakage and reunion of DNA.

4. A large portion of the genome, even in simple microorganisms, is concerned with the regulation of the activity of genes which determine the synthesis of proteins.

REFERENCES

1. Marmur, J., and Lane, D.: Strand separation and specific recombination in DNA: Biological studies. Proc. Nat. Acad. Sc. 46: 453, 1960.
2. Meselson, M. and Stahl, F. W.: The replication of DNA in Escherichia coli. Proc. Nat. Acad. Sc. 44: 671, 1958.

3. ———., AND WEIGLE, J. J.: Chromosome breakage accompanying genetic recombination in bacteriophage. Proc. Nat. Acad. Sc. 47: 857, 1961.

4. PARDEE, A. B., JACOB, F., AND MONOD, J.: The genetic control and cytoplasmic expression of inducibility in the synthesis of β-galactosidase by E. coli. J. Molec. Biol. 1: 165, 1959.

15

Discussion

Dr. H. Bentley Glass

I am much obliged to Prof. Lindegren for living up so well to my introductory comments. He has given us some fascinating insights into various possible theories regarding the nature and evolutionary history of the human cell structure.

Dr. Gordon Allen

Since an erroneous impression might be created if Prof. Lindegren's presentation were to remain without some reply, may I say that the mention of Richard Goldschmidt's name in this symposium has been entirely fitting. I am inclined to believe, however, that Goldschmidt would turn over in his grave if he knew the speculation which his name has been used to authenticate.

To judge from Prof. Lindegren's explanation of enzyme synthesis by genes, one gains the impression that he appreciates the tremendous complexity of information and the great fidelity of transmission of this information required for orderly development of an animal with a central nervous system. Such complexity and fidelity are beautifully and rather simply provided by the facts now known about DNA structure and DNA biosynthesis. This very stability of DNA implies virtual immunity from the feedback processes to which Dr. Lindegren refers.

Apparently, it is in search of the primary element in evolutionary change that cytoplasmic organelles have been brought into the picture. It is widely recognized that the more we learn about these organelles, the more complex may their structure prove to be. Compared to DNA, however, they have yielded no indication of similar capacities for information storage and replication. In considering the possible permutations of organelles in the egg and in the sperm, we introduce greater complexity, but we lose the required stability.

In view of these doubts, the following questions may be raised: (a) Are the other organelles assumed by Prof. Lindegren to have any capacity for reliable transmission of complex information which is comparable to that of DNA? If his answer is in the affirmative, how is this stability to be reconciled with susceptibility to modification by feedback? (b) Is the stability of the genome assumed to be so low that it can be readily influenced by the environment?

Dr. H. Bentley Glass

Before Prof. Lindegren's reply, may I make one brief statement on his behalf. As I understand his main point of emphasis, DNA normally conveys genetic information only as part of a total cellular system. What is stressed in this theory is the integrity and interaction of all cellular components.

Dr. Carl C. Lindegren

The first question raised by Dr. Allen can be answered most readily in relation to one cellular component, the mitochondrium, which is a perfect representative of a coacervate. It is indicated by several pieces of evidence that the mitochondrium, once it has disintegrated, can be reconstituted without the intervention of enzymes. Mitochondria are extremely ancient. Apart from minor variations, they are alike in bacteria, yeast, mice and humans, even in their smallest dimensions. Here we have then a hereditary apparatus which must have originated prior to the separation of the different phyla.

As to Dr. Allen's second question, may I say that the genome does not seem to be a really stable structure. In fact, its stability is so low as to render it susceptible to environmental influences. In the absence of sugar, for instance, the capacity of yeast for fermenting a certain sugar tends to be lost very readily. This capacity can be restored by treating the sugar, although the given treatment has nothing to do with the transformation process. In other words, the sugar itself is a mutagenic agent.

Dr. K. C. Atwood

Speaking for the "reactionary" molecular viewpoint, may I stress the fact, or near-fact, that the nature of the repressor is indicated by its production in the presence of a protein synthesis inhibitor. If one uses chloramphenacol to inhibit protein synthesis, the repressor made by that beta-galactosidase locus is being produced, suggesting that the repressor is not a protein.

As to the transcription of genetic information, we may keep in mind that in addition to the Kornberg enzyme, there is another enzyme, the so-called Horowitz enzyme, which replicates the DNA. By making RNA on a DNA template, this enzyme performs the biochemical act of transcribing the genetic information, which then goes out into the cytoplasm to do its work. Therefore, the question of what determines whether or not the gene is acting may be rephrased. The real question is which one of these enzymes is working along the chain. If it is the Kornberg enzyme, then it is replicating itself. If it is the Horowitz enzyme, then it is acting by creating a messenger.

We do not really know that these messengers do what they are supposed to do. The limited evidence which is available on this point is based on a recent report by Nirenberg and Matthaei about a cell-free system synthesizing protein (Proceedings of the National Academy of Science 47: 1588, 1961). For the purpose of protein synthesis, this system depends on RNA and a number of other substances. By adding different kinds of RNA, the investigators discovered a little fragment of the Rosetta stone, namely, some clue to the question of what kind of protein is turned out by that system.

If a synthetic polynucleotide is added to the system — a pure polyuridylic acid made by the true enzyme — one obtains a peculiar polypeptide which contains only one amino acid, 1-phenylalanine. Since the old enzyme does not just copy a template, but makes a certain chain depending on a certain type of monomer provided, the given finding means that the word spelling phenylalanine in the genetic code is composed purely of uridylic residues. Polycytidylic acid is another word which upon addition to the protein-synthesizing system, leads to the incorporation of only one amino acid, 1-proline. It is possible, however, that the proline is merely being added to pre-existing proteins.

At any rate, Nirenberg and Matthaei have furnished us with important clues to one of the coding mechanisms.

SECTION III: PROGRESS IN GENETIC STUDIES OF NEUROLOGICAL DISORDERS, DEAFNESS AND MENTAL DEFICIENCY

16

Introduction

CHARLES BUCKMAN, M.D.

As the outgoing president of the Eastern Psychiatric Research Association, which takes great pride in the annual genetic symposia arranged by Dr. Kallmann, and as the director of one of those many psychiatric hospitals in New York State, which have profited so much from their close contact with this dedicated research worker in the past 25 years, I consider it a great privilege to introduce the contributors to the third section of this first-class symposium. I undertake this gratifying task with the same degree of cordiality and appreciation with which we have always welcomed the regular research visits of Dr. Kallmann and his associates. It is due to the many data-collecting field trips of this research unit that the important principles and applications of human genetics have been brought into the understandable psychiatric atmosphere.

Further evidence of the remarkable productiveness of Dr. Kallmann's research group may be seen in the fact that all contributors to this section, dealing with the genetic aspects of *neurological disorders, deafness* and *mental deficiency,* either have been directly associated with this group at one time or another or have worked in close proximity to it. In the latter category is Dr. G. A. Jervis who is well known to us as one of the most proficient experts in the genetics of mental deficiency, his topic in this symposium. He is now Director of Psychiatric Research at Letchworth Village, but he was still a member of the staff of the Psychiatric Institute when he began his thorough investigation into the genetics of phenylpyruvic oligophrenia.

Similarly, Dr. W. Haberlandt is now conducting his genetic research at the Psychiatric University Clinic in Düsseldorf where he is associated with one of Dr. Kallmann's earliest collaborators in psychiatric population studies, Prof. F. Panse. Dr. Gordon Allen has returned to the National Institute of Mental Health in Bethesda, while Dr. George Baroff is now serving as Chief Psychologist of the Training School at Vineland. Despite these varied locations and professional activities, however, all the men mentioned became interested in the genetic studies to be reported here, while they were connected with the Department of Medical Genetics at the Psychiatric Institute. The work there is now being carried on by such experienced members of the department's current research staff as Drs. A. Falek and E. V. Glanville and Miss Diane Sank, whose well documented research reports are concerned with two of the main techniques in the departmental program, *twin studies* and *the detection of genetic carriers.*

It is widely appreciated by rank and file workers in clinical psychiatry that, as a result of painstaking investigations of this dedicated group, the genetic aspects of *mental deficiency* and *early total deafness* as well as the difficult problems encountered in genetic family counseling are presently receiving more and more attention.

17

Progress in Neurological Genetics

WALTER F. HABERLANDT, M.D., AND EDWARD V. GLANVILLE, PH.D.

As IN OTHER AREAS of medical genetics, recent progress in *neurological genetics* has been fast and highly diversified, with the main impetus coming from advances in neurophysiology, molecular biology and biochemical genetics. The net effect has been an increased confidence in the study of such differences as changes in enzyme activity, which are relatively close to the primary "informational" defect in neurological disorders. Clinically as well as genetically it is by no means surprising, however, that in the quest for the source of the "inappropriate information" which may lead to neuropathological sequelae, many different approaches have been followed.

Within the frame of this symposium, considerable *selectivity* in the choice of topics and techniques will be inevitable. The determinants for the processes of selection employed may be traceable partly to the different national and professional backgrounds of the two authors, and partly to certain predilections in the program of the joint session of the Seventh International Congress of Neurology and the Second International Conference of Human Genetics, held in Rome in September, 1961. Sponsored by the World Federation of Neurology and the Muscular Dystrophy Association of America, this memorable session was chaired by Professor van Bogaert and largely devoted to myopathies. It may be noted, however, that at the time when the final version of this report was prepared (January, 1962), only the abstracts of the papers presented at the joint Rome meeting were available in print.[29]

The main theme of the chairman's introductory address was that "analysis of normal and pathological muscle function must now turn to biochemistry without, however, neglecting clinical science. The morphological phase of genetics has almost passed, and we may hope to enter soon into a new phase of biochemical genetics."[29]

GENERAL GENETIC PRINCIPLES IN MAN

Since *the geneticist* studies the causes and origins of the differences observed among individuals and populations, the area of his investigative pursuits is almost boundless. His main objectives are (a) to identify the nature of the information given at conception and embodied in the *genetic* material; (b) to integrate this information with that which comes from without and is embodied in such ways as the concentrations of materials in *the environment;* and (c) to comprehend *the continuous interaction* between these varied sources of information during their realization in the life and development of the individual. The biochemical equivalents of this interaction have been described by Knox in another section of this volume.

126

The individual who is seen by *the neurologist* is the product of a long proc-ess of transformation. The genetic and environmental information has been translated into terms of protein structure, enzyme activity, nerve structure, muscle innervation, coordinated patterns of movement, and psychological moti-vations. Each of these interrelated elements represents a certain level of organ-ization.

Pathological symptoms may be studied at any level of organization. Ulti-mately, however, they are certain to have their source in the chemical and physical properties of the molecules which make up the human body. There is general agreement that the symptoms encountered by the medical specialist in disorders of the central nervous system encompass the most elaborate of all the differences observable among individuals. It is easy to understand, there-fore, why neurological genetics made relatively slow progress until very recently.

HEREDITARY MYOPATHIES IN ANIMALS

According to Hadlow's report at the Rome symposium on myopathies,[29] only a few of the muscular diseases occurring in animals are known to be hereditary, although some inbred strains tend to be more susceptible to myo-pathic afflictions of various kinds than others. Among the muscular dystrophies that have been shown to be inherited as autosomal recessive traits is a condi-tion found in *mice* and *chickens,* which has been described as primary myopa-thy and closely resembles muscular dystrophy in man. Another affection in this category is a form of dystrophy which arises in fetal life and is associated with multiple congenital arthrogryposis in *lambs.*

A muscular disorder, which is similar to myotonia congenita and has been observed in *goats,* is characterized by the inability of affected animals to move when startled. These attacks do not affect consciousness and occur only after periods of inactivity. The mode of inheritance remains undetermined, although the tendency to such seizures can be relieved or prevented by thymus extracts. Similar myotonic disturbances have been reported in young *Scottish terriers,* but their exact cause is also unknown.

Another anomaly called "double muscle" (Doppellender") is widespread among *cattle.* Affected calves have abnormally large muscle of the thighs, rump and back, making parturition difficult. The increased bulk of the muscles is due to hyperplasia rather than a true hypertrophy of muscle fibers, and dupli-cation of the muscles does not occur. The condition is inherited as a recessive trait with variable expressivity.

Some remarkable experiments were carried out by E. S. Russel in *mice* af-fected by muscular dystrophy. Although dystrophic mice of the type used do not normally reproduce, transplantation of ovaries from affected into normal mice produced viable offspring. The condition was found to be recessively in-herited, while experiments on parabiosis, in which the blood system of dys-trophic and normal mice were conjoined, yielded no evidence of a circulating factor responsible for, or preventing, muscle breakdown.[29]

THE GENETICS OF MUSCULAR DYSTROPHIES IN MAN

Classification of the muscular dystrophies has long been a matter of contro-versy. Ocular and distal varieties are clearly distinct, but much confusion surrounds the definition of the other forms. Morton and Chung [4, 22] have divided the myopathies into two major groups; the *pure muscular dystrophies* and *other myopathic forms* such as paramyotonia, myotonia congenita and dystrophia myotonica.

In the former group, four genetic types were distinguished:

1. *Duchenne:* sex-linked, occurring exclusively in males.
2. *Facioscapulohumeral:* autosomal dominant.
3. *Limb-girdle:* autosomal recessive form including most "sporadic" cases without known affected relatives.
4. *Limb-girdle:* etiologically undetermined. These cases cannot be explained by the hypothesis of a dominant mutation as the progeny are not affected, and on mathematical grounds they are unlikely to be due to recessive inheritance. It is possible that they represent occasional pathological expression in the heterozygote, or they may be phenocopies without a simple genetic etiology.

Morton and Chung's study is a good example of the manner in which statistical data may be used to delineate genetic entities and to distinguish between genetic and environmental effects. From a clinical standpoint, however, the disadvantages are that the distinction between the last two subgroups is largely theoretical, and that none of the four subgroups can be defined on clinical grounds alone.

There is now little doubt that a form of dystrophy exists which is clinically indistinguishable from the Duchenne type, but which can affect both boys and girls, and is inherited as an autosomal recessive, or possibly a dominant with incomplete penetrance.[31] This form can be distinguished without difficulty if both sexes are affected in the same family, but in isolated cases it may be impossible to distinguish the two types. Recognition is often important, however, as the disease inherited as a recessive is unlikely to reappear in later generations, but the sex-linked form will be expected to recur in 50 per cent of the male children of half the sisters of an affected boy.

A possible method of distinguishing between the two forms by clinical means was suggested by the fact that children with Duchenne dystrophy frequently die of congestive heart failure. Abnormalities in the ECG pattern were described in cases of Duchenne but not of facioscapulohumeral dystrophy.[21,28] This finding has been extended by Skyring and McKusick[31] in their study of two families, each with an affected boy and girl, affected with a form of dystrophy clinically indistinguishable from the sex-linked Duchenne form. Eighteen of the 23 cases with the sex-linked form showed ECG abnormalities, but none of the four cases with autosomally inherited dystrophy showed such symptoms. If these results can be substantiated, the ECG pattern will become an important clue in distinguishing between the two genetic entities.

The prevalence, mutation and fertility rates for the four genetically determined forms of muscular dystrophy tend to vary considerable.[22] While the *prevalence* of the Duchenne type has been reported as 66 living cases per million males, that of the facioscapulohumeral type is said to be 2 living cases per million; that of the autosomal recessive limb-girdle type, 12 living cases per million; and that of the sporadic limb-girdle type, 8 living cases per million. The corresponding *fertility* rates are (a) four per cent of normal; (b) nearly normal; and (c) and (d) 25 per cent of normal. The various *mutation* rates have been estimated at (a) 89 per million gametes; (b) 50 per million gametes; and (c) 31 per million loci.

Of the *serum enzymes* with a known tendency to increased activity in neuromuscular disease, aldolase has been found to be particularly increased in dystrophic patients. Other enzymes in this category are phosphohexose isomerase, lactic dehydrogenase, glutamic oxaloacetic transaminase and glutamic pyruvic transaminase. Increased aldolase activity seems most pronounced in rapidly progressing forms, especially in the early phases of Duchenne dystrophy, and may precede the onset of clinical symptoms. It is assumed that excess enzyme may leak into the serum from the muscles due to an abnormal permeability of the cell walls.[1]

Since creatine phosphokinase is generally more important in muscular contraction than is aldolase, its assay may prove to be of even greater value in the diagnosis of dystrophy. However, it is not yet certain whether and to what extent creatine phosphokinase may be useful in distinguishing the different forms of dystrophies.[25]

Enzyme assay techniques for identifying *the carriers* of muscular dystrophy, particularly the female carriers of the Duchenne anomaly, have not been consistently successful in the hands of different investigators. Recent reports varied from no increase to a slight increase in aldolase and creative phosphokinase activity in from a few to about one-third of known Duchenne dystrophy carriers,[4,19,25,27,33] while the results of tests for glutamic oxaloacetic transaminase and glutamic pyruvic transaminase were almost entirely negative. According to Dreyfus and coworkers,[29] a combination of measurements of aldolase and creatinekinase activity (revealing an anomaly in about 30 per cent of Duchenne carriers) and of circulation time (accelerated in nearly 60 per cent of these carriers) may eventually facilitate the detection of 80 per cent of the given type of carrier.

OTHER MYOPATHIES

In addition to the classic inherited forms of muscular dystrophies, each of which presents an independent genetic defect, several other related conditions can be distinguished genetically as well as histologically. Since a striated muscle has many enzymatic functions, it presents multiple possibilities for genetically determined dysfunctions. In particular, muscular dystrophy is to be sharply distinguished from McArdle's syndrome and muscle "core disease" as was emphasized by Denny-Brown at the Rome symposium.[29] While dystrophy is related to primary defects in the muscle nucleus, the other two conditions are related to defects in the mitochondrial enzymes and the structure of the myofibrils, respectively.

In *McArdle's syndrome* (myophosphorylase deficiency glycogenosis) which is inherited as an autosomal recessive, excessive amounts of glycogen are deposited in the muscles, without causing a severe disability. The presenting symptoms are weakness, pain and stiffness of the muscles after exercise, resulting from a deficiency in myophosphorylase. The enzyme appears to be completely inactive in the homozygote.[9]

By contrast, *muscle core disease,* described by Shy and Magee in 1956,[30] is a congenital non-progressive myopathy, in which no biochemical abnormality has as yet been discovered. It is probable, however, that the condition is inherited as a dominant and occurs in both sexes. Affected infants are hypotonic and "floppy" at birth, while adult patients are weak but not severely disabled. Biopsy reveals a highly abnormal muscle structure, with central areas of closely packed basophilic fibers which may contract independently of the peripheral fibers.[7]

Another type of defect, more directly concerned with the process of membrane excitability, is apparently responsible for the abnormal muscle contraction observed in *dystrophia myotonica.* The muscular symptoms in this dominantly inherited disease (autosomal with high penetrance) include a myotonic response which is induced either by volition or by mechanical or electrical stimulation. Progressive loss of muscle structure results in poor accommodation and repetitive discharges that can be demonstrated electromyographically. In fact, while the disease does usually not occur before adolescence in clinically recognizable form, Moldaver has found an abnormal response to continuous electrical stimulation which makes it possible to detect carriers in early childhood.[29]

According to Klein,[29] an association with cataract is typical of dystrophia myotonica (97.9 per cent) but not of congenital myotonia. Other frequently concurrent conditions include testicular atrophy (69.9 per cent) and goitre (50 per cent).

In *congenital myotonia,* a recent German study by Becker[29] revealed a fairly even distribution throughout the country, with a large proportion of sporadic cases in which exogenous factors such as cranial injury, infections or starvation seemed to be of etiological significance. The familial cases showed an earlier onset than the sporadic ones (before the age of 10 years) and were equally distributed between the dominant (no difference between the sexes) and recessive (excess of males) modes of inheritance.

NEUROPATHIES AND OTHER NEUROLOGICAL SYNDROMES

Among the neuropathies, *dystonia musculorum deformans* (torsion dystonia) is also characterized by the fact that some cases disclose familial accumulation, while others tend to follow infection (e.g., encephalitis). Zeman et al. [34] traced the condition through four generations and reported the occurrence of "formes frustes." Abortive forms lack the characteristic dystonic movements and postures, but show dyssynergias and hyperkinesias not usually related to dystonia, as well as a tendency to atypical postural abnormalities and contracture deformities. However, without a known biochemical defect and in the absence of positive pedigree data, it is still impossible to distinguish the hereditary form from the non-hereditary phenocopy (see next section). In other words, the genetic situation in regard to torsion dystonia is at present approximately the same as it is in such conditions as status dysraphicus, tuberous sclerosis or multiple sclerosis.

In *syringomyelia* (status dysraphicus) which is frequently familial but also tends to occur in sporadic form, the majority of symptoms are probably traceable to defective closure of the neural tube early in embryonic life. Common concomitants of the condition, observable also in relatives of affected individuals, include deformities of the sternum, kyphoscoliosis, asymmetrical development of the breasts and limbs, cyanosis of the extremities, clinodactyly, disturbances of cutaneous sensation, enuresis, cervical rib, spina bifida, pes cavus, acromegaly and defective heart development. The train of events set off by inappropriate information at an early stage of embryological development—either genetic or environmental — is still poorly understood.[23]

Abortive forms are particularly common in families affected by *tuberous sclerosis,* which in its classical symptomatology is characterized by mental deficiency, convulsions, adenoma sebaceum, and tumors in various tissues. Inherited as a dominant abnormality with a high penetrance, the condition has been followed through six generations.[14] The expressivity of the gene shows wide symptomatological variations within families, making the recognition of carriers ("formes frustes") an especially important task, if only because their children have a high probability of developing the disease in its severe form. According to Hudolin,[13] retinal phacoma may be the most specific diagnostic feature of all forms of the disease.

Genetically or otherwise, the etiology of *multiple sclerosis* remains in the undetermined category of neurological disorders, despite some recent reports which favor heredity as a predisposing factor.[2,8,24] This hypothesis is based on the finding that the relatives of verified patients with this illness are more frequently affected than is the population as a whole. In fact, in the opinion of some investigators[24] a plausible explanation would be that of a single recessive factor with a penetrance of less than 50 per cent in the homozygote. However, twin data have been inconclusive, possibly because of the small series available for analysis.

More productive from a genetic standpoint have been recent studies on two other syndromes, familial periodic paralysis (as distinguished from adynamia episodica) and Charcot's disease, an eponymous term which includes amyotrophic lateral sclerosis and progressive bulbar paralysis.

It has long been known that *familial periodic paralysis,* which usually follows the autosomal dominant mode of inheritance, is characterized by the periodic loss of the ability of the muscles to contract either voluntarily or in response to electrical stimulation. Attacks may occur spontaneously or may follow administration of salt-retaining adrenocortical steroids. While an increase in serum aldosterone and 17-ketosteroids tends to precede the attack, the serum potassium level is found to be decreased during the paralysis. Pathogenesis may be connected with a defective permeability of the muscle membrane which apparently results in an abnormal Na/K balance "triggering" hypersecretion of aldosterone.[6] Another possibility is that of an increased production of aldosterone which may induce the observed electrolytic imbalance. [12]

A genetically distinct but clinically similar variant is *adynamia episodica hereditaria,* which is also inherited as an autosomal dominant. The main differences consist in an increased serum potassium level during attacks, electrocardiographic abnormalities, and provocation of the episodes by hunger or KC1 administration.[5]

Extensive studies of the genetic and demographic aspects of *Charcot's dis-*

ease have been carried out in the United States, the Mariana Islands, and West Germany.[3,10,11,15,16,17,18] One of the reasons for the West German survey (population of Westphalia as registered by the Institute for Human Genetics at the University of Münster) was seen in the possible dangers arising from nuclear radiation and other mutagenic agents.

Of the 253 Westphalian cases diagnosed as Charcot's disease, 80 were regarded as exogenous in origin (trauma, infection, toxic agents) and therefore excluded from the statistical analysis. The remaining 173 probands included 19 patients (12 per cent) with other clinical cases in the family. The average age at onset was 45.5 years; the mean duration of the illness, 4.4 years; and the prevalence in the population, 2.5 per 100,000. Maternal age and the birth order of the index cases showed the expected distribution, and there was no increase either in the infant mortality rate of affected families or in the *parental consanguinity rate.*

It was concluded, therefore, that the familial form of Charcot's disease follows the autosomal dominant mode of inheritance (with incomplete penetrance and an approximately 50 per cent excess of affected males) and that there are numerous sporadic cases which cannot be definitely ascribed either to a genetic origin (mutation) or to definable environmental agents. Other pathological conditions which were found to be frequently associated with Charcot's disease were cerebellar ataxia, status dysraphicus, diabetes mellitus, and mental deficiency.

According to Kurland [17] and Tans, [32] it has not yet been possible to identify the basic enzymatic defect responsible for this type of neuropathy.

PHENOCOPIES IN NEUROLOGICAL GENETICS

The problem posed by the occurence of *phenocopies* (the same symptoms produced by different genetic or environmental causes) is particularly troublesome in neurological genetics. In the absence of a positive family history, it is often impossible to decide whether an isolated case is due to environmental causes or represents a dominant mutation or the fortuitous manifestation of a recessive homozygote. In some instances, it has become possible to make such a distinction. For example, electrocardiographic patterns may help in distinguishing between sex-linked and autosomally inherited forms of the Duchenne type of muscular dystrophy. However, situations of this kind are as yet very few.

Many of the difficulties of neurological genetics and the reasons for the frequently inconclusive nature of its genetic data stem from working with symptoms far removed from the primary informational defect. Without a firm basis for distinguishing between the categories under study, the value of any genetic investigation is bound to be limited.

Diagnosis of those diseases, in which an enzymatic defect can be recognized, rests on relatively secure foundations (e.g., McArdle's syndrome). In such others as "core disease," the histological picture may be characteristic. Frequently, however, no single character is sufficiently pathognomonic. For instance, the difficulty of distinguishing between myopathic and neurogenic forms of dystrophy was recently illustrated by a report on the histories of a mother and her two sons who had been initially diagnosed as cases of muscular dystrophy.

[20] Only after biopsy and electromyograph examination was it determined that their symptoms were those of a neurogenic disease simulating muscular dystrophy. This report confirmed the necessity of using in genetic studies the most precise diagnostic tools available.

CONCLUSIONS

One of the most challenging problems faced by the geneticist in neurological disorders is *to trace the transmission of pathogenic genes* from generation to generation through the population. The ability to recognize abnormal and mild forms ("formes frustes") of a disease such as tuberous sclerosis and that of detecting asymptomatic carriers of such conditions as Duchenne's dystrophy are of particular importance. Only then can we give warning of the increased probability of such carriers producing affected children, and relieve the anxiety of those individuals who belong to affected families but are not carriers themselves. Considerable success in detecting the female carriers of sex-linked Duchenne's dystrophy has been achieved through enzyme assay and the measurement of circulation time. Such encouraging results should spur the development of more precise means of detection in the future.

The discovery of a *detectable abnormality* close to the primary informational defect can supply a powerful tool for the diagnosis of affected persons as well as for the recognition of carriers. It may even lead to a cure for the disease. Taken alone, however, such a discovery no more explains a certain variety of pathological symptoms than that of a chromosomal aberration in Down's syndrome elucidated the mental deficiency and facial expression found in this condition. It has also been pointed out [26] that although the primary defect in phenylketonuria has been attributed to a deficiency of the enzyme phenylalanine dehydroxylase, this fact has thrown no light on the mechanism by which the central nervous system exhibits such severe disturbances. Embryological and developmental investigations will be needed before the varied symptoms can be explained.

In order to understand fully the pathogenesis of any condition, it is necessary not only to identify the nature of the primary informational defect, but also to understand how the defect may manifest itself at each of the various levels of organization in the body. We also have to know, of course, how the expression of the defect at each level may be modified by the genetic and environmental milieu in which it develops.

REFERENCES

1. ARONSON, S. M.: Enzyme determinations in neurologic and neuromuscular diseases of infancy and childhood. Pediat. Clin. N. Amer. 7: 527, 1960.
2. BAMMER, H., SCHALTENBRAND, G., and SOLCHER, H.: Studies on twins with multiple sclerosis. Deutsche Ztschr. Nervenh. 181: 261, 1960.
3. BOETERS, H.: Erbleiden des Nervensystems beim Menschen. In Just, G., Ed.: Handbuch der Erbbiologie des Menschen. Berlin, Springer, 1939, Vol. 1.
4. CHUNG, C. S., MORTON, N. E., and PETERS, H. A.: Serum enzymes and genetic carriers in muscular dystrophy. Am. J. Human Genet. 12: 52, 1960.
5. CONN, J. W., and STREETEN, D. H. P.: Adynamia episodica hereditaria. In Stanbury, J. B. Wyngaarden, J. B., and Fredrickson, D. S., Eds.: The Metabolic Basis of Inherited Disease. New York, McGraw-Hill, 1960.

6. CONN, J. W., and STREETEN, D. H. P.: Periodic paralysis. In Stanbury, J. B., Wyngaarden, J. B., and Fredrickson, D. S., Eds.: The Metabolic Basis of Inherited Disease. New York, McGraw-Hill, 1960.

7. CORNMAN, T., and SHY, G. M.: The prognostic value of the muscle biopsy in the "floppy infant." Brain 81: 461, 1958.

8. CURTIS, F.: Neue Ergebnisse der erbbiologischen Multiple Sklerose-Forschung. Fortschr. Neurol. Psychiat. 27: 161, 1959.

9. FIELD, R. A.: Glycogen disposition diseases. In Stanbury, J. B., Wyngaarden, J. B., and Fredrickson, D. S., Eds.: The Metabolic Basis of Inherited Disease. New York, McGraw-Hill, 1960.

10. GREEN, J. B.: Familial amyotrophic lateral sclerosis occurring in 4 generations. Report of a case. Neurology 10: 960, 1960.

11. HABERLANDT, W. F.: Genetic aspects of amyotrophic lateral sclerosis and progressive bulbar paralysis. A. Ge. Me. Ge. 8: 369, 1959.

12. HADDAD, C.: Variations of the electrolytes in periodic paralysis. Rev. méd. fr. Moyen-Orient 15: 503, 1959.

13. HUDOLIN, V.: Retinalne promjene kod tuberozne skleroze. Neuropsihijatrija 8: 30, 1960.

14. IWAMOTO, S., and TOMODA, H.: Über eine Sippschaft mit der tuberösen Hirnsklerose. Eine klinisch-erbbiologische Untersuchung. Kobe J. Med. Sci. 5: 11, 1959.

15. KURLAND, L. T.: Epidemiologic investigations of amyotrophic lateral sclerosis. III. A genetic interpretation of incidence and geographic distribution. Proc. Staff Meet. Mayo Clin. 32: 449, 1957.

16. ———: Descriptive epidemiology of selected neurologic and myopathic disorders with particular reference to a survey in Rochester, Minnesota. J. Chron. Dis. 8: 378, 1958.

17. ———, MULDER, D. W. and WESTLUND, K. B.: Multiple sclerosis and amyotrophic lateral sclerosis. N. England J. Med. 252: 649 and 697, 1955.

18. ———, et al.: Amyotrophic lateral sclerosis in the Mariana Islands. A. M. A. Arch. Neurol. & Psychiat. 75: 435, 1956.

19. LEYBURN, P., THOMSON, W. H. S., and WALTON, J. N.: An investigation of the carrier state in the Duchenne type muscular dystrophy. Ann. Human Genet. 25: 41, 1961.

20. MAGEE, K. R., and DE JONG, R. W.: Neurogenic muscular atrophy simulating muscular dystrophy. A. M. A. Arch. Neurol. 2: 677, 1960.

21. MANNING, G. W., and CROPP, G. J.: The electrocardiogram in progressive muscular dystrophy. Brit. Heart J. 20: 416, 1958.

22. MORTON, N. E., and CHUNG, C. S.: Formal genetics of muscular dystrophy. Am. J. Human Genet. 11: 360, 1960.

23. MURAKAMI, U.: Clinico-genetic study of hereditary disorders of the nervous system. Fol. Psychiat. Neurol. Jap. (suppl. I), 1958.

24. MYRIANTHOPOULOS, N. C., and MACKAY, R. P.: Multiple sclerosis in twins and their relatives. Genetic analysis of family histories. Acta Genet. 10: 33, 1960.

25. OKINAKA, S., et al.: Serum creatine phosphokinase. Arch. Neurol. 4: 520, 1961.

26. POSER, C. M., and VAN BOGAERT, L.: Neuropathologic observations in phenylketonuria. Brain 82: 1, 1959.

27. SCHAPIRA, F., et al.: Etude de l'aldolase et de la créatine kinase du serum chez les mères de myopathes. Rev. fr. clin. biol. 5: 990, 1960.

28. SCHOTT, J., JACOBI, M., and WALD, M. A.: Electrocardiographic patterns in the differential diagnosis of progressive muscular dystrophy. Am. J. Md. Sc. 229: 517, 1955.

29. Second International Conference of Human Genetics (Rome 1961). Amsterdam, Excerpta Medica, 1961.

30. SHY, G. M., and MAGEE, K. R.: A new congenital non-progressive myopathy. Brain 79: 610, 1956.

31. SKYRING, A. P., and MCKUSICK, V. A.: Clinical genetics and electrocardiography

in childhood muscular dystrophy. Am. J. M. Sc. 242: 534, 1961.

32. TANS, J. M. J.: Amyotrophische Lateraalsklerose (een klinischanatomische studie). Diss. Amsterdam, 1950.

33. THOMSON, W. H. S., LEYBURN, P., and WALTON, J. N.: Serum enzyme activity in muscular dystrophy. Brit. M. J. 2: 1276, 1960.

34. ZEMAN, W., KAEBLING, R., and PASAMANICK, B.: Idiopathic dystonia musculorum deformans II. The formes frustes. Neurology 10: 1068, 1960.

18

Investigation of Genetic Carriers

ARTHUR FALEK, Ph.D., and EDWARD V. GLANVILLE, Ph.D.

THE DETECTION of clinically asymptomatic carriers of genetically determined abnormalities can be of value to the diagnostic, therapeutic and preventive programs of medical and public health specialists, while early diagnosis and treatment may be beneficial to persons predisposed to the development of some gene-specific disease. Genetic counseling of members of affected families prior to marriage or parenthood is concerned with the advisability of reducing the number of children who may carry hereditary defects. For the purposes of this report which will be limited to neuropsychiatric disorders, carriers are defined as individuals who transmit the genic determinants of a specific hereditary disease, but never display clinical symptoms, as well as those who show no obvious clinical symptoms at the time of examination, but develop the illness in later life. The extensive literature on the biochemical and other methods of carrier detection has been recently reviewed by Hsia,[12-14] Knox[23] and Neel [32-34] and in a well documented book edited by Stanbury, Wyngaarden and Frederickson.[39]

As long as the search for possible carriers usable in experimental studies has to proceed along conventional lines, that is, through an investigation of the members of affected family units, it is likely, by and large, to remain a hit and miss affair. Regardless of the mode of transmission involved, it is the immediate relatives of an affected person who have the greatest chance to be identifiable carriers of the trait in question. With regard to recessive inheritance, it has long been stressed by Kallmann[18] that it is only in the children of two affected parents or in the partners of one-egg twin index cases that one can be certain of dealing with genetic carriers despite the absence of clinical symptoms.

Groups of people known to carry, or merely suspected of carrying, the genetic potentialities for a particular pathological condition can be investigated with a battery of tests which may reveal some subclinical signs of the disorder. To be indicative of the carrier state, of course, the observed changes should differ either quantitatively or qualitatively from the phenotypes of normal persons, while they may or may not differ from those seen in fully established cases.

The neuropsychiatric disorders to be discussed may be conveniently grouped as follows: (1) mental deficiency states, (2) predominantly neurological conditions and (3) mental disorders.

MENTAL DEFICIENCY STATES

Phenylketonuria is the classic example of a disease inherited as an autosomal recessive for which sensitive methods are available for detecting the heterozygote as well as the homozygote. The clinical symptoms result from a deficiency of the enzyme phenylalanine dehydroxylase produced in the liver. Under standardized dietary conditions, the level of phenylalanine in the plasma is quantitatively characteristic of both symptomless carrier states and the fully established syndrome. It is known, however, that the homozygous carrier remains undetectable until two or three weeks after birth. It is only at that stage of development that the liver becomes biochemically differentiated and the enzyme deficiency becomes apparent. Yet, if infants with phenylketonuria are fed a diet low in phenylalanine from a sufficiently early stage, all major biochemical deviations may be either prevented or reversed. In this manner, intellectual impairment can be controlled.[24]

As to the various phenylalanine tolerance tests available for the identification of the three genotypes, it may be noted that the overlap between the normal and the heterozygote is still considerable. The proportion of cases in which standard tests fail to distinguish carriers from genotypically normal individuals is close to 15 per cent. More recently, however, a modified technique has been developed by Wang and his co-workers,[42] supposed to reduce the error to approximately 4 per cent.

Galactosemia is another example of a gene-specific enzyme deficiency that gives rise to intellectual impairment. According to family studies, the defect probably follows the autosomal recessive mode of inheritance, with a deficiency in the enzyme galactose 1-phosphate uridyl transferase resulting in the inability to convert galactose to glucose. If uncontrolled, the defect leads to cataract formation, hepatosplenomegaly and cirrhosis of the liver in addition to mental retardation, with the first symptoms occurring shortly after birth. Symptoms of galactosemia can be prevented by the elimination of both lactose and galactose from the diet. A specific test for the diagnosis of galactosemia has been devised by Anderson[2] and is based on a transferase assay in red blood cells.

In his first attempt to detect the heterozygote with this technique, Hsia [15] observed a decrease of transferase activity from normal controls to heterozygotes. However, the difference was not large enough to detect individual carriers with any degree of certainty. More recently, several investigators claimed to have been successful in segregating galactosemia patients from both heterozygous and normal subjects using more refined assay techniques. In appraising the effectiveness of four of these methods, however, Hsia's group [16] found that although the mean values for carriers were significantly lower than those for the homozygous normal control subjects, there was still considerable overlap between the two groups in all tests.

NEUROLOGICAL DISORDERS

The infantile and juvenile forms of *familial amaurotic idiocy* are among the neurological disorders distinguished by an accumulation of lipids within the central nervous system. According to the results of pedigree studies, these two forms of amaurotic idiocy are probably genetically distinct syndromes.

Usually referred to as *Tay-Sachs' disease* and almost always associated with mental defect and convulsions, the infantile form of the disorder is recessively inherited and tends to end fatally at about 30 months of age. The mean age of onset is around 6 months.

Of the two methods which have been proposed for the detection of heterozygotes, the one used by Spiegel-Adolf[38] is based on the vacuolization of lymphocytes as observed in a series of affected infants and some of their parents. The other has been recommended by Dowben[7] who described a quantitative increase in the rate of oxidation of phenylenediamine in some relatives of affected infants. The oxidation of this compound in presumed heterozygotes seems to be intermediate between the values found in normal children and clinical Tay-Sachs' cases. The basic biochemical defect is still unknown.

In the *juvenile form of familial amaurotic idiocy,* the illness begins around the age of 7 years and leads to death around the age of 16. Otherwise, there is much similarity between the juvenile and infantile forms, not only clinically and histopathologically, but also in their mode of transmission. Vacuolated lymphocytes have likewise been observed in the near relatives of children showing the juvenile type of disease.[41]

At present, no cytological or biochemical techniques are available to distinguish between the infantile and juvenile forms of amaurotic idiocy. Two questions in need of clarification are (a) whether these two forms of the disease are consequences of the same mutant gene acting upon different background genotypes or (b) whether the two disorders are due to different genes which may be either allelic or nonallelic.

Wilson's disease (hepatolenticular degeneration) is another neurological disorder raising various unanswered questions from the standpoint of carrier detection. This syndrome is characterized by cirrhosis of the liver and bilateral changes in the lenticular nucleus due to an abnormality in copper metabolism. Its onset tends to fall into the period of adolescence, and death usually follows a few years later. Transmitted as an autosomal recessive, the disease presents a general picture of an extrapyramidal disorder with a moderate degree of intellectual impairment and a consistently observed deficiency of the plasma protein ceruloplasmin. According to Bearn,[4] however, ceruloplasmin may not be the primary gene product, and Sass-Kortsak[36] believes that a more basic defect may be traceable to a decrease in the rate of copper incorporation into ceruloplasmin. While attempts to detect carriers by quantitative assays of ceruloplasmin have met with only limited success,[4,14] recent work by Sternlieb and his associates on the rate of Cu^{64} incorporation into ceruloplasmin [40] has led to the development of a satisfactory technique for distinguishing many of the heterozygous carriers from homozygous normal individuals.

Genetically even less clear and homogeneous is the group of *convulsive disorders* which may develop as a consequence of congenital or acquired cerebral dysfunction. Some cases of convulsions are known to follow detectable trauma but others seem to manifest themselves without a precipitating agent. The latter cases are still described as having the "idiopathic" form of epilepsy.

According to twin data, concordance for clinical symptoms of epilepsy varies from 67 to 85 per cent in one-egg pairs, and from 3 to 24 per cent in two-egg pairs.[6,27,35] For the detection of carriers some use has been made of comparative electroencephalographic recordings in normal and epileptic twin partners. The given findings were interpreted as evidence for a genetically controlled brain wave pattern. In one-egg pairs, the concordance rate for dysrhythmia reported by both Lennox[26,27] and Inouye[17] exceeded 75 per cent, while the corresponding rate for two-egg twins varied from 4 to 22 per cent.

Supportive evidence for the hypothesis that genetic elements may play a significant part in the development of convulsive disorder, has also been derived from family studies of dysrhythmic patients with idiopathic epilepsy.[11,25] Of particular interest was the observation that over 10 per cent of normal control subjects showed abnormal EEG patterns. On the other hand, in Harvald's[11] electroencephalographic study of 23 clinically asymptomatic persons who were suspected carriers of epilepsy, at least 12 were found to have normal recordings.

It may be concluded, therefore, that many carriers of a convulsive disorder can be detected by their EEG patterns, although it would be incorrect to say that all persons with dysrhythmia are transmitters of the disease. By the same token, some individuals with normal patterns may be carriers of the disorder that can not yet be detected with our present laboratory equipment.

Similar technical difficulties are encountered in *Huntington's chorea,* which usually begins at the age of 35 and clinically shows progressive choreiform movements, mental disorganization and early death. In line with the principles of the dominant mode of inheritance, each child of an affected parent has a 50 per cent chance of eventually developing the disorder, while affected children will, in turn, pass the disease potential to one-half of their offspring. With unaffected children and their offspring being expected to remain forever free of pathological symptoms, it is essential that the disease be diagnosed prior to the age of clinical onset. No prodromal symptoms are known, and to date no method for the early detection of carriers has been discovered, although various attempts have been made in this direction. In our own studies, paper and column chromatography failed to reveal abnormal protein concentrations in affected individuals, and the chromosome counts made of one patient showed no irregularity.

In another attempt to detect subtle signs of the illness prior to its overt onset, tests of coordination, motor control and steadiness (degree of tremor) were administered to a series of siblings and children of affected individuals as well as to normal control subjects.[3] Among the tests used in this study were Bender Gestalt, Heath rail-walking, finger-tapping, pegboard, turnbuckle and punchboard. This battery proved to be effective in distinguishing between normal and affected individuals, but it did not result in the identification of potential cases of Huntington's chorea in the families investigated.

Our present efforts to detect carriers of this disorder are aimed at developing more sensitive instruments for motor movement evaluation. In this new investigation which is being carried out with the cooperation and laboratory facilities of Drs. F. J. Agate and L. J. Doshay of our Medical Center, the electronic equipment employed measures both displacement and acceleration. This is a modification of the method devised by Agate and his colleagues[1] to study tremor and movement in Parkinson's disease. Transducers, strain gauge and accelerometer are utilized in the graphic recording of fine hand, foot and face movements.

In this preliminary report, only the vertical acceleration of a point on the hand will be considered. Our main finding has been that the recordings of all 5 chorea patients examined to date show intermittent bursts (duration of one or two seconds) which are considerably above the usual level of ordinary types of tremor. In contrast, nearly all of the 54 normal controls have been found to have a pattern which clearly differs from that of clinical cases. Only very few have acceleration bursts which might be confused with those of choreic patients. A similar statement can be made with regard to the records of patients with Parkinson's disease. For purposes of genetic counseling, however, it is seldom necessary to distinguish between the different abnormal movement patterns. Usually, it may suffice that in a family known to be afflicted with Huntington's chorea, an abnormal movement pattern can or cannot be recognized in another family member before the clinical onset of his illness.

The upper graph in figure 1 is an example of the hand recording pattern of a normal control subject. This person is in her mid-thirties and has no known family history of a neurological disorder. The lower recording is that of a clinical case of Huntington's chorea, being distinguishable by intermittent bursts of excessive acceleration.

In figure 2, the hand recordings are presented of a family which includes a choreic mother and two clinically asymptomatic children aged 14 and 19 years. The record of the younger child is of special interest as it resembles that of his ill mother, while the older son's record is patterned like the one of the normal control shown previously.

Needless to say, much further work will be necessary before this refined diagnostic technique can be used with any degree of confidence. In our future testing program, a study of various other neurological disorders will be combined with that of a larger series of Huntington's chorea cases and their families. Of course, the clinically asymptomatic relatives with abnormal recordings in this sample will require a long-term follow-up. At present, there is still a possibility that the acceleration bursts observed may be the result of some artifact, although such an explanation would seem to be highly implausible in view of the consistent difference between affected and clinically asymptomatic individuals.

If fully confirmed, the tremometer test will be a useful tool, not only for purposes of genetic counseling, but also in the search for the elusive metabolic defect at the root of this clearly gene-borne neurological disorder. In our own counseling work, only very few persons have been found among the children of choreic patients who proved to be sufficiently informed about the clinical and genetic aspects of the disease, or had received adequate guidance in relation to their special marriage and parenthood problems. What can at present be offered as a minimum program to members of Huntington's chorea families seeking advice and help is a thorough neurological examination to establish or preclude the presence of early clinical symptoms. Under appropriate circumstances, the examination should be followed by a personal discussion of the given morbidity risk potential.[20] In line with Kallmann's long standing recommendations,[19] such counseling should primarily be aimed at reducing anxiety and tension.

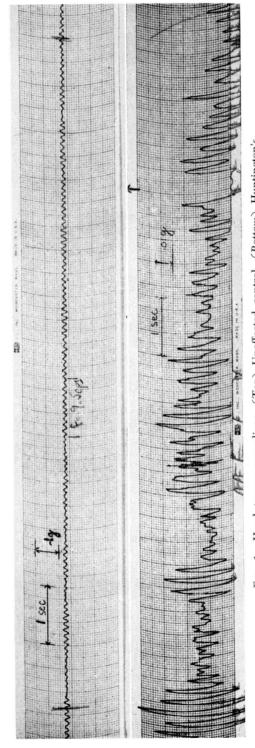

Fig. 1. Hand tremor recordings. (*Top*) Unaffected control. (*Bottom*) Huntington's chorea patient.

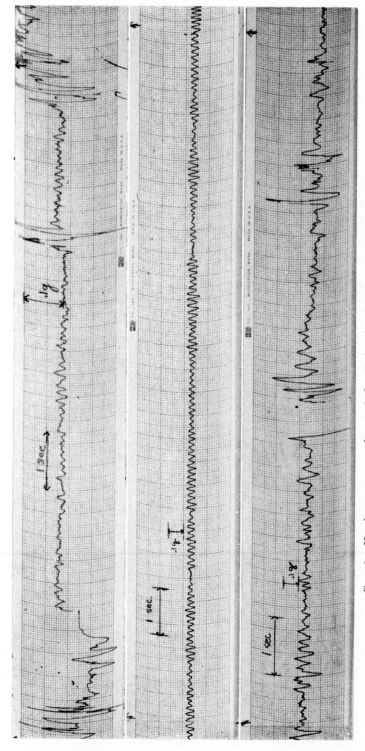

Fig. 2. Hand tremor recordings of the K family. (*Top*) Mother with Huntigton's chorea. (*Center*) Son, age 19. (*Bottom*) Son, age 14.

Obviously, the adequacy of this kind of guidance program for Huntington's chorea families would be greatly enhanced by a readily available tool for heterozygote detection. Furthermore, long-term studies on phenotypically normal persons with the mutant gene should aid in the development of methods to control the progress of the disease. At present, a Damoclean sword hangs over the head of all direct descendants of choreic patients, whether they carry the dominant mutant or not.

MENTAL ILLNESS

In the group of the major psychoses, the discussion of potential advantages of carrier state detection will be limited to the most common type of psychosis, schizophrenia. It was at this institute, of course, where Kallmann and his colleagues collected family and twin data on the mode of inheritance of schizophrenia during the past 25 years. It would seem, therefore, that this is not the right time or place for rehashing the relative contributions made by genetic and nongenetic factors to the etiology of this disorder. According to Kallmann's work,[18] however, the following points call for special attention in regard to the inheritance of schizophrenia:

a. Penetrance is less than 100 per cent, varying from 68 per cent in the children of 2 schizophrenic parents to 86 per cent in the one-egg partners of schizophrenic twins.

b. As some heterozygotes seem to be capable of developing psychotic symptoms under particular stress conditions, there are two types of carrier in this group of disorders: that of the homozygote without a clinical breakdown and that of the heterozygote who may or may not be schizoid in his appearance.

Of the immediate relatives of schizophrenics to be considered as a source of possible carriers, it is especially the children of 2 schizophrenic parents who provide us with a well defined population for investigative purposes. Although such marriages (dual matings) are rare, all children authentically derived from them represent a more promising group of asymptomatic persons for carrier state detection than do one-egg twin pairs still discordant for schizophrenia. Since most twins of this type become psychotic at about the same time, and are available for preclinical studies only after the breakdown of one partner, discordant cases are extremely difficult to ascertain.

Fortunately, research into the detection of carriers does not have to await the identification of the type or types of defect which may lead to schizophrenic phenomena in genetically vulnerable persons. The only supposition necessary to justify such research is that some physical or chemical change precedes the onset of the psychosis.

To identify metabolic changes in the clinical stage of the disease, the emphasis during the past 10 years has been placed on drug studies combined with new biochemical methods. Despite improved techniques, however, the results of most of these studies have fallen short of expectation in that they produced either inconclusive or contradictory findings. [22,37]

Among the more promising approaches (table 1) have been those investigating the effects of serum from schizophrenics on the metabolism of adrena-

TABLE 1.   SOME PROMISING METHODS TO DETECT AN ABNORMALITY
IN SCHIZOPHRENIC PATIENTS

Procedure	Results
Patient's serum injected into sensitized guinea pig	Anaphylactic shock
Patient's plasma injected into trained rat	Delayed climbing time
Precipitate from patient's urine injected into rabbit	Hyperglycemia
Chicken red blood cells suspended in patient's serum	Altered lactate/pyruvate ratio
Serum injected into rabbit, epinephrine placed on exposed brain	Inhibition of epinephrine induced hypertension
Antigen introduced into patient	Decreased antibody response

line and related compounds.[30] Others attempted to assess the toxic effects produced in rodents by plasma[5] or urine[31] from schizophrenic patients. Of particular interest was Frohman's[9] discovery of a factor in the serum of schizophrenic patients, which seemed to alter significantly the metabolism as measured by lactate-pyruvate ratios in the chicken erythrocyte. Also, an anaphylactic test for the detection of abnormal antigens in the serum of schizophrenics was described by Malis,[28] and successfully repeated by Haddad and Rabe.[10] In this work it was found that the serum of chronic schizophrenics contains an antigen capable of producing symptoms of anaphylactic shock in previously sensitized guinea pigs. More recently, Kerbikov[21] described a decrease in the immunological postvaccination response of patients with some forms of schizophrenia. While such a decrease in antibody formation was observed in catatonic patients, the response of paranoid schizophrenics was not distinguishable from that of normal controls.

With respect to most of the experiments designed to detect chemical changes in schizophrenia, it may be noted that they were conducted only in chronic cases. One of the consequences of this procedure was the inability to distinguish between primary and secondary changes. On the other hand, it was pointed out by Kety,[22] in his comprehensive review of the biochemical theories of schizophrenia, that even in acute cases the period of emotional turmoil prior to hospitalization would not be conducive to normal metabolic function. Technical difficulties of this kind are greatly reduced in studies of asymptomatic carriers. It would seem to be desirable, therefore, that tests which have given conflicting results in psychotic individuals be repeated on carriers.

For this purpose, our own departmental program is currently focused on ascertaining families in which both husband and wife were hospitalized for schizophrenia. By using chromatographic, electrophoretic, cytological and immunological techniques on the series of over 150 children produced by 75 dual matings of this kind, we hope to avoid the secondary complications produced by the metabolic upheaval following the onset of a psychotic episode. Definitive results of this work are not yet available.

In conclusion, it may be stated that a survey of some of the more promising attempts at carrier state detection in neuropsychiatric disorders has uncovered

TABLE 2.   CARRIER DETECTION IN NEUROPSYCHIATRIC DISORDERS

Method	Disease	Abnormalities Reported in Carriers
Biochemical	Phenylketonuria	Increased serum phenylalanine
	Galactosemia	Decreased galactose transferase
	Infantile amaurotic idiocy	Increased rate of phenylenediamine oxidation
	Wilson's disease	Ceruloplasmin deficiency
		Decreased serum copper levels
Cytological	Infantile amaurotic idiocy Juvenile amaurotic idiocy	Vacuolization of lymphocytes
Physiological	Idiopathic epilepsy	Deviant electroencephalogram
	Huntington's chorea	Deviant tremor pattern

no more than limited success (table 2). Only in phenylketonuria is a method already available which distinguishes sharply between the unaffected and the heterozygous carrier. In galactosemia, the abnormal homozygote has been largely identified, but the heterozygous carrier can not yet be detected with any degree of certainty. In other neuropsychiatric disorders with an apparently gene-specific basis, it is still impossible to recognize the basic defect.

In many instances, the inability to identify the genetically deviant individual is due to the relative inaccuracy of current procedures. In others, it may be due to the fact that heterozygous individuals fail to show a quantitative or qualitative difference from the unaffected homozygote at all times. The former difficulty can be overcome by more sensitive techniques, while the latter may in some instances be resolved by one of two possible approaches, linkage studies or cytogenetic techniques.

That knowledge gained from the construction of linkage maps may be useful in the detection of carriers needs no particular emphasis here. In this procedure, genes which are detectable in the heterozygote may prove to be useful as markers to trace the transmission of a pathogenic gene linked to them. However, it was pointed out by Neel[32] over a decade ago that there are some serious theoretical limitations to this method. As yet, very few cases of linkage have been recognized in man, not only because of the relatively large number of his chromosomes and the lack of suitable marker genes, but also because of the enormous amount of work involved in collecting adequate pedigree data.

Cytogenetic studies offer a more hopeful approach, although present techniques are not yet sufficiently precise to detect other than gross chromosomal changes. Since the ensuing phenotypes are usually so abnormal that they seldom reproduce, the given chromosomal irregularities tend to express themselves like lethal or semilethal dominant genes. It is worth mentioning, therefore, that in recent months some apparently normal individuals have been observed who have abnormal chromosomal complements.[8,29]

Nevertheless, with the majority of defects resulting from point mutations, more refined techniques will have to be developed for tracing by cytological means the path of transmission of the mutant gene in affected families. One promising approach involving both linkage studies and cytogenetic techniques is based on the discovery that the size of the satellites found on the five pairs of acrocentric human chromosomes may vary in size in normal individuals, and that any given pair may be asymmetrical in this respect. According to Miller,[29] giant satellites are transmitted with the chromosomes carrying them, so that they may conceivably serve as chromosomal markers and aid in the localization of specific genes on specific chromosomes.

Once adequate methods become available for the detection of carriers, the work of the genetic counselor will be greatly facilitated. Data based on morbidity risk figures mean little to those not familiar with probability theory, and they do little to relieve the anxiety of persons directly concerned. If the carrier of a particular disorder can be reliably recognized, the genetic counselor would be able to remove doubt and anxiety from the minds of those family members found to be free of the trait in question. On the other hand, clearly established carriers would have the benefit of concentrated preventive measures.

In families where carriers are expected to transmit the disorder without ever developing clinical symptoms themselves, guidance of a different sort is needed. Such people can be informed that everyone is a carrier of several genes which, if homozygous, would be seriously detrimental to the individual's state of health. It should be understood, therefore, that the fact of being a carrier is in itself no reason for concern, but in premarital counseling, the inadvisability of marrying another individual carrying the same abnormality should be pointed out. If both mates are found to be carriers of such a trait, a realistic discussion of the given risk aspects would seem to be indicated.

On the whole, there can be no doubt that the treatment and prevention of hereditary disease are two of the most challenging problems facing medical science today. While much success has been achieved in the control of infectious disease, only a few hereditary disorders can as yet be prevented or remedied. Carrier detection combined with genetic counseling would help materially to reduce the number of affected individuals in the population; and in diseases with late onset, carrier detection would serve to identify for study a group of individuals where clinical symptoms of the underlying defect can be followed from preclinical stages to the final outcome.

REFERENCES

1. Agate, F. J., Jr., Doshay, L. J., and Curtis, F. K.: Quantitative measurement of therapy in paralysis agitans J.A.M.A. 160: 352, 1956.
2. Anderson, E. P., et al.: A specific enzymatic assay for the diagnosis of congenital galactosemia. J. Lab. & Clin. Med. 50: 469, 1957.
3. Baroff, G. S., Falek, A., and Haberlandt, W.: Impairment of psychomotor function in the early diagnosis of Huntington's chorea. Wien. Ztschr. Nervenh. 15: 28, 1958.
4. Bearn, A. G.: Wilson's disease. In Stanbury, J. B. Wyngaarden, J. B., and Frederickson, D. S., Eds.: The Metabolic Basis of Hereditary Disease. New York, McGraw-Hill, 1960.
5. Bergen, J. R., et al.: Rat behavior changes in response to a blood factor from normal and psychotic persons. A.M.A. Arch. Neurol. & Psychiat. 2: 146, 1960.
6 Conrad, C.: Die erbliche Fallsucht. In Guett, A., Ed.: Handbuch der Erbkrankheiten. Leipzig, Thieme, 1940, vol. 3, pt. 2.
7. Dowben, R. M.: Increased oxidation of p-phenylenediamine by serum of patients with Tay-Sachs disease. Quart. Bull., Northwestern Univ. M. School 33: 15, 1959.
8. Forssman, H., and Lehmann, O.: Translocation-carrying phenotypically normal males and the Down syndrome. Lancet 1: 1286, 1961.

9. FROHMAN, C., et al.: Steps toward the isolation of a serum factor in schizophrenia. Am. J. Psychiat. 117: 401, 1960.
10. HADDAD, R. K., AND RABE, A.: Abstracts: Third World Congr. Psychiat. Montreal, 1961.
11. HARVALD, B.: Heredity in Epilepsy. Copenhagen, Munksgaard, 1954.
12. HSIA, D. Y. Y.: The laboratory detection of heterozygotes. Am. J. Human Genet. 9: 98, 1957.
13. ———: Medical genetics. N. England J. Med. 262: 1172, 1222, 1273 and 1318, 1960.
14. ———: Recent advances in biochemical detection of heterozygous carriers in hereditary diseases. Metabolism 9: 301, 1960.
15. ———: HUANG, I., AND DRISCOLL, S. G.: The heterozygous carrier in galactosemia. Nature 16: 1389, 1958.
16. ———, et al.: Further studies on the heterozygous carrier in galactosemia. J. Lab. & Clin. Med. 56: 368, 1960.
17 INOUYE, E.: Observations on 40 twin index cases with chronic epilepsy and their co-twins. J. Nerv. & Ment. Dis. 130: 401, 1960.
18. KALLMANN, F. J.: Heredity in Health and Mental Disorder. New York, Norton, 1953.
19. ———: New goals and perspectives in human genetics. A. Ge. Me. Ge. 10: 377, 1961.
20. ———, AND RAINER, J. D.: Psychotherapeutically oriented counseling techniques in the setting of a medical genetics department. Fifth Internat. Congr. for Psychother. (Vienna 1961), in press.
21. KERBIOV, O. V.: Immunological reactivity in schizophrenia as influenced by some modern drugs. Ann. N.Y. Acad. Sc. 92: 1098, 1961.
22. KETY, S. S.: Biochemical theories of schizophrenia. Science 129: 1528 and 1590, 1959.
23. KNOX, W. E.: Sir Archibald Garrod's "inborn errors of metabolism," Parts 1-4. Am. J. Human Genet. 10: 3, 95, 249 and 385, 1958.
24. KNOX, W. E.: Phenylketonuria. In Stanbury, J. B., Wyngaarden, J. B., and Frederickson, D. S., Eds.: The Metabolic Basis of Inherited Disease. New York, McGraw-Hill, 1960.
25. LENNOX, W. G.: The heredity of epilepsy as told by relatives and twins. J.A.M.A. 146: 529, 1951.
26. ———, GIBBS, E. L., AND GIBBS, F. A..: The brain wave pattern; an hereditary trait. J. Hered. 36: 233, 1945.
27. ———, AND JOLLY, D. H.: Seizures, brain waves and intelligence scores of epileptic twins. In Hooker, D., and Hare, C., Eds.: Genetics and the Inheritance of Integrated Neurological and Psychiatric Patterns. Baltimore, Williams & Wilkins, 1954, Vol. 38.
28. MALIS, G.: Iu, K etiologii schizofrenii (Etiology of Schizophrenia). Moscow, Medgiz, 1959.
29. MILLER, O. J., COOPER, H. L., AND HIRSCHHORN, K.: Recent developments in human cytogenetics. Eugenics Quart. 8: 23, 1961.
30. MINZ, B., AND WALASZEK, E. J.: Effects of serum from schizophrenics on epinephrine sensitive elements in the rabbit brain. J. Nerv. & Ment. Dis. 130: 420, 1960.
31. MOYA, F., et al.: Hyperglycemic action and toxicity of the urine of schizophrenic patients. Canad. J. Biochem. Physiol. 36: 505, 1958.
32. NEEL, J. V.: The detection of the genetic carriers of hereditary disease. Am. J. Human Genet. 1: 19, 1949.
33. ———: The detection of genetic carriers of inherited disease. In Sorsby, A., Ed.: Clinical Genetics. London, Butterworth, 1953.
34. ———: The clinical detection of the genetic carriers of inherited disease. Medicine 26: 115, 1957.

35. ROSANOFF, A. J. HANDY, L. M., AND ROSANOFF, A.: Etiology of epilepsy with special reference to its occurrence in twins. Arch. Neurol. & Psychiat. 31: 1165, 1934.
36. SASS-KORTSAK, A., et al.: A study of heterozygosity in Wilson's disease. Proc. Ann. Meet. Soc. Pediat. Res. 29: 62, 1959.
37. SMYTH ES, J. B.: Recent advances in the biochemistry of psychosis. Lancet 1: 1287, 1960.
38. SPIEGEL-ADOLF, M., et. al.: Cerebrospinal fluid, serum and blood investigations in amaurotic family idiocy. Am. J. Dis. Child. 97: 676, 1959.
39. STANBURY, J. B., WYNGAARDEN, J. B., AND FREDERICKSON, D. S. (Eds.): The Metabolic Basis of Inherited Disease. New York, McGraw-Hill, 1960.
40. STERNLIEB, I., et al.: Detection of the heterozygous carrier of the Wilson's disease gene. J. Clin. Invest. 40: 707, 1961.
41. v. BAGH, K., AND HORTLING, H.: Blodfynd vid juvenil amaurotisk idioti. Nord. Med. 38: 1072, 1948.
42. WANG, H. L., MORTON, N. E., AND WAISMAN, H. A.: Increased reliability for the determination of the carrier state in phenylketonuria. Am. J. Human Genet. 13: 255, 1961.

19

The Genetic and Adjustive Aspects of Early

Total Deafness

DIANE SANK, M.S.

THE GENETIC DATA presented here are based on a comprehensive study of total deafness in the State of New York, conducted by various research teams of the Department of Medical Genetics (1955-1962). The study included a special investigation of deaf twins designed to yield comparative information about the etiology and psychological (developmental) corollaries of deafness. Among other subgroups, which were chosen from a statewide (demographic) census for the exploration of problems of particular psychiatric or genetic interest, were especially those connected with the adjustive potentials, emotional reaction types, intrafamily relations and reproductive trends of the deaf.

In line with long-standing usage, the term "total deafness" denotes a condition characterized by the absence of normal response to sounds, usually resulting in the absence of normal speech patterns, in a child who is otherwise healthy and has normal intelligence. Within such a totally deaf population, our genetic investigation has been limited to that nuclear group which is best described as "congenital total deafness" and to those deaf who developed their affliction after birth but early in childhood. The latter cases will be referred to as "early-onset total deafness."

In addition to twins and an analysis of mating and fertility patterns in an adult deaf population,[16] the following subgroups were used for special investigative purposes:

1. Deaf persons with outstanding professional achievements.

2. Deaf persons with criminal records or other forms of deviant behavior.

3. Deaf patients with a history of suicidal tendencies or serious accidents as well as those institutionalized in state schools or mental hospitals.

4. Emotionally disturbed members of deaf families who sought guidance or treatment in our Mental Health Clinic for the Deaf.

5. Index families with a history of schizophrenia.

This report is the twenty-fifth on the progress of the department's Mental Health Project for the Deaf, sponsored by the Office of Vocational Rehabilitation, U. S. Department of Health, Education, and Welfare. The financial aid provided for the entire project and the generous scientific guidance received in this special study from Professors F. J. Kallmann, H. Levene and J. D. Rainer as well as Dr. I. L. Firschein (all of Columbia University) are gratefully acknowledged.

CLINICAL AND DEMOGRAPHIC DATA ON THE ADJUSTIVE
ASPECTS OF DEAFNESS

According to earlier reports,[1,14,17] nearly 11,000 deaf persons in the adult range formed the basis for the total population study. Approximately 500 of them presented clinical evidence of psychiatric illness or intellectual subnormalcy, and were or had been institutionalized. Furthermore, over 800 deaf children below the age of 14 were reported to be in special schools for the deaf, with the majority remaining there until early adulthood.

To determine the total range of *adjustive problems of the deaf,* and to assess the unusual difficulties confronting deaf persons and *their families,* detailed accounts of the stressful conditions that the deaf are subject to at all stages of development have been given in previous reports and will again be reviewed in the final monograph which is now being prepared.[15] Early parent-child relations are known to be distorted by severe flaws in communication. Many of the young children (before reaching the age of 3 or 4 years) are placed in residential schools where the possible advantage of growing up with similarly afflicted youngsters may be more than offset by certain adverse factors, especially by limitations in personal contact with the outside world to which they must eventually return.

In line with generally accepted psychiatric concepts, the combination of handicap-induced dependence, prolonged cloistered living and segregation by sexes—with the consequent lack of opportunity for developing normal social relationships—are apt to contribute materially to disturbances in adjustment, including psychosexual identification. Reflecting these shortcomings as well as deficiencies in the school programs of sex education and the older students' preparation for marriage are (a) the decreased marriage rate and the relatively high number of divorced persons among the deaf as disclosed by mating and fertility statistics and (b) the observation that the frequency of homosexuality seems to be increased in dependent, handicapped and sequestered groups such as the deaf.[15]

While the total schizophrenia risk in the deaf has not been found to be significantly increased, an unusually high proportion of the hospitalized deaf (25 per cent) tend to be diagnosed as "psychosis with mental deficiency."[1] This tendency persists, although examination by psychiatrists skilled in communicating with the deaf frequently fails to yield evidence for the presence of mental retardation. Hence, the given diagnostic category would seem to represent "a convenient but indefinite classification for emotionally disturbed individuals with unintelligible speech or disordered language."

Of the types of maladjustment seen in our series of clinic patients,[14] passive-aggressive personality disorders (with a preponderance of the passive-dependent type) have been reported to be second only to schizophrenia (16 and 18 per cent, respectively). Overt homosexuality in a dependent personality structure has been observed as the predominant feature in some 10 per cent of the entire clinic population. Other common reasons for referral are poor work adjustment, intellectual subnormalcy, acute situational and antisocial reaction syndromes, and family conflicts associated with the handicap. It may be noted, however, that the assortment of patients seen in a special Mental Health Clinic for the Deaf is to a great extent determined by the attitudes and considerations of the referring agencies.[15]

Family problems encountered in a deaf community (marriage and parenthood counseling) may be presented by hearing members of deaf families as well as by the deaf themselves. Not infrequently, guidance is sought by hearing men who want to know whether it would be advisable to marry a hearing woman with deaf parents, or vice versa. It has been pointed out that counseling in such cases cannot confine itself to estimates of the statistical risk of deafness in the couple's future children.[14] What should also be taken into account are the emotional stability of the two persons involved, their attitude toward acquiring deaf relatives with the attendant possibility of social stigma, and any other genetic health risks for the children of the given mating.

Equally complex are the problems posed by a deaf person who wishes to marry a hearing one. While our clinic data include the records of several good marriages between exceptionally successful deaf men and hearing women, they also provide evidence of potential pitfalls in marital adjustment that may eventually result in broken homes. Other important questions are related to the optimal conditions for rearing a deaf child in a hearing family or, conversely, a hearing child of deaf parents.

Most certainly, counseling services of this kind call not only for specially trained staffs who are familiar with the life, language and particular adjustive norms of the deaf, but also for a knowledge of the *genetic aspects* of deafness.

GENERAL POPULATION DATA ON THE GENETIC ASPECTS OF DEAFNESS

In the total population study, various sets of data have been collected which are useful in investigating the role of genetic factors in the causation of early total deafness.

Soon after the activation of the project in 1955, an *introductory questionnaire* was mailed to every known deaf resident of New York State over 12 years of age, mainly to establish contact with this part of the deaf population. The list of names available at that time numbered 8200.

Aside from information regarding name and address, the form contained only one crucial question: "Are you a twin?" Approximately 1700 deaf persons replied to this questionnaire, while 2000 letters were returned by the post office as undeliverable.

A few years later (1958), *a second questionnaire* was sent out to the original respondents and, for purposes other than those of the present analysis, to a weighted sample of persons who had not answered. While primarily designed to yield marriage and fertility rates, the given form provided material which was easily translated into genetically pertinent information.

At the same time, every conceivable effort was made to establish personal contact with *the twins* in this group. In this manner, we obtained from the deaf population of New York State an almost completely ascertained sample of twins who met the following criteria: (a) total deafness of the perception type (inner ear nerve deafness) in one or both partners and (b) either congenital or early-onset total deafness. Omitted from the twin study were persons with a conductive type of hearing loss and those with a partial nerve-type hearing impairment (hard of hearing).

Excluded from the population study were those cases whose deafness had reportedly been acquired after the age of four years; that is, at a time when some speech pattern has usually been formed, placing such persons into the category "hearing during early childhood." This procedure was adopted in order to facilitate a comparison of our data with the results of previous studies of "hereditary total deafness," especially with that of Stevenson and Cheeseman [21] in Northern Ireland (1956). The Irish sample consisted only of persons assumed to have been born deaf or to have been recognized as deaf before the development of a speech pattern and in the absence of any other known cause of deafness (other than heredity). In our study, therefore, we also discounted the replies of respondents who volunteered the information that their hearing loss had resulted from some viral infection or was otherwise acquired and apparently not specifically genetic in origin (scarlet fever, spinal meningitis, trauma, etc.). In this manner, we were able in our genetic analysis to combine data collected with a demographic procedure (census method) with data obtained by means of Kallmann's twin-family method.

Although a total of 968 properly executed replies were received in response to the second questionnaire, only 688 respondents were acceptable *deaf index cases* (adults of marriageable age) and used in the genetic analysis. The family histories of these 688 cases revealed the following distribution:

a.   501 index cases were the only deaf members of their families; more specifically, they were known to have had parents with normal hearing;

b.   95 index cases had deaf siblings, although the parent had no hearing impairment;

c.   92 index cases had other deaf relatives, regardless of whether or not they had deaf siblings; namely, deafness in one or both parents (45 cases) or in a cousin, grandparent or a sibling of parents who themselves had normal hearing (47 cases).

The sibship size (including the index cases) and the reported ages of onset in the 501 index cases without deaf relatives are tabulated in table 1. Only 40 per cent of these isolated cases believed that they had been born deaf. In another 40 per cent, deafness presumably occurred after the first and before the fifth year of life. The remaining 20 per cent of the cases had a reported age of onset "within the first year," but they probably include a considerable number of congenitally deaf cases, whose hearing impairment was erroneously ascribed to some coincidental event in early life (e.g., viral infection, trauma and so forth). In fact, similar reservations would seem to be justified in some of the 194 index cases with apparently acquired deafness in the second, third or fourth year of life. Without adequate clinical criteria for pinpointing the onset of deafness in a child's development in retrospect, the distinction between congenital and early-onset types of deafness in a large population study such as the present cannot possibly be expected to be clearly defined.

Similar difficulties are encountered in distinguishing between truly hereditary and ostensibly acquired forms of total deafness, especially in cases in which it

TABLE 1. AGE OF ONSET AND SIBSHIP SIZE IN 501 INDEX CASES
WITHOUT DEAF RELATIVES

Size Sibship	Reported Age of Onset			
	At birth	First year	Second to fourth year	Total
1	41	22	18	81
2	55	26	41	122
3	34	15	36	85
4	25	11	36	72
5	18	12	26	56
6	9	7	19	35
7	10	5	6	21
8	3	3	5	11
9	5	3	5	13
10	—	—	1	1
11	—	3	1	4
Total	200	107	194	501

may be hypothesized that a noxious exogenous factor acted before or during birth. For practical purposes, an expedient procedure for the classification of hereditary deafness is based on the presence of another case of deafness in the index families (in addition to the index case) as a principal requirement. While it will be shown in the analysis of our population data that families with sibships comprising more than one deaf sib most probably represent instances of *recessive deafness,* it may be presumed that the 92 index families with deaf members other than affected sibs of index cases exemplify the *dominant* mode of inheritance. Consequently, isolated cases of total deafness, although they form the bulk of this affliction in any given population, cannot with certainty be categorized as either hereditary or nonhereditary (acquired).

The distribution of the 95 index sibships with at least one other deaf sib and unaffected parents is shown in table 2 according to sibship size and the number of deaf per sibship. Although some families have four or five deaf sibs

TABLE 2. SIBSHIPS WITH ONE OR MORE DEAF SIBS
OTHER THAN INDEX CASE

Total Sibship Size	Number of Deaf Per Sibship				
	2	3	4	5	Total
2	13	—	—	—	13
3	7	4	—	—	11
4	11	4	—	—	15
5	13	1	—	1	15
6	8	2	2	1	13
7	5	2	2	—	9
8	3	7	2	—	12
9	2	1	2	—	5
10	—	—	—	—	—
11	—	—	—	1	1
12	—	—	—	1	1
Total	62	21	8	4	95

in one sibship (8 and 4 families, respectively), it may be noted that detailed information about age of onset is available only for the index cases themselves and not for their deaf sibs. Of the hearing losses of the index cases, 71.6 per cent were classified as congenital, 9.5 per cent as having developed during the first year, and 18.9 per cent as "acquired" during the second, third or fourth year of life. Omitted from the analysis were 5 index cases, whose deafness occurred at the ages of 6 (2 cases) and 7 years (3 cases).

In order to determine whether our data fit *a hypothesis of recessive inheritance,* it is necessary to estimate the probability of a recessively inherited form of deafness in those index cases, whose hearing loss was neither known to be exogenous nor due to the effect of a dominant gene. This segment of our deaf sample consists of the 501 isolated index cases and the 95 index cases who had at least one affected sib, although the parents and other relatives were not deaf.

For purposes of this estimate, certain statistical tests were needed which could at least in part overcome the procedural difficulties encountered in extracting genetic information from pedigrees. In collecting a series of hereditary deafness cases assumed to follow the recessive mode of inheritance, we were able to include only those family units which had at least one affected child. Obviously, we could not identify those families where fertile parents, although heterozygous carriers of the gene for deafness, failed by chance to produce a deaf child. Only by taking into account this type of parental mating in analyzing a recessive trait can we obtain the expected 3:1 ratio of unaffected to affected children (in this case, 75 per cent hearing and 25 per cent deaf children).

Another bias which may be present in our data stems from the fact that our index families were ascertained through a deaf person. Since we do not claim to have identified every deaf individual in the State of New York (complete ascertainment where all affected individuals are registered independently), we have to assume that our sampling procedure favored families with more than one affected sib. In other words, families with two, three or four deaf sibs are more likely to be represented in our sample than families with only one deaf child.

In dealing with this statistical problem, we might postulate, without impairing the genetic information obtained, that every deaf individual that came to our attention had an equal chance to be included in the questionnaire mailing list. An alternative procedure recommended by Haldane[8] would be to estimate our data twice, once assuming complete ascertainment and then assuming minimum ascertainment. Actually, the only disadvantage arising from an erroneous assumption of complete ascertainment would be an inflated proportion of affected children in the sample, leading to an overestimation of the value of p, the probability of deafness in the child of two heterozygous parents. Hence, by assuming complete ascertainment and then computing the relative proportions of hereditary and nonhereditary cases of deafness in our sample, we would underestimate the latter and merely obtain a minimum value for them.

In our test for recessiveness, we used Haldane's method[7] which corrects for the fact that identification of specific matings and sibs is possible only through an affected child. Our goal was to estimate the probability (p) of having a deaf child from matings between two heterozygous parents, considering the fact that each sibship was represented by at least one deaf child. If the criteria for the given mating type are met, the expected probability (p) would be 25 per cent. However, the observed p value would be below 25 per cent, if some of the deaf children in the sample lost their hearing through an exogenous factor occurring with a frequency of less than 25 per cent.

In investigating families with at least one affected child, we can represent the probability that a family of size s will have at least one affected child as $1 - q^s$, where q^s is the probability of no affected children. The formula that expresses the expected number r_s of affected children to be found in families of sibship size s is

$$r_s = \frac{sp}{1 - q^s}$$

and the expected total number of affected children in a sample of s-child families is

$$R = \sum_s \frac{sp}{1 - q^s} n_s$$

where n_s is the number of families of size s.

In employing this formula, we may estimate p by specifying trial values of p, simplifying the computation by means of Lejeune's tables.[11] Following the calculation, by trial, of two values of R (total expected number of affected children in s-child families) that bracket our observed number of affected children, we can, by linear interpolation, derive an estimated p value. The standard error of $\hat{p}$ may be taken from Finney's tabulations.[4]

In the test of our data for *recessiveness* (table 3), the following distribution is observed if the families of the isolated cases of congenital deafness (table 1) are combined with those of the 95 index cases who have at least one additional sib despite the absence of deafness in the parents or other relatives (table 2):

TABLE 3.   TEST FOR RECESSIVE HYPOTHESIS

Sibship Size	Number of Sibships	Number of Children	Number of Deaf	Expected Number of Deaf	
				p= .25	p= .275
2	68	136	81	77.724	78.812
3	45	135	60	58.365	59.985
4	40	160	59	58.520	60.800
5	33	165	52	54.087	56.727
6	22	132	44	40.150	42.460
7	19	133	34	38.380	40.888
8	15	120	38	33.345	35.730
9	10	90	20	24.330	26.200
10	—	—	—	—	—
11	1	11	5	2.871	3.116
12	1	12	5	3.098	3.371
Total	254	1094	398	390.870	408.089

Data from index cases deaf at birth and having no deaf relatives, and from index cases deaf before age 4 and with only deaf siblings.

In 254 sibships which are formed by two or more sibs and include at least one case of total deafness, we find 398 deaf subjects among altogether 1094 persons. A trial value of p = .25 gives 390.9 for R, the expected total number of deaf subjects. Using a value of p = .275, we should expect 408.1 deaf subjects. By linear interpolation the estimate of p for our sample is .260* with a standard error of ± .017.

This value of p is a good fit for the recessive hypothesis, provided that our category of isolated cases of "congenital deafness" is no artefact. If it is correct that congenital cases cannot be distinguished from those with a reported onset during the first year of life, and if the latter cases are therefore included in the analysis, we find that p equals .206 ± .014 (with a minimum estimate of .129 ± .010). In this instance, we obtain an excess of isolated cases of nongenetic origin. A similar excess (p = .15 ± .01) is observed if the analysis is extended to all isolated index cases (501), including those who reportedly lost their hearing after the first and before the fifth year of life.

The *double case method* of Bruno Schulz[19] may be used to test the *representativeness* of those 95 sibships with more than one deaf sib which have been assumed to be recessive cases of deafness. If only sibships with at least three members and two deaf sibs are included, the statistical procedure described previously yields the following values

$$r_s = \frac{sp\ (1-q^{s-1})}{(1-q^s) - (spq^{s-1})} \text{ and } R = \sum_s \frac{sp\ (1-q^{s-1})}{(1-q^s) - (spq^{s-1})}\ n_s$$

The use of trial values of p for this population gives $\hat{p}$ equal to .310 ± .031. As previously pointed out, this value is probably an overestimate because it assumes complete ascertainment. Moreover, it is not much larger than the theoretical value of .25. Hence, our data seem to be in accord with the hypothesis that the families with more than one affected sib represent recessive cases of deafness.

In another test for recessiveness, we asked a certain proportion of the index cases whether their parents were *cousins*. Of the 247 replies, 30 (over 12 per cent) were in the affirmative. Further analysis confirmed the finding of Stevenson and Cheeseman[21] that consanguineous marriages give a good fit to the recessive hypothesis, while nonconsanguineous marriages show an excess of isolated cases. The estimated p value for our series of 26 sibships with two or more children from cousin marriages is in accordance with expectation; namely, .25 ± .04.

Another important question is whether early total deafness may be caused by one, two, or more independent recessive genes. According to our data, at least one out of 10 cases of deafness occurring before the age of 5 years is

---

*In order to minimize the value of $\hat{p}$, incomplete ascertainment of the affected in our sample would have to be assumed. In this case, the probability that a given family is represented in the test sample is directly proportional to the number of affected in the family. The recessive proportion (p) of affected individuals in the sibship may be simply counted by subtraction of one recessive member from each observed sibship (i.e., the index case that brought the family to our attention). The minimum estimate of p now becomes .171 ± .013.

known to come from the consanguineous mating of two hearing persons. This finding alone indicates that there are certainly more than two independent recessive genes for deafness. Generally speaking, the rarer a recessive gene is in a given population, the more frequent will be the cases springing from cousin marriages.

According to Stevenson and Cheeseman,[21] the population frequency of recessive deafness approximates 20 per 100,000 (.02 per cent), while Chung et al.[3] estimated, on the basis of Stevenson's first-cousin marriage data, that no less than 36 different recessive genes (provided that all of them are equal in frequency) may be expected to cause congenital total deafness. In the State of New York, the expectancy of recessive deafness cases from first-cousin matings would be .4 per cent, if the frequency of first-cousin marriage is assumed to be .1 per cent. Even if the New York consanguinity rate were ten times as high (1 per cent), we should not expect more than 4 per cent of the deaf to be the children of first-cousin marriages, while the observed rate is over 10 per cent. It may be concluded, therefore, that in the New York State population, too, there are *many different recessive genes* which may cause total deafness in a homozygous condition. In other words, although the deaf tend to practice *assortative mating,* we cannot expect to find a 100 per cent deafness rate among the children of dual matings even if there were no cases of deafness of nongenetic origin in the given group of parents.

In our sample, the analysis of different mating types discloses a total of 310 dual matings with altogether 441 children, 62 of whom are deaf. Of this total of dual matings, 62 have remained childless and 116 united two index cases.

Of the 248 reproductive dual matings, 10 produced only one child each that is deaf; 14 produced 34 children, all of whom are deaf (10 matings with two deaf children each, 3 matings with three, and 1 mating with five deaf children); 15 produced children of both varieties (18 deaf, 23 hearing); and 209 produced 356 children, all of whom have normal hearing.

In general genetic terms, the following possibilities exist for the children of *dual matings* in a deaf population:

1. All children may be *deaf,* because their parents carry the same type of recessive gene.

2. Only *some* of the children may be deaf, because:

a. One parent is a homozygote for recessive deafness, and the other, in addition to being afflicted with an exogenous form of deafness, happens to be a heterozygous carrier of the same recessive gene.

b. One parent has a recessive, and the other a dominant type of deafness.

c. One parent is both a heterozygote for the recessive gene for which his mate is homozygous, and a homozygote for another type of recessive gene.

With respect to the last possibility it may be noted that in the absence of linkage, a deaf person who is homozygous for one recessive gene has virtually the same chance of being heterozygous for another recessive gene as hearing persons in the general population.

3. All children may be *hearing,* because:

a. Their parents are homozygous for different recessive genes.

b. One or both parents have an exogenous type of deafness.

In conclusion, it may be stated that inasmuch as early total deafness can apparently be caused by homozygosity for one of a large number of recessive genes, it is to be expected that many hearing people are heterozygous for at least one of these genes. With each individual gene being rare, it is also in accordance with expectation that the consanguinity rate for the hearing parents of deaf subjects is high, and that the majority of totally deaf people come from matings of heterozygous carriers with normal hearing.

In addition, there are dominantly inherited forms of deafness, estimated by Chung et al.[3] at 15 to 22 per cent of all hereditary cases, and probably a few cases of sex-linked deafness.[13,18] The latter variety seems to be very rare, affecting no more than eight men per one million males.

TWIN DATA WITH SOME PEDIGREES OF TWIN FAMILIES

Corroborative evidence for the genetic determinants in the etiology of early total deafness is furnished by pedigree studies as well as by twin data. It is by means of the twin-family method that these two investigative procedures can be fruitfully combined.

This *twin study* was set up in such a manner that apart from supplying much-needed control data for the census of the deaf population of New York State, it could readily be extended to the metropolitan districts of Washington, D. C. and Philadelphia. The need for this extension stemmed from the relative infrequency of the condition to be investigated, but it caused no procedural difficulty through the introduction of major inconsistencies either in ascertaining or in studying the twin index cases. On the whole, it can be said that the centrally organized screening systems for the three geographical areas functioned with comparable effectiveness. What is more, there were no significant differences in the degree or over-all lack of cooperativeness received from deaf twins in the various districts.

Of the originally reported total series of 114 pairs of twins with deafness in one or both partners, only those pairs were regarded as adequately investigated where both twins were alive, available for all essential tests, and sufficiently cooperative. These restrictive criteria reduced our fully studied series to 39 pairs including one set of triplets counted as two pairs, and the incompletely studied series to 48 pairs. Based on a comparison of same-sex and opposite-sex pairs, the two series do not differ in the distribution of concordance and discordance rates for deafness.

The *zygosity diagnosis* in the fully studied series was based on the principles of the probability method devised by Smith and Penrose.[20] In addition to the usual physical characteristics, it included an extensive analysis of blood groups and total fingerprint ridge counts according to the methods of Nixon [12] and Brodhage and Wendt.[2] While same-sex pairs with a difference in a major blood group system, a DZ rating on the ridge count or a Smith-Penrose DZ probability of more than 93 per cent were classified as dizygotic, the majority of pairs diagnosed as monozygotic (12 out of 17 pairs) had a Smith-Penrose MZ probability of more than 99 per cent, and the remainder, of more than 90 per cent. Curiously, the ratio of monozygotic to dizygotic pairs obtained in this manner (17:22) is precisely the same as the one estimated according to Weinberg's differential method.

The *deafness concordance rates* for the 17 MZ and 22 DZ pairs of the fully studied series (table 4) are 59 per cent and 23 per cent, respectively, showing

TABLE 4. CONCORDANCE FOR TOTAL DEAFNESS IN 39 TWIN PAIRS

Zygosity	Concordant Pairs	Discordant Pairs	Total
Monozygotic	10	7	17
Dizygotic	5	17	22
Total	15	24	39

a statistically significant difference at the .05 level. These differential rates are in agreement with the previously discussed theories on the genetic aspects of early total deafness.

The collection of sizable proportions of *discordant* pairs in both categories (MZ and DZ) proved to be of particular value not only in the search for clearly definable anamnestic, clinical, biochemical or cytological concomitants of deafness, but also for the quantifying purposes of audiometric and psychometric comparisons. For instance, the extent of intellectual or maturational intrapair differences as measured by psychological tests in discordant MZ twins provides a useful estimate of the retarding effect of total deafness on the various components of personality development.

While it is planned to present the detailed psychological and audiometric test results in connection with another departmental report,[15] it is essential to mention here that despite some observable trends toward intrapair similarity in the *audiometric responses,* or lack of responses, of concordant twins ("familial signatures"), it is not yet possible with current techniques to identify specific audiometric patterns with the effect of any particular gene. What can be said is that the "no or minimal response" pattern, shown in figure 1 as an example of bilateral similarity in a completely concordant MZ pair, is typical of many genetically determined deafness cases, especially of the recessive ones, and that the more variable expressivity pattern illustrated by the comparative audiometric twin records in figures 2 and 3 (clinically discordant, but audiometrically partly concordant MZ pair and clinically as well as audiometrically concordant DZ pair, respectively) seems to occur particularly in the dominant types of deafness. According to Fisch,[5] the "no or minimal response" pattern with bilateral residual hearing at some of the tested frequencies is found in approximately one-fourth of all hereditary cases of deafness.

The bilateral twin audiograms compared in figures 1-3 represent the responses to pure tone sounds at 11 different sound frequencies with a range from 125 to 8000 cycles per second (cps) as recorded on the horizontal axis of the audiograms. The degrees of hearing loss noted on the vertical axis were measured in decibels (db) according to the intensity of sound and varied from −10 to +100, although responses above normal hearing (−1 to −10) were eliminated here for the sake of clarity. Like all other audiometric records in this twin study, the audiograms shown were taken with a standard portable Bell-Tone audiometer.

Clinically as well as genetically, it would seem to be of particular significance that of the 7 MZ pairs classified as discordant for deafness according to standard criteria (table 4), only 2 proved audiometrically to be *completely discordant* (table 5). In the remaining 5 pairs, the presumably "hearing" co-twins were found to have some hearing impairment beyond the range of variability

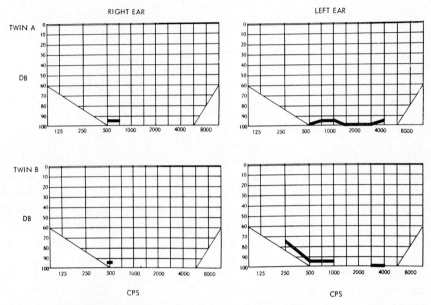

FIG. 1. Audiometrically similar, female MZ twins concordant for the recessive type of early total deafness (A. twins).

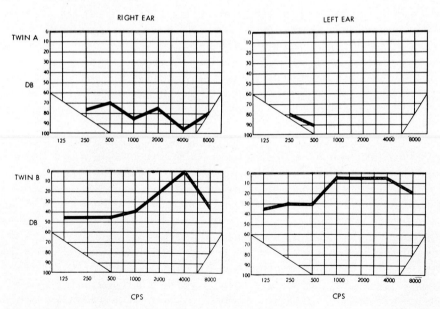

FIG. 2. Clinically and audiometrically dissimilar, female MZ twins partly concordant for the dominant type of early total deafness (R. twins).

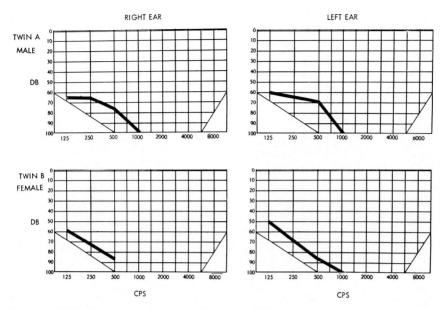

Fig. 3. Clinically and audiometrically similar DZ twins of opposite sex completely concordant for dominant type of deafness (E. twins).

TABLE 5.   DEGREES OF CONCORDANCE BASED ON AUDIOGRAMS

Zygosity and Sex		Concordance as to Deafness			
		Completely concordant	Partly concordant	Completely discordant	Total
Monozygotic pairs	Male	6	—	—	6
	Female	4	5	2	11
Dizygotic pairs	Male	—	—	3	3
	Female	1	2	5	8
	Opposite sex	4	1	6	11
Total		15	8	16	39

observed in a population with normal hearing. Peculiarly, all of the 5 one-egg co-twins reclassified as "partly concordant" belonged to the *female sex,* and it may not be a mere coincidence that there was the same sex preference in those two pairs in the group of discordant same-sex DZ twins (10 pairs), which were not completely discordant.

It may also be noted that of the 10 completely concordant MZ pairs, 9 were classified as *congenital* (table 6) and as apparently recessive in type, while of the other 7 MZ pairs which were either completely discordant or only partly concordant, all seemed exogenous in origin. By comparison, the total series of 39 pairs considered as adequately investigated (including 33 pairs with congenital or first-year deafness) showed the following distribution: 20 were classified as recessive, 5 as dominant and 14 as exogenous.

In the relatively small group of *dominantly* inherited forms, important clues to further inquiries into the etiology of early total deafness may be seen not

TABLE 6. DISTRIBUTION OF TWIN INDEX PAIRS ACCORDING
TO AGE OF ONSET

Zygosity and Concordance		Age of Onset			
		At birth	First year	Second to fourth year	Over four years
Monozygotic pairs	Completely concordant	9	—	—	1
	Partly concordant	1	2	1	1
	Completely discordant	1	1	—	—
Dizygotic pairs	Completely concordant	3	1	—	1
	Partly concordant	2	1	—	—
	Completely discordant	8	4	—	2
Total		24	9	1	5

only in its marked variability in penetrance and clinical expression extending from discordance in some one-egg pairs of twins to unilaterality in some individuals, but also in its tendency to associate itself with pigmentary and other pathological symptoms outside of the auditory system, including the syndromes described by Klein[10] and Waardenburg.[23] On the other hand, association

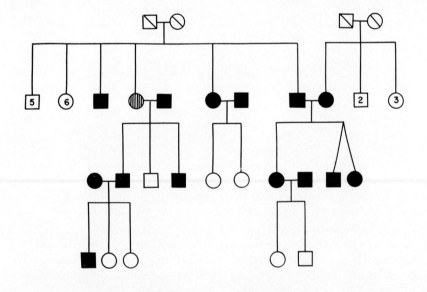

FIG. 4. Apparently dominant form of early total deafness in E. family with concordant pair of twins.

with additional disorders has also been observed in nondominant forms of deafness. In this category are Usher's syndrome combining total deafness with retinitis pigmentosa[9] and the D trisomy syndrome reported by Therman et al.,[22] combining deafness with a definable chromosomal aberration.

The pedigrees of two interesting twin families may serve to illustrate the variable degrees of expressivity in apparently dominant forms of early total deafness. As used here, the term "incomplete expressivity" denotes hearing losses which are either of limited extent or expressed only unilaterally or later than in early life.

In the E. family (fig. 4) which includes a concordant pair of opposite-sex twins, all 9 cases of deafness that occurred in consanguineously related members were *fully expressed,* with the exception of one case of partial hearing loss in a paternal aunt of the twins. Of the three dual matings in this family, one gave rise to deaf offspring only, one to hearing offspring only, and one to a combination of deaf and hearing children.

The pedigree of the R. family (fig. 5) exemplifies *various degrees of*

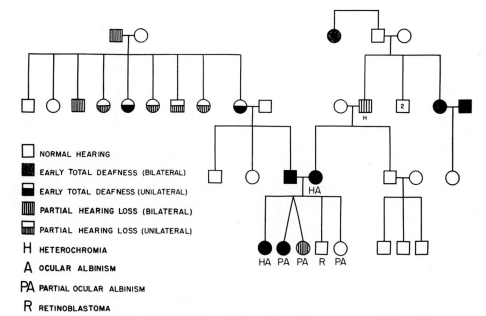

FIG. 5. Apparently dominant form of early total deafness showing incomplete expressivity and association with ocular albinism, heterochromia and retinoblastoma in the R. family.

expressivity as well as an association with such diverse *eye conditions* as retinoblastoma, heterochromia, and ocular albinism (unilateral and bilateral). This family includes not only the dual mating unit shown in figure 6, but also among the five children of this unit (four daughters, one son) a rather unique pair of MZ twins concordant for partial ocular albinism and clinically discordant for early total deafness. Audiometrically, however, the twins had to be

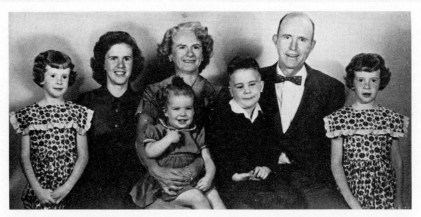

FIG. 6.   The R. twins with their parents and sibs.

classified as partly concordant for an early hearing loss. Their audiograms* are compared in figure 2.

Of the three sibs of these twins, the oldest sister is deaf and heterochromic, like the mother and the maternal grandfather, but the hearing loss of the latter is only incomplete. The two younger sibs have normal hearing, although the girl has partial ocular albinism, and the boy had one eye enucleated because of a histopathologically verified retinoblastoma. *Cytological* and other *laboratory* techniques contributed no tangible clue to the etiology of this particular syndrome.

CONCLUSIONS

1.   Early total deafness is an extremely stressful disability, which in the State of New York occurs with a frequency of approximately 0.1 per cent (one deaf per 1000 persons in the general population) and often tends to be associated with a severe degree of maladjustment.

2.   Family problems encountered in a deaf community extend to both hearing and deaf persons within afflicted families and urgently call for specialized counseling services. Such services require specially trained personnel familiar with the adjustive as well as the genetic aspects of deafness. In fact, the availability of adequate services of this kind may be considered to represent a definitive yardstick of a sound and benevolent system of general population policies, deserving this name in an enlightened twentieth-century society.[15]

---

*Since this set of audiograms was taken at the laboratories of the Department of Otolaryngology of Columbia-Presbyterian Medical Center, in conjunction with the thorough otological examinations of the whole R. family, the author wishes to acknowledge our indebtedness to Professor E. P. Fowler, Jr. and his staff for the generous assistance rendered in this study. At the same time, we should like to express our gratitude to Professor A. G. De Voe and his associates of the Institute of Ophthalmology for having helped us with the ophthalmological part of the study, and to Dr. Ernest Chu of the Biology Division of the Oak Ridge National Laboratory for his painstaking cytological work. The author is also obliged to Mrs. L. Ruut and Mrs. C. Wolff for their efficient help in preparing the bibliography and illustrations for this report.

3. The diagnostic category called early total deafness is not a homogeneous one from an etiological standpoint. Genetic and nongenetic forms contribute to this category in approximately equal proportions. The genetically determined group includes, apart from a few rare sex-linked forms, both dominant and recessive cases, approximately in a 1:4 ratio.

4. Our genetic data derived from a New York State population sample of 688 deaf persons of marriageable age are in agreement with the theory, based on the results of an earlier Irish study,[21] that the majority of genetically determined deafness cases follow the recessive mode of inheritance. They also indicate that there are many rare recessive genes in the gene pool of a large population such as that of the State of New York. This conclusion is based on the finding of a relatively high consanguinity rate for the hearing parents of deaf index cases. It is safe to state, therefore, that early total deafness may be caused by homozygosity for any one of these different recessive genes, and that many hearing people in the general population are to be expected to be heterozygous carriers of at least one of these genes.

5. Corroborative evidence for the partly genetic and partly nongenetic etiology of early total deafness has been obtained by a comprehensive study of a consecutive series of 39 twin pairs (with two living and sufficiently cooperative members) and their families. The clinically observed concordance rates in this series are 23 per cent for two-egg twins of the same or opposite sex, and 59 per cent for one-egg twins. In an additional 30 per cent of the one-egg pairs, audiometric examinations have established the presence of a partial hearing loss in those co-twins classified clinically as having no total deafness ("hearing" in terms of this study). It may be noted that all "hearing" co-twins who have been found in this series to have a partial hearing loss belong to the female sex.

6. Clinically as well as genetically, it is of particular interest that a more variable expressivity pattern apparently occurs especially in the dominant and not in the recessive forms of early total deafness.

7. The deaf population of the State of New York is distinguished by a decreased marriage rate with a relatively high proportion of divorces. [15, 16] Within the present sample, information has been obtained about 310 dual matings, 62 of which have remained childless. The 248 reproductive dual matings have produced a total of 441 children, 62 of whom are deaf. In 15 matings of this kind, children of both varieties have been produced (18 deaf, 23 hearing).

REFERENCES

1. ALTSHULER, K. Z., AND RAINER, J. D.: Patterns and course of schizophrenia in the deaf. J. Nerv. Ment. Dis. 127: 77, 1958.
2. BRODHAGE, G., AND WENDT, G. G.: Die Verwendung qualitativer Fingerleistenmerkmale in Vaterschaftsgutachten. Ztschr. menschl. Vererb. u.-Konstitutionslehre 30: 212 and 221, 1951.
3. CHUNG, C. S., ROBISON, O. W., AND MORTON, N. S.: A note on deaf mutism. Ann. Human Genet. 23: 357, 1959.
4. FINNEY, D. J.: The truncated binomial distribution. Ann. Eugenics 14: 319, 1949.
5. FISCH, L.: The aetiology of congenital deafness and audiometric patterns. J. Laryng. Otol. 69: 479, 1955.

6. ——, AND NORMAN, A. P.: Hyperbilirubinaemia and perceptive deafness. Brit. Med. J. 2: 142, 1961.

7. HALDANE, J. B. S.: A method for investigating recessive characters in man. J. Genetics 25: 251, 1932.

8. ——: The estimation of the frequencies of recessive conditions in man. Ann. Eugenics 8: 255, 1938.

9. HALLGREN, B.: Retinitis pigmentosa combined with congenital deafness. Acta psychiat. et neurol. (suppl. 138,) 1959.

10. KLEIN, J.: Albinisme partiel (leucisme) avec surdi-mutité, blépharophimosis et dysplasie myo-osteo-articulaire. Helvet. paediat. acta 5: 38, 1950.

11. LEJEUNE, J.: Sur une solution "a priori" de la methode "a posteriori" de Haldane. Biometrics 14: 513, 1958.

12. NIXON, W. L. B.: On the diagnosis of twin-pair ovularity and the use of dermatoglyphic data. In Gedda, L., Ed.: Novant'anni delle Leggi Mendeliane. Rome, Istituto Gregorio Mendel, 1956.

13. PARKER, N.: Congenital deafness due to a sex-linked recessive gene. Am. J. Human Genet. 10: 196, 1958.

14. RAINER, J. D., ALTSHULER, K. Z., AND KALLMANN, F. J.: Psychotherapy for the deaf. In Stokvis, B., Ed.: Advances in Psychosomatic Medicine. Basel, S. Karger, 1962, Vol. iii, in press. Fifth Internat. Congr. Psychother. (Rome 1961). Amsterdam, Excerpta Medica, 1961.

15. ——, ——, AND ——, (Eds.): Family and Mental Health Problems in a Deaf Population, in preparation.

16. RAINER, J. D., AND FIRSCHEIN, I. L.: Mating and fertility patterns in families with early total deafness. Eugenics Quart. 6: 117, 1959.

17. ——, AND KALLMANN, F. J.: A constructive psychiatric program for a deaf population. Proc. 38th Conv., Am. Instr. Deaf, Senate Document No. 66. Washington, D. C., U. S. Govt. Printing Office, 1958.

18. SATALOFF, J., PASTORE, P. N., AND BLOOM, E.: Sex-linked hereditary deafness. Am. J. Human Genet. 7: 201, 1955.

19. SCHULZ, B.: Methodik der medizinischen Erbforschung. Leipzig, Thieme, 1936.

20. SMITH, A. M., AND PENROSE, L. S.: Monozygotic and dizygotic twin diagnosis. Ann. Human Genet. 19: 273, 1955.

21. STEVENSON, A. C., AND CHEESEMAN, E. A.: Hereditary deaf mutism, with particular reference to Northern Ireland. Ann. Human Genet. 20: 177, 1956.

22. THERMAN, E., et al.: The D trisomy syndrome and XO gonadal dysgenesis in two sisters. Am. J. Human Genet. 13: 193, 1961.

23. WAARDENBURG, P. J.: A new syndrome combining developmental anomalies of the eyelids, eyebrows, and nose root with pigmentary defects of the iris and the head, hair, and with congenital deafness. Am. J. Human Genet. 3: 195, 1951.

20

Genetic Aspects of Mental Deficiency

GEORGE A. JERVIS, M.D.

IT SEEMS APPROPRIATE to discuss some problems of the influence of heredity on mental deficiency in this symposium devoted to the expanding goals of psychiatric genetics. It was, in fact, in the field of mental deficiency that much original work was done by the early medical geneticists, and one may confidently expect new important developments in the future, albeit with considerable changes on emphases.

This necessarily limited discussion will be confined to brief comments on three different problems: (1) the genetics of so-called simple mental deficiency, (2) the problem of congenital malformations of the central nervous system in their relation to genetics, and (3) the implications of biochemical genetics with respect to mental deficiency.

SIMPLE MENTAL DEFICIENCY

The term simple (or undifferentiated) mental deficiency is used extensively by workers in the field. It originates from the assumption that when the long process of singling out distinct entities from the large heterogeneous group of mental subnormality will ultimately be completed, a residual group of defectives will remain. These individuals show no pathological lesions, either structural or chemical in nature, and no clinical manifestations other than subnormal intelligence. They appear to be the counterpart of the "gifted" group. Statistics tend to support such an assumption. The distribution curve of intelligence test scores, as is well known, theoretically approximates the Gaussian curve, but it is actually skewed on the negative side. The skewness is particularly seen in the segment of the curve below IQ 50, where it probably represents the specific pathological entities exogenous or genetic in origin. Above IQ 50, the difference between expectation and observation is less apparent. It is in this segment of the curve that the "simple" defectives usually do fit, thus being part of the normal distribution curve of intelligence in the general population to the same extent as gifted children are part of it.

If this assumption is correct, it follows that the etiological determinants of the simple type of mental deficiency are of the same order as those responsible for variations of intelligence in the general population. It is not the place here to expand on the lively controversy, almost a century old, between geneticists and environmentalists concerning the determinants of intelligence.

Perhaps one may summarize the present status of the problem by stating that there is no consensus of opinion as to the nature of intelligence. However, regardless of whether one accepts the concept of a "general ability" which mainly determines intellectual efficiency or prefers other concepts, one may base an operational definition of intelligence on the plain fact that what is measured by reliable intelligence tests is a trait which under standard conditions may be confidently correlated with both hereditary and environmental factors. Pedigree records, family correlation data, the study of twins, animal experimentation and the results of necessarily limited human experiments suggest that genetic factors determine this "intelligence" trait to a considerable extent.[2] An attempt to state in exact percentages the degree of this influence is apt to be meaningless because of the extreme complexity of the interaction between genetic and environmental factors. Genetic influences are most likely the result of the action of multiple genes, the effects of which yield continuously distributed frequency curves.

In line with these few basic assumptions it would appear that the problem of the influence of heredity upon "simple" mental deficiency is somewhat clarified. It is probably safe to conclude that the diverse genetic contributions play a larger part than the environment in determining that variance in brain functioning which is at the basis of the "simple" form of mental deficiency.

However, in transposing data from general population studies of intelligence to the investigation of "simple" mental deficiency, considerable difficulties are encountered. In studying the influence of heredity on intelligence, much emphasis has been placed on *correlation techniques*. Correlation close to the theoretical .50 for parent-child or sib-sib regression of IQ have been reported in extensive population surveys, suggesting the importance of hereditary factors.[6] Similar figures have been reported with respect to "simple" mental deficiency. However, when data of this type are related to "simple" defectives, they may be viewed with some criticism on various *statistical* grounds including the following: (a) Samples are usually too small to be conclusive; (b) since considerable resistance is often encountered in testing the intelligence of adults in families with "simple" mental retardation, many samples are incomplete; (c) random mating, a necessary theoretical premise for the validity of these correlations, rarely prevails in families of "simple" mental defectives; (d) the random effect of environmental factors, another theoretical premise, is obviously difficult to prove in families with "simple" retardation; and (e) data on correlations between relatives other than sibs or parents are extremely limited in number and usually based on very small samples. It may be noted that Penrose's correlation figures for cousins of defectives show a value of 0.28, which is more than double the value of 0.125, theoretically expected on the basis of the genetic hypothesis.[6]

The main objection to the statistical treatment of the problem may be raised on purely *clinical grounds*. Since the clinical diagnosis of "simple" mental retardation is generally made by exclusion, it requires a painstaking evaluation of all pertinent anamnestic data and a comprehensive examination of each individual by means of all available clinical and laboratory methods. Obviously, it would be impossible to apply such rigid diagnostic criteria to a sample of the size required for statistical purposes. The only positive element in the diagnosis of "simple" mental retardation is familial incidence of the defect. However, if one relies on this datum in the selection of cases, the sample would be seriously biased.

In conclusion, it may be said that the classic problem of the influence of inheritance on "simple" mental deficiency is still unsolved after more than half a century of investigative efforts. The clinical delineation of this group appears more difficult, and the diagnostic distinction between the "simple" defective and the defective with minimal exogenously determined brain damage is less clear than was previously thought. Even if highly refined statistical methods are used in evaluating representative sets of data, the main obstacle will still be the ascertainment of unselected samples.

CONGENITAL MALFORMATIONS

The second topic in this brief review concerns congenital malformation of the central nervous system, a subject which has recently attracted wide attention. The magnitude of the problem in terms of loss of life is appalling. According to present estimates, 30 per cent of all pregnancies fail to survive in utero, and about one-half of these losses may be due to congenital malformations. More specifically, congenital malformations of the central nervous system are responsible for about one-third of all deaths from congenital malformations during the first two years of life. In terms of persons afflicted with mental retardation, it may be said that some 30 per cent of low-grade defectives show malformation of the central nervous system demonstrable by autopsy and apparently directly connected with the failure of mental development. Down's syndrome (mongolism) is one of the most striking malformations. Also, it is one of the most common causes of mental retardation, its frequency in the general population being close to two per thousand.

The problem of the relative pertinence of genetic or environmental factors in the etiology of malformations associated with mental deficiency has been disputed by many investigators, but with unimpressive results. Genetically oriented workers have convincingly demonstrated that some of these conditions are due to the effect of single genes. For instance, tuberous sclerosis and certain syndromes of mental defect associated with skeletal malformations seem to be caused by single dominant genes.[4] Similarly, a number of ocular malformations with mental defect and certain forms of both microcephaly and hydrocephaly have been shown to be clearly genetic in origin. However, these conditions are rare, their proportion not being above 2 to 3 per cent of all malformations of the central nervous system.

On the environmental side, experimental teratology data lend considerable support to the theory of exogenous influences. It should be noted, however, that the rigorous man-made conditions enforceable in animal experimentation cannot readily be matched in human pathology. Hence, the large majority of malformations associated with mental defect remained unexplained until in 1959 the discovery of chromosomal abnormalities in Down's syndrome opened an entirely new field of investigation and led to the rapid accumulation of significant pieces of information about other congenital malformations. Pertinent to mental deficiency are, besides Down's syndrome, the D and E syndromes and some aneuploid states characterized by various malformations and mental subnormalities; also, certain Klinefelter cases and other sex-chromosomal irregularities where, with few exceptions, mental defect is an outstanding feature.

Other participants in this symposium are discussing with more authority the various implications of these discoveries. Before an audience of clinicians it may be appropriate to stress how important the finding of chromosomal anomalies in Down's syndrome has been to the clinical worker. Until recently, very little was known about the causation of what had long been referred to as mongolism. We had to be resigned to the discouraging task of adding periodically a new hypothesis to the long list of unproved etiological theories. As a consequence, genetic family counseling, so often requested in relation to the risk of having another mongoloid child, was a difficult if not impossible task. It is now known that many cases of Down's syndrome are associated with trisomy of chromosome No. 21, the extra chromosome probably being the result of nondisjunction. This finding is consistent with some well established and heretofore unexplained observations about the disease: (a) its usually random occurrence in the population; (b) the tendency of one-egg twins to be concordant and that of two-egg twins to be usually discordant[1]; and (c) the presence of the condition in about one-half of the children of mongoloid mothers, with the other half being unaffected.

Trisomy itself would not explain the well known fact that nearly 75 per cent of mongoloid births are statistically correlated with advanced maternal age of the mother. However, it seems that old ova may be more prone to nondisjunction than younger ones, and this fact may explain the puzzling influence of maternal age in this syndrome.

The cause or causes of nondisjunction are not yet clear. It is known only that several agents producing mutations, such as radiations and certain chemical substances, may also be instrumental in producing nondisjunction. It may also be significant that animal viruses seem to be responsible for chromosomal aberrations in certain lines of mammalian tissue cultures.[3] Apparently, karyotype anomalies represent one stage of the mutagenic process caused by physical, chemical or viral agents. Whatever the cause, the effect may be a random effect in the majority of cases. It is safe to state, therefore, that in a family with a mongoloid child distinguished by trisomy, the risk of an unaffected mother having a second mongoloid child is comparatively slight.

There are, however, some 20 to 25 per cent of mongoloid births which do not depend on maternal age. Some of these cases are certain to be trisomic and may be associated with a genetically determined predisposition to nondisjunction in the mother. In fact, it cannot be excluded that such predisposition may occasionally occur in older mothers whose mongoloid children are trisomic. However, a substantial number of cases which do not depend on maternal age show various types of translocation, while their chromosomal complement is normal. In such cases, either the mother and other maternal relatives or, exceptionally, the father would reveal evidence of chromosomal translocation, thus being identifiable as carriers of the trait. In these families, the risk of multiple mongoloid births is obviously high. Hence, the newly acquired knowledge about the etiology of Down's syndrome offers a solid basis for genetic counseling.

The main problem of the mechanisms, by which karyotypic aberration may bring about mental subnormality, remains to be clarified. On the basis of our present fragmentary knowledge of the strict relations between genes and enzymes, one may suspect that some still largely unknown metabolic changes may result from alterations of genic material.

BIOCHEMICAL GENETICS AND MENTAL DEFICIENCY

The last topic to be touched upon here is biochemical genetics in relation to mental deficiency. Those who took an interest in these problems some 25 years ago could not possibly have foreseen the astonishing growth of this branch of human genetics. In this area, as well as in that of chromosomal abnormalities, it is clear that mental deficiency occupies a central position. The large majority of conditions, in fact, that have been investigated by the biochemical geneticist are characterized by mental subnormality.

At our present state of knowledge, there are some 38 types of mental deficiency associated with biochemical abnormalities. Metabolism of proteins and that of carbohydrates, lipids, pigments and minerals are involved in this assortment of admittedly rare diseases, with wide variations of the mental defect in each disease and among the various diseases. However, the deviation in intelligence is usually sharp enough to show a reasonably clear-cut segregation from the continuously distributed variations of intelligence observed in the general population. Moreover, the metabolic alteration which is basic to the condition can be measured exactly by laboratory methods and tends to segregate quite sharply. In the genetic investigation of these conditions, therefore, one is on more solid grounds than in the study of "simple" mental retardation discussed in the first part of this report.

In almost every condition thus far described there is some evidence suggestive of a genetic mechanism. Even in those diseases where only a few cases have been reported—i.e., congenital amaurotic idiocy, "maple sugar urine" disease, non-hemolytic hyperbilirubinemia or argininosuccinic aciduria—the given cases tend to show evidence of familial incidence. Because of the rarity of most of these diseases, statistical genetic analysis has not been possible so that the exact mode of inheritance is still not clearly understood. In some conditions, however, sufficient data are available for statistical evaluation. For instance, in Tay-Sachs' disease, juvenile amaurotic idiocy, gargoylism, phenylketonuria or galactosemia the available evidence indicates clearly enough that the disorder is inherited as a recessive trait which is determined by a single autosomal gene. Sex-linkage is noted only in certain forms of gargoylism and in pitressin-resistant diabetes insipidus. In all other conditions in this group, family data, although limited to a few families, are consistent with the hypothesis of recessive inheritance.

The discovery of these forms of mental retardation with defective metabolism inevitably led to attempts at demonstrating the lack of a specific enzyme in other conditions, following the classic postulate of Garrod that the immediate cause of a congenital metabolic abnormality may have to be sought in the defect of an enzyme essential for the normal metabolism of the substance involved in the biochemical disorder. The defect of a specific enzyme has been conclusively demonstrated in galactosemia (phosphogalacto-uridyl-transferase), phenylketonuria (phenylalanine-hydroxylase), constitutional hyperbilirubinemia (glucuronyl-transferase), and in some forms of nonendemic cretinism (deiodi-nase). In many other conditions it may be presumed that a defective enzymatic system is at the base of the metabolic defect, but adequate evidence is still lacking. For instance, present knowledge about the enzymatic systems catalyz-ing the normal steps in the metabolisms of the substances involved in the cerebral lipidoses or in gargoylism is rather fragmentary.

In some forms of mental deficiency, the interaction between altered gene and enzymatic defect is now somewhat clearer. The work of Pauling and his collaborators and that of later investigators[7] on inheritable differences in the structure of the globin position of the hemoglobin molecule has clarified the manner in which genetic information may control the activity of an enzyme by altering its structure. One may then visualize how changes in the activity of the enzymatic protein molecules, phenylalanine hydroxylase (to use the example of phenylketonuria), may be effected under genetic control by minor changes in molecular structure.

The relation between metabolic disorders (enzyme deficiency) and deviant intelligence is apparently much more complex. The effects of the enzymatic defect vary in the various conditions, and the mechanisms by which the biochemical alteration brings about brain function impairment are certainly different from disease to disease.

In the cerebral lipidoses, abnormal amounts of lipids accumulate in the central nervous system either within the neurons, as in the amaurotic idiocies, or within the white matter, as in metachromatic leukodystrophy. Striking morphological changes result, and the defect in intellectual functioning is obviously the correlate of extensive pathological lesions in the brain. Mental defect in gargoylism, a disease of carbohydrate metabolism, may be similarly explained. In the various forms of hypothyroidism, characterized by a genetical-ly determined enzymatic deficiency in the synthesis of thyroid hormones, the ensuing lack of thyroxine is directly responsible for retarded mental develop-ment in a manner similar to that observed in common types of cretinism. A direct toxic action of the abnormal metabolite upon the nervous system may be assumed to take place in constitutional nonhemolytic hyperbilirubinemia where the nonconjugated bilirubins directly damage the neurons.

In other diseases, the damaging effect upon the brain seems to be mediated through a known secondary mechanism; for instance, through hypoglycemia in hypoglycemosis or through repeated dehydration and electrolyte imbalance in pitressin-resistant diabetes insipidus. More subtle biochemical mechanisms resulting in brain damage probably act in galactosemia. In view of certain experimental findings, galactose-1-phosphate, the metabolite which accumulates in the body fluid as the result of a specific enzymatic deficiency, is assumed to inhibit competitively phosphoglucomutase, an enzymatic system of impor-tance for the metabolism of the brain. Apparently, similar enzymatic interfer-ences are operating in phenylketonuria, thus explaining the delay in brain development. Further investigations along these lines will lead to a considerable increase in our knowledge of the effects which genetically determined meta-bolic abnormality exerts upon brain functions.

SUMMARY

It is clear from the program of this symposium that problems of mental deficiency still hold a prominent place in psychiatric genetics. Emphases may have shifted, and old problems such as the influence of heredity on "simple" mental deficiency, which 25 years ago were sharply in focus, would seem to have lost some meaning. However, fresh problems have arisen to keep very much alive the genetic investigation of mental subnormality.[5]

REFERENCES

1. ALLEN, G., AND KALLMANN, F. J.: Mongolism in twin sibships. Acta Genet. 7: 385, 1957.
2. FULLER, J. L., AND THOMPSON, W. R.: Behavior Genetics. New York, Wiley, 1960.
3. HAMPAR, B., AND ELLISON, S. A.: Chromosomal aberrations induced by an animal virus. Nature 192: 145, 1961.
4. KALLMANN, F. J.: Heredity in Health and Mental Disorder. New York, Norton, 1953.
5. KOLB, L. C., MASLAND, R. L., AND COOKE, R. E. (Eds.): Mental Retardation. Baltimore, William & Wilkins, 1920, Vol. 39.
6. PENROSE, L. S.: The Biology of Mental Defect. London, Sidgwick & Jackson, 1954.
7. RUCKNAGEL, D. L., AND NEEL, J. V.: The hemoglobinopathies. In Steinberg, A. G., Ed.: Progress in Medical Genetics. New York, Grune & Stratton, 1961.

21

Etiology of Mental Subnormality in Twins

GORDON ALLEN, M.D., AND FRANZ J. KALLMANN, M.D.

With the Collaboration of
George S. Baroff, Ph.D., and Diane Sank, M.S.

ONLY A SMALL PROPORTION of the mentally subnormal can be confidently classified by etiology. Patients with a clear history of early trauma or infection are probably the largest group, although they present diverse clinical pictures. A little less frequent and more homogeneous is Down's syndrome (mongolism), now known to result from an abnormal chromosome complement. The types of mental defect attributable to known simple genetic factors comprise, in the aggregate, not more than 2 per cent of institutionalized defectives. The preponderance of mental subnormality, not yet explained, may be due to hereditary or environmental factors, and probably often to both.

Among institutionalized mental subnormals the frequency of twins is known to be greater than in the general population. While Pasamanick and Lilienfeld [16] reported that twins constituted 3.2 per cent of a series of 1107 subnormal children, we have found 3.1 per cent for one group of the institutions that cooperated in the present investigation. [4] These figures are to be compared with a twin frequency of about 2.2 per cent at birth and 1.9 per cent among children surviving infancy. [2] The abnormal circumstances of gestation in twins, and particularly the high incidence of prematurity, would explain some excess of mental handicap. In our earlier analysis, however, increased twin rates were not restricted to the diagnostic groups commonly associated with a history of trauma. A general increase among twins may reflect either a sociocultural handicap, for which there is substantial evidence, [9,20] or a greater likelihood of placement in public institutions for twin, as compared with single-born, subnormals. It is thus possible that the observed 50 per cent excess of twins in institutions exaggerates the difference, and that most cases of subnormality in twins, excepting instances of obvious twin-birth sequelae, are comparable to cases in single-born children.

In the hope, therefore, of advancing knowledge of mental subnormality in general, we will present the etiological evidence afforded by the circumstances of twinship in the cases we have studied. There have been several major twin studies in mental deficiency. [7,11,13,19,22] The present report may be justified either because it amplifies the earlier data or because it analyzes the twin data in ways not previously attempted. The principal contribution of past twin studies to medicine has been the demonstration of significant genetic factors in many conditions with a complex etiology. Mental subnormality offers a wider scope for the application of twin studies in two respects. First, mental

174

subnormality is composite, and any population of patients from a state school, for example, will contain many types with many different causes. This compositeness permits the use of internal comparisons, and such relative statistics are often more reliable, possibly more informative, than estimates of absolute parameters in single diagnostic categories.

The second advantage of twin studies in this area is that, by definition and by common observation, the causes of mental subnormality operate early in ontogeny. Twinning is intimately involved with the same early period of life, and affords various means for distinguishing among possible causes. Hence, in addition to demonstrating genetic influences, a twin study of mental subnormality can provide unique evidence that should assist in the differentiation of etiological groups. We have attempted to make maximum use of this potential in the present study.

DEFINITIONS AND CRITERIA

For the most part, we shall follow the terminology proposed by the World Health Organization.[25] *Mental subnormality* will refer to any general insufficiency of mental development; *mental defect,* to conditions in which mental capacities are diminished as a result of assumed physical causes; and *mental retardation,* to states in which educational and social performances are markedly below what would be expected from known intellectual abilities.

Division of subjects into three categories, moron, imbecile and idiot (or mild, moderate and severe), is useful for educational and clinical purposes, but is less meaningful in an etiological analysis. It seems preferable to differentiate only high-grade and low-grade patients. The former can nearly all be accounted for statistically on the basis of normal variation, while most of the low-grade patients exceed the expected frequency and require special etiological explanation. In this report, no sharp dividing line is made between high and low grades of defect, and in the IQ range from 40 to 50, classification is based on developmental history and other considerations. An upper IQ limit of 79 is chosen to coincide as nearly as possible with the limit for patients retained in the state schools (State of New York).

A further subdivision cuts across all intelligence levels according to presence or absence of relevant clinical pathology. This separation, like the preceding, is arbitrary, but it yields groups that differ in apparent frequencies of etiological types. The examples given below will sufficiently define our criteria of "clinical pathology" as applied to the case studies in the Appendix.

Cases were further classified according to five clinical diagnoses:

1. *Cerebral palsy* was used to signify spasticity associated with impaired coordination. In a few cases, the diagnosis was based on chorea, athetosis or general motor retardation when out of proportion to the severity of mental defect.

2. *Convulsive disorder* was considered as substantiated by a history of three or more convulsions in infancy or any convulsion after the age of four.

3. *Microcephaly* was diagnosed whenever the maximum head circumference, measured above the brow ridges, was 2.5 standard deviations or more below the mean for the patient's age and sex. Defined in this way, microcephaly is, of course, etiologically diverse.

4. *Other cranial anomalies* included any major abnormality of the brain case other than microcephaly. "Macrocephaly" was applied to patients whose head circumference exceeded 58 cm. without history of rapid head growth. "Hypertelorism" was defined in terms of the index proposed and standardized by Romanus, [15] values below 300 being regarded as pathological.

5. *Other major anomalies* were defects apparently present from birth and having a plausible relation to mental deficiency. In some instances the diagnosis was applied to minor anomalies if several occurred together (see, for example, case No. 2012).

Minor or secondary defects and disorders were disregarded in the etiological analysis. For example, retrolental fibroplasia was not regarded as etiologically relevant. Although it is often associated with mental defect, [14,23] oxygen damage to the retina in premature babies may be unrelated to brain damage. Prematurity itself is given first importance as an etiological factor in our analysis of birth weights.

The application of the above principles is illustrated in the classification of the following three pairs of twins:

Monozygotic twin sisters (Nos. 1803, 1804), described as the M twins in another report, [1] were regarded as discordant with respect to pathology. Although both were mentally subnormal as a probable result of erythroblastosis, one had a mild case of cerebral palsy and the other had only equivocal neurological signs.

In another identical set (Nos. 863, 864) both twins were severely defective with increased deep reflexes and marked pectus carinatum; one was unable to stand without support. However, there was no neurological asymmetry or muscular atrophy beyond that of disuse, and their mental age was commensurate with or below their motor development. These twins were classified as low-grade, undifferentiated, i.e., not having clinical pathology.

The dizygotic twins, Nos. 1495 and 1496, had moron intelligence and a mild hearing loss and A was born with cleft lip and palate. Though commonly not associated with mental subnormality, this anomaly was regarded as possibly relevant to the observed mental subnormality because of its anatomical proximity to the brain case. The pair was classified as discordant with respect to clinical pathology.

These cases illustrate another convention that was observed in our analysis. The primary criteria for classification were psychological and clinical observations in the individual patient, without reference to possible etiology. With the exception of epilepsy, in which seizure history was accepted as equivalent to clinical observation, information from the medical history or about the twin partner or the family was reserved for later use in the statistical analysis of the primary groups. This procedure would, of course, be inappropriate in clinical practice, in which all available information must be brought to bear on the individual diagnosis.

ASCERTAINMENT OF TWIN CASES

Twins used in this study were reported to the New York State Psychiatric Institute, Department of Medical Genetics, in the years 1937 through 1955. The total series (table 1, Appendix) consisted of 592 sets of twins, triplets and quadruplets. However, since 61 of them were never admitted to any of the state schools for mental defectives, they will not be included in the analysis. Another 11 sets (12 cases) were found upon investigation or upon later testing to have attained intelligence quotients of at least 80 on a standard intelligence test. There are thus 520 sets of twins, triplets and quadruplets, represented by valid index cases, i.e., by patients who were mentally subnormal and who had been admitted to a state school. Table 1 shows the distribution

TABLE 1. FISCAL YEAR OF ADMISSION OF 656 INDEX CASES
AND ESTIMATED TWIN RATES

	Before 1940	1940-1944	1945-1949	1950-1955	1956
Twins reported	149	94	166	234	13
All first admissions		6299	6476	9268	
Twin rate		1.49	2.56	2.52	

of these cases by year of admission for the period 1940-1955, together with first admissions of all patients excepting those subsequently classified as not defective.

Many of the patients admitted before 1945 and nearly all of those admitted before 1940 were reported as resident patients rather than as new admissions. Therefore, twins admitted in those years and discharged before the beginning of the study were generally unknown to us. This fact probably explains the low twin rate of 1.49 per cent in the 1940-1944 period. The early cases included a higher proportion of double-index pairs (see table 2, Appendix), that is, index twins whose partners were also admitted and reported, possibly because such twins stay in residence longer or because they are more readily discovered. A few patients who were originally admitted to a state school were reported to us only on transfer or readmission, and in some of these cases the original diagnosis could only be inferred.

The five- and six-year periods between 1944 and 1956 show similar twin rates. Because these admission years provide sufficient numbers (60 per cent of the twin cases) and because reporting here was apparently constant and maximal, the analysis of diagnostic class frequencies (table 3) will be restricted to this period.

Despite the high and apparently constant twin rate from 1945 to 1955, reporting was not complete. This fact was determined by direct file searches in two of the state schools. In a school reporting one of the highest twin rates, examination of a block of 657 resident case histories revealed 27 twins of whom 24, or about 90 per cent, were already known to us. Many were early admissions, and one of the three new cases had been admitted before 1945. In a school that had reported only 6 twin admissions in the three-year period between 1947 and 1950, search of the corresponding files brought to light a total of 23 twins (21 pairs) among 909 new admissions. Of the 6 cases previously reported, 4 belonged to two pairs; of the 17 new cases found, none belonged to a double-index set, and 3 had lost their twin partners at birth or in infancy.

Upon search of the records, therefore, twins were found to constitute at least 2.5 per cent of *admissions* in one school and 4.0 per cent of the *resident population* in another, with rather wide possible sampling errors in these estimates. Completeness of twin reporting through the regular channels was probably less than 90 per cent but more than 60 per cent between 1945 and 1955. The lower limit of 60 per cent is obtained from the ratio of the overall twin rate for these years to the maximum observed twin rate after search of records.

Pairs in which one or both members were dead at the beginning of our intensive study (July, 1952) were not considered for zygosity diagnosis or clinical evaluation. There were 156 such cases (table 1, Appendix). The proportion of exclusions exhibited no overall trend in the period covered, but more of the earlier cases would probably have been excluded if all deaths of discharged patients had been known. Cases not known to have died, and pairs in which death occurred after commencement of the study, were considered potential study material and thus were included in the defined population from which the sample was drawn.

While the defined twin population comprised 500 cases and 376 sets, only 261 cases and 177 sets were located and adequately studied. Selective factors that appear to have influenced the sample composition have been analyzed in some detail; the most significant effects are summarized in table 2, and more

TABLE 2.   EFFECTS OF SELECTION ON COMPOSITION
OF THE STUDIED SAMPLE

	One Twin Admitted		Both Admitted	
	Same sex	Opposite sex	Same sex	Opposite sex
All cases from live pairs	139	115	207	39
Cases studied	49	46	145	21
Proportion studied	35%	40%	70%	54%
	37%		68%	

detail is given in tables 4-6 (Appendix). It will be noted that 68 per cent of double-index cases and only 37 per cent of single-index cases were studied. Since the latter group contained nearly all discordant pairs, the studied sample will tend to exaggerate the extent of concordance, possibly to a different degree for different diagnostic categories. However, such exaggeration is likely to affect dizygotic concordance rates as much as, or more than, monozygotic concordance rates; more, in categories where the true monozygotic rate is already close to 100 per cent.

The sample ratios for same-sex and opposite-sex pairs are not significantly different in either half of table 2, nor are these differences large enough to account for any of the findings that will be discussed.

The selection effects seen in tables I and 2 warn against quantitative interpretation of concordance rates. However, observational facts and certain internal qualitative comparisons are not invalidated. Concordance rates of both types of twins may be informative when very high or very low. Within the dizygotic class, differences between same-sex and opposite-sex twins provide what appears to be significant evidence. Among monozygotic twins, the discordant pairs yield much information as might be expected.

Basic information was obtained on all index cases from the state school records. Additional data on many of the cases selected for study were gathered by visits to the home or to the hospital of birth. Clinical findings of the institutions were supplemented in all but four of the studied twin sets with a complete physical examination of at least one institutionalized twin by one of the authors or by Dr. Lucille Ross. Of the partners who were not institutionalized, most received screening neurological examinations in the home and some were brought to the Psychiatric Institute as outpatients for special examinations. In order to decide difficult questions of zygosity, reciprocal skin grafts were performed upon two pairs at the Psychiatric Institute[16] and on one pair, case No. 2156, at the patient's institution, Wassaic State School.

Although the state schools routinely test urine of new admissions for phenylpyruvic acid, nearly all patients still in residence were tested again in the course of this study, with negative results. In the five schools equipped for x-ray diagnosis, sufficiently cooperative twin patients were given postero-anterior and lateral skull x-rays that were interpreted at the Psychiatric Institute (Dr. Juan Taveras). Electroencephalograms were obtained on many patients at Letchworth Village (Dr. George Jervis). The following blood studies were carried out in selected cases, with negative results: hemoglobin electrophoresis (Dr. Helen Ranney), dye test for toxoplasmosis (Dr. Harry Feldman), indirect Coombs and other tests for maternal Rh antibodies (Columbia-Presbyterian Blood Bank). In addition, of course, results of many earlier clinical or laboratory examinations were made available to us by state schools and by hospitals in which patients had been examined.

Same-sex pairs were classified as to zygosity mainly on the basis of sequential blood grouping; tests for the minor factors were carried out only when differences failed to appear in the major factors. In three pairs blood could not be obtained; one pair (No. 1958) was hemophilic, and in the other two pairs one partner refused to cooperate beyond letting us take fingerprints. Other observations were used to confirm or to supplement the results of blood grouping. Dermatoglyphics were analyzed by several methods[14,21,23] including, in many pairs, qualitative comparison of palmar main-line formulas. In some sets with similar blood cell antigens, pigmentation differences proved decisive. Three cases were decided with the aid of skin grafts. When partners were similar clinically, a definite diagnosis of monozygosity was not made unless there was a close physical resemblance. The greatest facial dissimilarity in a concordant pair classified as monozygotic occurred in the twin sisters listed as Nos. 878 and 879.

Zygosity of 10 cases (8 pairs) appeared doubtful prior to analysis of clinical data; blood groups and pigmentation were similar, but dermatoglyphics and physical features were conflicting or indeterminate. Four pairs that were clinically discordant (Nos. 794, 1944, 1946, 2347) had similar fingerprints, while another pair (Nos. 1968, 1978), clinically concordant, appeared to be dizygotic on the basis of fingerprints. Acceptance of the dermatoglyphic evidence without regard to other morphological traits therefore proved to be the conservative course with respect to any genetic etiological explanation. In the other three doubtful pairs the fingerprints were indeterminate, and no attempt was made to classify them (Nos. 1974, 2351, 2441-2442).

Nine sets of triplets and one of quadruplets were included with the twin material. In most sets only two members survived infancy, permitting them to be dealt with like twins in the analysis. Two complete sets of triplets contributed one index case each (No. 2301 and No. 2302), the second and third members having much higher and similar IQ's. The first set, with male and female partners at home, was classified with the opposite-sex twins. In the second set, all male, the partners at home were possibly an identical pair, and the set was placed, for the analysis, with same-sex dizygotic twins. Two other sets of triplets contributed six index cases. Triplets Nos. 1765, 1766 and 1767 were excluded from the concordance analysis, because they were trizygotic and of mixed sex; no statistical method seems even approximately correct for incorporation of such a set into twin calculations. The last set (Nos. 1524, 1525 and 1526) consisted of three boys of low grade, two from one zygote and one from a second; in the pair-wise analysis of concordance (table 6) this set was counted once as monozygotic, once as dizygotic.

Intelligence tests, usually Stanford-Binet or Kuhlman-Binet, were made available by the state schools on almost all patients, except for a few severely defective ones. Nevertheless, to provide a consistent system of intrapair comparisons, many patients who had scored in the moron range were retested with either the W.I.S.C. or the W.A.I.S. In the case histories (Appendix) and for psychological classification of pairs, patients were assigned the highest IQ obtained on a standard test, with the following exceptions: When the patient's highest IQ represented an equivalent mental age below 2.5 years, any later test at a higher equivalent mental age was regarded as more informative. In a few pairs, the highest IQ's were identical and concealed differences found consistently on other occasions; in these instances, more representative IQ's are cited in the case histories.

Psychomotor and projective tests were administered only in selected cases. As noted in the histories, a few patients had severe personality disorders or seemed psychotic, but such symptoms were not considered evidence of clinical pathology as defined in this study.

Some noninstitutionalized co-twins had been tested by an outside agency. Where such a test result was not readily available, the subject was given a screening examination, usually the W.I.S.C. vocabulary, followed by a full-scale test when the first result was borderline or doubtful. In some cases the co-twin could not be contacted, but results of group tests were available from schools. When the co-twin's IQ could not be obtained at all, statements from the family or from social workers to the effect that he was normal were accepted.

RELATIVE FREQUENCY OF SUBNORMALITY IN TWINS

The simplest fact to ascertain about mentally subnormal twins, and one of the most useful, is their relative frequency. Twin individuals are expected to constitute about 2 per cent of a normal American White population. The small proportion of Negroes in this series, about 14 per cent, would not alter that expectancy. A higher frequency of twins in a mentally subnormal population implies that twins are in some way more prone to subnormality. This finding would point to etiological factors that are accentuated in twins by circumstances of gestation, birth, or the postnatal environment. It is well known, for example, that birth trauma is frequent in twins because of prematurity and complications of delivery.[8] It is also widely assumed that such trauma may produce both cerebral palsy and mental defect in surviving infants. This assumption would be supported by the finding of a high frequency of twins diagnosed as "cerebral palsy" or "due to birth trauma."

Table 3 shows diagnoses of twins and single-born admissions for the years 1945 through 1955. The diagnostic terms used by the state schools have been abridged for our purposes (see table 2, Appendix), and cases diagnosed as "not defective" are omitted. The first two categories are combined because concordant twins with no subnormal relatives are occasionally diagnosed as "familial" rather than as "undifferentiated," complicating comparison with the single-born.

TABLE 3.   FREQUENCY OF DIAGNOSES IN TWIN
AND SINGLE-BORN PATIENTS
(New York State Schools 1945-1955)

Diagnosis*	Single-Born	Twins	Twin Rate
Familial or undifferentiated	10,147	250	.024
Down's syndrome	1426	27	.019
Birth trauma	882	46	.050
Cranial anomaly	847	25	.029
Cerebral palsy	722	27	.036
Epilepsy	320	8	.024
Other forms	998	16	.016
Total	15,342	399	.025

*Designations are explained in table 2, Appendix.

As expected, the highest twin rates in table 3 are associated with the diagnoses "birth trauma" and "cerebral palsy." However, in absolute numbers, more than half of the excess over 2 per cent occurred in the familial and undifferentiated groups. This finding tends to confirm and amplify the observation of Illingworth and Woods, [10] that the proportion of twins is high among mentally subnormal patients even after exclusion of those with cerebral palsy. Some clues to the possible meaning of this observation emerge from the fully studied sample.

HIGH-GRADE, UNDIFFERENTIATED CASES

Nearly all of the institutions' "familial" cases and a large proportion of their "differentiated" twins fall within our high-grade, undifferentiated group. In this group, 80 per cent of twins were diagnosed as "familial" by the admitting schools. Excluded from the group are nine high-grade, undifferentiated patients with low-grade or clinically abnormal partners, to be discussed in subsequent sections, because they are neither concordant nor discordant as the terms are applied to the other sets.

As shown in table 4, all the monozygotic sets of the high-grade, undiffer-

TABLE 4.   CONCORDANCE AND DISCORDANCE IN HIGH-GRADE,
UNDIFFERENTIATED CASES

		Concordant	Discordant
	Double-index	40	—
Monozygotic	Single-index	1	0
	Total	41	0
Dizygotic,	Double-index	32	—
same sex	Single-index	3	4
	Total	35	4
Dizygotic,	Double-index	10	—
opposite sex	Single-index	8	3
	Total	18	3

entiated variety were concordant, and in all but one pair both partners have been institutionalized. However, dizygotic twins in this group also have a high concordance rate, with 53 of the 60 cases belonging to concordant pairs. While this rate is undoubtedly exaggerated by the sampling inequalities in favor of double-index pairs, a majority even among the single-index cases belong to concordant pairs. To explain such a high concordance figure in dizygotic twins, one must invoke environmental determinants rather than, or in addition to, genetic factors. At least one inference can be drawn regarding the nature of these environmental determinants. In cases with documented physical trauma (see below), monozygotic twins are generally discordant. The fact that none of the monozygotic sets in table 4 is discordant seems to rule out slight physical trauma as an important cause in this type of subnormality.

Another significant finding is the uneven distribution of same-sex and opposite-sex dizygotic twins. While one-half of the dizygotic twins are expected to be of same sex and one-half of opposite sex, more than three-quarters of the double-index pairs shown in table 4 are of the same sex. A higher sampling ratio in opposite-sex pairs — i.e., 70 per cent instead of 54 per cent (see table 2) — would be expected to add only 3 cases to the 10 studied, and there would still be significantly fewer than the 32 same-sex pairs. The deficit of opposite-sex, double-index pairs is therefore a characteristic of the population, not merely of the sample. At the same time, in opposite-sex and same-sex dizygotic twins, the concordance rates are similar. When the number of double-index cases is divided by two in the required manner, [2] the resulting ratios of concordant pairs to total pairs are, in the same-sex and opposite-sex dizygotic twins, respectively,

$$\frac{16 + 3}{16 + 3 + 4} = .83, \text{ and} \qquad \frac{5 + 8}{5 + 8 + 3} = .81$$

Hence, there is no evidence that same-sex dizygotic twins have a higher concordance rate than opposite-sex pairs with respect to high-grade, undifferentiated subnormality.

However, while parents tend to institutionalize only one member of a concordant, opposite-sex pair, they usually send away both members of a same-sex pair. If parents had kept at home the second member of same-six pairs as often as the second member of opposite-sex pairs, our sample would contain 20 fewer cases in the high-grade, undifferentiated group. A similar 26 per cent reduction in all familial and undifferentiated cases in table 3 would lower the twin rate in those groups (combined) to less than the 2 per cent found in the general population. Thus, institutionalization, rather than intellectual handicap, may explain the observed frequency of high-grade twins. This is true only if members of opposite-sex twin pairs have the same likelihood of placement as single-born children.

The tendency to institutionalize both members of same-sex pairs may apply only to male sets. Of the 16 double-index, same-sex, dizygotic pairs, 11 were male, and of the 20 double-index monozygotic pairs, 12 were male. However, the corresponding excess of females among single-index, same-sex pairs is not in evidence: two of the three dizygotic pairs are female, and the one monozygotic pair is male, so that the total is two pairs of each sex.

LOW-GRADE, UNDIFFERENTIATED CASES

It has sometimes been assumed that many or most patients in this group represent rare recessive metabolic diseases. If this assumption were correct, there should be a noticeable proportion of consanguineous marriages among the parents of such cases. Although failure to find an increased rate of cousin marriages in this type of study is not conclusive, it is interesting that only one among 178 "undifferentiated" patients in the entire series of twins was found to have parents related as first cousins. This case, No. 838, lost her partner in infancy and was not in the studied sample. Two other patients with first-cousin parents, also omitted from the detailed study, had institutional diagnoses of Down's syndrome and cerebral palsy (Nos. 866 and 2470, respectively).

Concordance data on the low-grade, undifferentiated cases in our studied sample are presented in table 5. Cases belonging to concordant pairs appear in the left column and those from discordant cases are on the right. In the middle column are 2 cases whose partners are mentally subnormal, but not comparable to the severely affected index cases.

Same-sex dizygotic twins are similar to the monozygotic pairs with respect to concordance, while opposite-sex pairs have a distribution that differs significantly ($P < .01$). Part of this difference can be attributed to unequal sampling ratios (see table 2); among double-index, concordant cases, same-sex pairs were more fully sampled than opposite-sex pairs, while among single-index cases (mainly discordant), the ratio was slightly in favor of opposite-sex sets. However, the sampling difference was small compared with the difference in table 5, and it has no bearing on the similarity of concordance ratios in the monozygotic and same-sex dizygotic series.

Although the difference between opposite-sex and all same-sex twins in table 5 is highly significant, that between opposite-sex and same-sex dizygotic twins is

TABLE 5.   CONCORDANCE IN LOW-GRADE, UNDIFFERENTIATED CASES

| | Co-twin's Intelligence | | |
	IQ under 45	IQ 45-70	Normal
Monozygotic	19	0	2
Dizygotic, same sex	10	2	1
Dizygotic, opposite sex	4	0	7

significant at the .02 probability level only if the two high-grade cases are counted as concordant with their low-grade partners. This equivocal finding would be interesting if it could be confirmed, because it points to some social interaction after birth, such as parental rejection, as a significant cause in certain cases. Only such an influence can readily explain the isolated occurrence of defect in four male and three female members of opposite-sex pairs and in both members of most same-sex pairs. Confirmation might be sought in the case histories (Appendix) and indeed some of the cases do present evidence of severe neglect or of striking psychiatric symptomatology (see, for example, Nos. 819, 1980-1981, 2154-2155). However, similar cases occur in the high-grade series, where concordance rates were similar in same-sex and opposite-sex pairs. Social causation of severe mental defect in some cases may nevertheless be a possibility.

CLINICAL CASES

This group consists of 68 pairs in which one or both partners, not necessarily the index case, had one or more of the five diagnoses already defined: *cerebral palsy, convulsive disorder, microcephaly, other cranial anomalies,* or *other major anomalies.* We have excluded case No. 2250, whose history clearly indicates a traumatic etiology at the age of 4 years, and 17 cases of Down's syndrome reported previously.[3,5]

Table 6 shows the distribution of pairs — not index cases — by zygosity, concordance, and clinical classification. Most of the concordant and some of

TABLE 6.   CONCORDANCE AND DISCORDANCE, BY PAIRS, WITH RESPECT TO
MENTAL SUBNORMALITY COMBINED WITH CLINICAL PATHOLOGY

| | Monozygotic | | Dizygotic | |
	Concordant	Discordant	Concordant	Discordant
Cerebral palsy alone	1	1*	1	7*
Convulsive disorder alone	0	3†	0	7
Microcephaly alone	3	0	0	5
Other cranial anomalies	0	2‡	1	4
Cerebral palsy with other pathology	0	8	0	14
Other major anomalies or combinations	3	3‡	1§	5

*One pair concordant for moron intelligence.
†Two pairs concordant for low-grade mental defect.
‡One pair concordant for low-grade mental defect.
§Both epileptic but with differences in intelligence and in physical defects.

the discordant pairs consist of 2 index cases. The table reveals that clinical pathology rarely affected both members of a dizygotic pair as would be expected if the causes resided in the general environment, either pre- or postnatal. The rather frequent occurrence of discordance in monozygotic twins, especially those with convulsive disorder or with complicated cerebral palsy, points to within-pair environmental differences with respect to important contributing causes. Even here, however, one discordant monozygotic pair with hemophilia (case No. 1958) illustrates the potential importance of genetic susceptibility. The most likely immediate causes that would readily explain discordance in monozygotic twins are birth trauma and developmental accidents, i.e., chance deviations of embryonic differentiation.

Discordance as listed in table 6 refers either to mental subnormality or to the associated clinical pathology. Taking into account all ancillary information that was excluded from the clinical classification, we can further elucidate the etiology of the mental defects concerned. First we shall make use of the clinical findings in the partner of each case, then we shall consider trauma in the medical history. The next section will consider the relationship of prematurity to concordance and diagnosis in the low-grade clinical group.

Four of the monozygotic pairs shown as discordant in table 6 are actually concordant with respect to low-grade mental defect (Nos. 767-768, 812-813, 1988-1989, 2211-2212). If a clinical finding in one of these twins is etiologically related to his mental defect, it would seem to be similarly related to the co-twin's defect. It is reasonable, therefore, to classify these pairs, like the clinically concordant twins, as having a common etiology. Although a specific etiology is not known for any of these four pairs with severe mental defect, one high-grade pair already referred to (Nos. 1803-1804) illustrates how one cause may explain concordance with respect to mental defect in twins who are discordant with respect to neurological manifestations of the etiology. These girls both had erythroblastosis followed by similar mental impairment, but only one, for reasons possibly related to a greater birth weight, developed definite cerebral palsy.

With respect to concordance, index cases in a sample are expected to represent the population distribution more accurately than are pairs. The monozygotic twins listed by cases in the left half of table 7 belong to pairs in which both partners have the given clinical entity or, if only one twin is thus affected, the partners are at least similar as to low-grade mental defect.

Except for twins with clinical cerebral palsy, nearly all the one-egg pairs in table 7 are concordant with respect to mental defect. They seem to have been subjected as pairs to whatever agents caused clinical pathology in one or both partners. The main etiological factor usually affected both partners mentally, although the appearance of clinical signs such as convulsions evidently may be influenced by minor, perhaps accidental differences.

With respect to cerebral palsy, however, the high proportion of cases from discordant monozygotic pairs makes it doubtful that heredity and the general environment could have caused the associated mental defects. Both the clinical pathology and the mental subnormality may be attributable to accidental phenomena of development or birth. Some confirmation of the traumatic etiol-

TABLE 7. COMPARISON OF MONOZYGOTIC TWIN CONCORDANCE AND
HISTORY OF TRAUMA IN THE SAME CLINICAL GROUPS

	Monozygotic Twins		All Twins: History of Trauma	
	Concordant	Discordant	Negative	Positive
Cerebral palsy with or without other pathology	2	10	15	21
Convulsive disorder alone	4	1	7	2
Microcephaly alone	6	0	8	3
Other cranial anomalies, alone	2	1	4	4
Other major anomalies or combinations	8	2	15	0

ogy of mental defect associated with cerebral palsy may be found in the right half of table 7. Here, all clinical cases are tabulated according to the presence or absence of trauma in the individual's history. A history is considered positive, for example, if it mentions prolapse of an umbilical cord, neonatal signs of brain damage together with difficult delivery, or severe infectious diseases in the first year. Many such histories may be etiologically irrelevant, since they were also recorded in eight of the 45 low-grade, undifferentiated cases and are certainly not uncommon in normal children. On the other hand, some negative histories are doubtless in error.

Despite such uncertainties in the individual medical histories, the two right-hand columns of table 7 show a highly significant excess of positive histories in the cerebral palsy group (chi-square 10.1 for one degree of freedom) and of negative histories in the "other . . . . combinations" category (chi-square 9.5 for one degree of freedom). When each extreme group is compared with the three intermediate groups, the differences are less significant, and the first falls below the 0.5 probability level after correction for continuity. It nevertheless appears that, at least in mentally subnormal twins, accidental factors causing cerebral palsy are mostly of the kind likely to be recorded in medical histories.

BIRTH WEIGHTS OF LOW-GRADE AND CLINICAL CASES

Birth weight warrants special analysis as the variable in the medical history that is best suited to quantitative treatment. Moreover, it is often an indicator of abnormal development and, when low, of susceptibility to trauma. Birth weights are known for 83 of 113 twin pairs classified by zygosity and having low-grade or clinical mental defects. Of these birth weights, 32 are based on hospital records and 51 on the parents' statements. Intrapair differences are slightly larger and more frequent in the hospital reports than in the parental accounts, but the two sets of data are in close enough agreement to be combined.

The mean weights, standard errors of the means, and standard deviations are given in tables 8 and 9. The cases of Down's syndrome in discordant, dizygotic pairs have been analyzed separately because in this condition low birth weight is known to be a consequence, not a cause. It is noteworthy that the data in the last line of table 8 provide no evidence of shortened gesta-

TABLE 8. BIRTH WEIGHTS IN DISCORDANT PAIRS (IN POUNDS)

	N	Index Case (Low-grade or Clinical)			Partner (High-grade or normal)		
		Mean	Standard error	Standard deviation	Mean	Standard error	Standard deviation
Monozygotic	12	4.2	.30	1.04	5.1	.28	.97
Dizygotic	40	4.7	.13	.79	5.0	.14	.86
Down's syndrome (DZ)	7	4.4	.61	1.61	5.2	.70	1.73

TABLE 9. BIRTH WEIGHTS IN CONCORDANT PAIRS (IN POUNDS)

	N	Lighter Twin			Heavier Twin		
		Mean	Standard error	Standard deviation	Mean	Standard error	Standard deviation
Monozygotic	15	4.9	.39	1.50	5.3	.39	1.51
Dizygotic	9	4.4	.33	1.00	5.0	.43	1.30

tion time when prematurity is measured by birth weight of the normal partner. Rather, it appears that the average prematurity associated with Down's syndrome [6] is another reflection of developmental retardation. The weights of the normal partners are close to the mean for all twins, 5.25 lbs., as reported by Karn. [12]

The largest average intrapair difference shown in tables 8 and 9 is that for the discordant, monozygotic twins. Furthermore, it is the only difference that is more than twice its standard error. In the monozygotic (MZ) twins, the severely affected partner had an average birth weight handicap of .94 lbs., as against an average handicap of .32 lbs. in the dizygotic (DZ) twins. This comparison is more meaningful when expressed as the relative frequency of large birth weight differences. In seven of the 12 MZ pairs the defective partner weighed less than 90 per cent as much as his co-twin, while such a handicap was found in only 16 of the 40 DZ pairs.

Equally instructive are those few pairs in which the higher-grade or normal partner had the disadvantage in birth weight. There were three such pairs in the MZ group. In one pair (No. 2466) the heavier twin had a traumatic delivery and subsequently developed hydrocephalus; both birth weights were greater than five pounds and probably had no relation to the trauma. In the other two MZ pairs (Nos. 1803-1804 and 2454) the lighter partner also had moron intelligence of presumably traumatic origin, so that they do not really oppose the general trend.

Among the 40 discordant DZ twins, the severely affected partner was heavier in ten instances. In 9 of these 10 pairs (5 out of 6 who had at least a 10 per cent handicap), the lighter twin developed normally, in clear opposition to the general trend.

It may be concluded that among twins discordant for severe mental defect or for clinical types of defect, birth weight is causally implicated in a majority of MZ cases and in a minority of DZ cases. This finding favors the inference that nongenetic causes of low-grade or clinical mental defect, as seen in the discordant, monozygotic pairs, are commonly expressed in low birth weight, either secondary to prenatal growth disturbance or as a factor predisposing to birth injury. In contrast, dizygotic twins may differ in their genetic potentialities and, as a result, defects due to a genetic handicap in one partner contribute enough additional discordant pairs to make birth weight a minor cause. This conclusion is strikingly supported by the five DZ sets in which one twin became defective despite at least a ten per cent birth weight advantage over his normal partner.

Another informative comparison of birth weights is that between concordant and discordant pairs within the monozygotic series. In contrast to the discordant MZ twins, the concordant pairs show inappreciable differences in birth weight, even when all the lighter twins are compared with all the heavier ones (table 9). In only 3 of 15 pairs did one twin weigh less than 90 per cent as much as his partner and, in one of them, both twins had Down's syndrome where birth weight is of no etiological significance. In a second pair, the lighter twin was more severely defective although both were in the low-grade range (No. 2395).

The discordant MZ series provides some estimate, for twins, of the range of birth weights that are likely to cause, or to be related to the cause of, severe mental defect. In the 7 discordant MZ pairs with a significant handicap in the affected partner, the low birth weights ranged from 2.69 to 4.25 pounds with the median at 3.25. If weights in this range be considered etiologically significant, only 6 of 28 birth weights in concordant pairs excluding Down's syndrome were significantly low, and 3 of these 6 were above 4 pounds. It therefore seems that concordant MZ twins are almost entirely different, etiologically, from discordant MZ pairs. Apparently, birth weight and related trauma played a minor role in one group, a major role in the other.

In dizygotic twins there is little or no difference between discordant and concordant pairs with respect to birth weight handicaps. The discordant DZ series (low-grade or clinical) includes some cases attributable to birth weight handicap or trauma and apparently also many cases due to genetic factors. The concordant DZ twins are not distinguished with respect to birth weight and are predominantly undifferentiated; only 3 pairs had clinical pathology out of 11 low-grade or clinical pairs. This combination of findings in concordant DZ twins points to the postnatal environment, including the social environment, as the cause in some cases of low-grade, undifferentiated mental defect.

A final problem that can be elucidated by these data is whether low birth weight is more often a primary factor predisposing to trauma, or whether it is usually a secondary effect of abnormal development. As already noted, the latter alternative is indicated with respect to Down's syndrome. Certain of our twin pairs provide relevant information about other clinical types of defect. Our entire sample of discordant twins, MZ and DZ taken together, includes 10 pairs in which the more severely affected partner had a birth weight handicap, both absolutely and relatively: less than 4 pounds and less than 90 per cent of his partner's weight. One set of triplets, No. 2302, is omitted here because each of them weighed less than four pounds. Of the other 10 patients, only one (No. 2435) failed to show major clinical pathology, and this girl had retrolental fibroplasia as did her normal co-twin to a minimal degree.

In another female MZ pair (No. 1977) with a much greater weight difference, the lighter twin had not only retrolental fibroplasia, but also cerebral palsy, convulsive disorder and microcephaly. The association of microcephaly with cerebral palsy or convulsions or both was seen in three other twins with the history of a birth weight handicap (Nos. 794, 1946 and 2178). One patient had severe cerebral palsy alone (No. 2033) and one had only microcephaly (No. 1529). In three cases (Nos. 1810, 2270, and 2348) there were major anomalies, or multiple minor anomalies, of an embryological or developmental nature.

In the last 3 or 4 cases, the low birth weight may reflect a prenatal growth defect as in Down's syndrome rather than susceptibility to natal or postnatal trauma. In the other 6 or 7 cases of absolute and relative birth weight handicap, it is highly probable that prematurity was an important contributory cause, if not the primary cause, of susceptibility to subsequent trauma.

SUMMARY

A series of 177 sets of twins, triplets and quadruplets, each with one or more members institutionalized for mental subnormality, have been classified by zygosity and studied clinically. Sampling difficulties preclude useful estimates of absolute statistical parameters, but permit many significant internal comparisons.

There is an appreciable excess of twins among institutionalized subnormals, not only in types attributable to special birth handicaps in twins, but also in high-grade, undifferentiated patients. Another finding in high-grade, undifferentiated patients may be sufficient to explain the excess of twins in this category. Parents seem to be inclined to institutionalize same-sex twins and especially boy-twins together when both are subnormal, and to keep one member of opposite-sex pairs at home. Intrapair concordance with respect to subnormality is very high even among opposite-sex pairs in this diagnostic group, while monozygotic pairs are completely concordant.

In twins with low-grade, undifferentiated subnormality, concordance was high in all same-sex pairs and significantly lower in opposite-sex pairs. This finding suggests that, in addition to genetic and traumatic types, this group may include cases in which social factors such as parental rejection are of etiological significance. Near-normal birth weights in all but one concordant, dizygotic pair in this category afford further evidence of postnatal environmental causation in some cases.

Major clinical findings were generally confined to one member of dizygotic pairs, effectively ruling out general environmental influences as common causes of such pathology. As a rule, such discordance was also seen in monozygotic twins, at least with respect to cerebral palsy and convulsive disorder, thus militating against genetic explanations in these entities and suggesting accidental agents. However, when low-grade mental defect was associated with clinical pathology other than cerebral palsy, monozygotic twins were nearly always *concordant* for mental defect, if not for the other clinical findings.

If all of the clinically differentiated twins are taken as one series, only cerebral palsy, with or without other pathology, shows a significant relation to elicited history of *birth trauma*. In cerebral palsy, the association is strong enough to suggest recognizable trauma as the usual etiology. Since the other clinical types of subnormality are nearly always concordant in monozygotic twins and discordant in dizygotic twins, most of them appear to be due to *genetic* factors. The importance of genetic factors in this group is confirmed by birth weight data. A birth weight handicap is commonly found for the defective member of a discordant, monozygotic pair, infrequently for either member of concordant, monozygotic pairs, and in only a minority of discordant, dizygotic pairs.

In dizygotic twins with Down's syndrome (mongolism) in one member, the affected children have an average birth weight handicap that seems to be traceable to retarded growth, because it is not associated with prematurity in the normal partners. A similar relation of birth weight to the primary disorder is found in a few cases of other major developmental abnormalities. In general, however, birth weight handicaps in low-grade or clinical mental defectives appear to stand in a *primary* rather than a secondary relation to the pathogenesis.

REFERENCES

1. ALLEN, G.: Cases of cerebral palsy in a series of mentally defective twins. Am. J. Ment. Deficiency 59: 629, 1955.
2. ———: Comments on the analysis of twin samples. A. Ge. Me. Ge. 4: 143, 1955.
3. ———, AND BAROFF, G. S.: Mongoloid twins and their siblings. Acta Genet. 5: 294, 1955.
4. ———, AND KALLMANN, F. J.: Frequency and types of mental retardation in twins. Am. J. Human Genet. 7: 15, 1955.
5. ———, AND ———: Mongolism in twin sibships. Acta Genet. 7: 385, 1957.
6. BENDA, C. E.: The Child with Mongolism. New York, Grune & Stratton, 1960.
7. BERG, J. J., AND KIRMAN, B. H.: The mentally defective twin. Brit. Med J. 1: 1911, 1960.
8. GUTTMACHER, A. F.: Multiple pregnancy: clinical aspects. Gen. Pract. 13: 97, 1956.
9. HUSÉN, T.: Abilities of twins. Scand. J. Psychol. 1: 125, 1960.
10. ILLINGWORTH, R. S., AND WOODS, G. E.: The incidence of twins in cerebral palsy and mental retardation. Arch. Dis. Childhood 35: 332, 1960.
11. JUDA, A.: Neue psychiatrisch-genealogische Untersuchungen an Hilfsschulzwillingen und ihren Familien. Ztschr. Neurol. 166: 365, 1939 and 168: 448 and 804, 1940.
12. KARN, M. N.: Birthweight and length of gestation of twins, together with maternal age, parity and survival rate. Ann. Eugen. 16: 365, 1952.
13. LOOFT, C.: L'évolution de l'intelligence des jumeaux. Acta paediat. 12: 41, 1931.
14. NIXON, W. L. B.: On the diagnosis of twin-pair ovularity and the use of dermatoglyphic data. In Gedda, L., Ed.: Novant'anni delle Leggi Mendeliane. Rome, Istituto Gregorio Mendel, 1956.
15. PARMELEE, A. H., JR., et al.: The development of ten children with blindness as a result of retrolental fibroplasia. Dis. Child. 98: 198, 1959.
16. PASAMANICK, B., AND LILIENFELD, A. M.: Association of maternal and fetal factors with development of mental deficiency. J.A.M.A. 159: 155, 1955.
17. ROGERS, B. O., AND ALLEN, G.: Intolerance of dizygotic human twins to reciprocal skin homografts. Science 122: 158, 1955.
18. ROMANUS, T.: Interocular-biorbital index. Acta Genet. 4: 117, 1953.
19. ROSANOFF, A. J., HANDY, L. M., AND PLESSET, I. R.: The etiology of mental deficiency with special reference to its occurrence in twins. Psychol. Monogr. 48, No. 216, 1937.
20. SANDON, F.: The relative numbers and abilities of some ten-year-old twins. J. Roy. Stat. Soc. 120: 440, 1957.

21. SLATER, E.: Psychotic and Neurotic Illnesses in Twins. Med. Res. Council Special Report Series No. 278. London, Her Majesty's Stationery Office, 1953.

22. SMITH, J. C.: Das Ursachenverhältnis des Schwachsinns beleuchtet durch Untersuchungen von Zwillingen. Ztschr. Neurol. 125: 678, 1930.

23. WENDT, G. G.: Der individuelle Musterwert der Fingerleisten und seine Vererbung. A. Ge. Me. Ge. 4: 330, 1955.

24. WILLIAMS, C. E.: Retrolental fibroplasia in association with mental defect. Brit. J. Ophth. 42: 549, 1958.

25. World Health Organization Joint Expert Committee: The Mentally Subnormal Child. World Health Organization Technical Report Series No. 75, 1954.

22

Appendix

INDIVIDUAL CASE HISTORIES

THE CASE NUMBER or numbers at the beginning of each case description are those assigned in the departmental register, and do not necessarily indicate the sequence in which cases were detected or reported. When both partners were subnormal and admitted to a state school, two case numbers were given.

The case numbers are followed by the sex, the first referring to the index case or, if both are index cases, to the twin with lower IQ. In same-sex pairs, zygosity follows sex, together with the principal evidence relevant to the zygosity classification. The terms *Wendt, Nixon,* and *Slater* refer to the fingerprint scoring methods used by Wendt, [23] Nixon [14] and Slater and Shields, [21] respectively. Negative Nixon or Slater scores favor a monozygotic diagnosis; positive scores, a dizygotic diagnosis. The remainder of each heading gives race if not White, month and year of birth, state school, month and year of first admission (of each twin if admitted separately), admission diagnosis (see table 2), and highest standard IQ attained. When not specified, and with the exception of dermatoglyphics, information on the two twins is given in the same sequence as sex and IQ.

Each history begins with whatever significant data are available about the family. If subnormality is suspected in parents or siblings, this fact is given. Full siblings, but not half-siblings, are mentioned if known to have survived infancy, and are described as normal if they were reported to be in an appropriate grade at school, regularly employed, or successfully married.

Since birth order of twins was not always recorded, "A" is used in the text of each report to designate the index case or, in double-index sets, the one with lower IQ. Medical history and physical findings apply to the index case or cases unless otherwise specified. Birth order is given for twin A, whether first or second, if it is known. Birth weights, appearing in the original units, were reported by parents or the state school unless followed by "hosp." to indicate hospital records.

Cases of Down's syndrome (mongolism) are not described here. In this group, 17 twin pairs, studied in detail, were included in two previous reports (3, 5), the first of which provided zygosity data on each pair. The numbers of these cases are as follows: 1528, 1550, 1551, 1554, 1963, 1973, 1994, 2059, 2133, 2140, 2144, 2153, 2156, 2179, 2327, 2366, 2369.

414, 415. Female-female, DZ: blood cells A, D+ C+ E— / O, D+ C— E+; b. 2/21, adm. Syracuse 10/35 and 12/36. Familial. IQ's 52, 76.

Mother reportedly subnormal. Illegitimate, raised by maternal grandparents. Birth order, A second; weights 4 lb., 4½ lb. Hyperreflexia in both, A has speech and hearing defect, B has convulsions, defective vision and severe emotional disorder. Concordant high-grade, discordant clinical: convulsive disorder.

420. Male-female; b. 1/26, adm. Syracuse 9/34. Familial. IQ's 63, 92.

Mother's IQ 55. Five sibs. Birth weights 4 lb. 12 oz., 5½ lb. Physically normal. Discordant high-grade.

659. Female-male; b. 12/10, adm. Letchworth 11/24. Familial. IQ's 40, 136.

Father deserted in 1916. One normal sib. Difficult instrumental delivery. Physically normal. B hospitalized as schizophrenic. Discordant high-grade.

741, 742. Male-male, MZ: ridge counts 177/154, Wendt 45/43, Nixon —3.57; b. 4/27, adm. Newark 10/41. Familial. IQ's 42, 49.

Mother and one sister have IQ's of approximately 100, father's IQ 73. Two maternal uncles and a brother institutionalized with moron intelligence, nephew microcephalic. Birth weights, both 4½ lb. Minor neurological signs, hyperopia, thick skulls. Concordant high-grade.

747, 748. Male-male, MZ: ridge counts 134/124, Wendt 43/38, Nixon +1.26, Slater —2.20, stature 167 and 174 cm; b. 10/33, adm. Newark 4/39. Familial. IQ's 51, 53.

Mother's IQ 59, maternal aunt and uncle institutionalized with mental subnormality. One sib. Raised in institutions. Severe myopia. B's head circumference 578 mm., metopic suture, hearing loss. A's head 533 mm. Concordant high-grade.

754, 755. Male-male, DZ: blood types D+ C— E+ / D— C— E—; b. 5/20, adm. Wassaic 1/32. Cranial anomaly. IQ's 24, 26.

Mother died of pernicious anemia about 1927. Both have oxycephaly, malocclusion, marked funnel-chest; A, ptosis of eyelids. Concordant low-grade clinical: other cranial anomaly.

767, 768. Male-male, MZ: ridge counts 216/208, Wendt 58/57, Nixon —2.30; b. 2/34, adm. Wassaic 6/42. Undifferentiated. IQ's 13, 14.

Two normal sibs, older and younger. Birth order, A second. A, convulsive disorder and hyperostosis frontalis, otherwise normal physically. Concordant low-grade, discordant clinical; convulsive disorder.

769, 770. Female-female, MZ: ridge counts 148/142, Wendt 54/47, Nixon —1.49, Slater —1.47; b. 8/01, adm. Rome 7/24. Undifferentiated. IQ's 44, 46.

Mother apparently subnormal. Three sibs. Cataracts and hyperostosis frontalis. Concordant high-grade.

784, 785. Male-male, MZ: ridge counts 231/224, Wendt 63/62, Nixon —3.91; b. 12/28, adm. Wassaic 12/36. Undifferentiated. IQ's both 52 in 1936; 19 to 32 on several retests.

No sibs. Birth order, A second; weights 6 lb, 7 lb. Retardation recognized in infancy. Little speech. Obese. A had hematuria, anemia and hepatosplenomegaly at age 22, the last persisting. Concordant low-grade.

791. Male-female; b. 4/19, adm. Wassaic 10/37. Familial. IQ's 19, 93.

One sib, IQ 22. Birth order, A second. A resuscitated with difficulty. Possibly normal prior to mastoid operations and repeated surgery about age 7. Physically normal. Discordant low-grade. History of trauma.

794. Male-male, MZ (?): dermatoglyphics adjusted for 18 fingers: ridge counts 158/144, Wendt 39/38, Nixon —3.32, Slater —1.45, eye colors slightly different; incomparable physically; b. 7/38, adm. Wassaic 11/42. Cranial anomaly. IQ's 39, 92.

Four normal sibs. Birth order, A second; weights 3 lb. 3 oz, 5 lb. A had convulsions from age 4. Head circumference 508 mm., dorsal scoliosis, contractures of left hand, retinal pigmentary changes. Discordant low-grade clinical: microcephaly and convulsive disorder.

796. Male-female; b. 1/34, adm. Wassaic 6/42. Cerebral palsy. IQ's 5, 99.

Parents first cousins. One normal sib. Birth weights 6 lb., 6½ lb. Congenital cataracts; convulsions started neonatally. Spastic with some symmetrical involuntary movements. Wrists in ulnar deviation. Head circumference 504 mm. Discordant low-grade clinical: cerebral palsy, convulsive disorder, microcephaly, other major anomalies.

810, 811. Male-male, MZ: ridge counts 166/142, Wendt 43/40, Nixon —3.90; b. 1/18, adm. Syracuse 6/28. Familial. IQ's 59, 60.

Father alcoholic, abusive. Two sibs normal and one with IQ 33. Birth order, A first; weights 4½ lb., 5 lb. Internal strabismus. A, slight intention tremor, herniorrhaphy. Concordant high-grade.

812, 813. Male-male, MZ: ridge counts 205/190, Wendt 47/40, Nixon —1.95; b. 8/22, adm. Wassaic 9/37. IQ's 14, 30.

One sib subnormal, now dead, one has IQ 97. Birth order, A first, breech, at home. B born in hospital with assistance. High-arched palates, atrophic pectoral muscles. A, increased reflexes, scoliosis, right sternomastoid muscular contracture and marked cranial asymmetry, occasional seizures. Concordant low-grade, discordant clinical: convulsive disorder and other major anomalies.

819. Male-female; b. 2/26, adm. Wassaic 4/37. Familial. IQ 33, B unknown.

One sib, IQ 21. Birth order, A second. Physically normal; talkative with possible psychosis. B nearly finished high school; hospitalized once at age 20 with diagnosis of schizophrenia. Discordant low-grade.

824, 825. Male-male, MZ: ridge counts 172/164, Wendt 59/55, Nixon —3.42; b. 2/19, adm. Syracuse 3/28. Undifferentiated. IQ's 31, 33.

Father alcoholic. Two normal sibs. Birth weights 5 lb., 4½ lb. Strabismus, slight intention tremor. B, bilateral varicocele. Concordant low-grade.

835. Female-male; b. 11/31, adm. Letchworth 11/43. Familial. IQ's 56, 70.

Parents reportedly subnormal. One full sib. A removed as neglected at age 12. Birth order, A first, breech. Physically normal. Concordant high-grade.

836, 837. Female-female, MZ: ridge counts 140/138, Wendt 43/40, Nixon —1.31; b. 12/15, adm. Letchworth 6/25. Cerebral palsy. IQ's 58, 60.

Previously reported as the "B" twins (2). Three normal sibs. Child of B by brother essentially normal. Birth order, B first; both less than 2 lbs., at home. Spastic paraparesis. Concordant high-grade clinical: cerebral palsy.

855. Male-female; b. 3/30, adm. Letchworth 9/38. Familial. IQ's 62, 55.

Mother reportedly subnormal, father jailed and deported. One sib, IQ 79. Birth order, A first. Placed in institution at 6 months, B for 2 months and A longer. Hyperopia and restricted digital movements. Concordant high-grade.

856. Female-female, DZ: blood cells AB, D+ C+ E— c— / B, D+ C+ E— c+; b. 5/35, adm. Letchworth 4/39. Infection. IQ's 21, 105.

One normal sib. Birth order, A second, more than an hour after B; weights 6 lb., 6 lb. 6 oz. Positive Wassermann not confirmed. Excitable, self-destructive; skull very thick and sinuses large. Discordant low-grade clinical: other cranial anomaly. History of trauma.

863, 864. Male-male, MZ: ridge counts 152/146, Wendt 60/57, Nixon —3.39; b. 12/37, adm. Letchworth 7/40. Undifferentiated. IQ's 4,5.

Two normal sibs. Birth order, A second; weights 2380, 2680 gm (hosp.). Signs in A of fetal distress before delivery, but both cried spontaneously. Increased reflexes, disuse atrophy of muscles and pectus carinatum, all more marked in A. Concordant low-grade.

869, 870. Male-female; b. 4/27, adm. Letchworth 2/34. IQ's 58, 58.

Three of seven surviving sibs institutionalized as subnormal, one of the three with tremor and slight ataxia. Birth order, A first; weights 6 lb. 6 oz., 6 lb. Heavily freckled, A hyperopic, B has had seizures since age 18. Concordant high-grade, discordant clinical: convulsive disorder.

871, 872. Male-male, DZ: blood groups B/A; b. 3/27, adm. Letchworth 9/35. IQ's 45, 47.

Parents reportedly inadequate. Younger sib, IQ 94. Maternal age 37 at first delivery. Birth order, A first, both breech; weights 4 lb., 5 lb. A schizophrenic from age 17. B fine horizontal nystagmus. Concordant high-grade.

873, 874. Male-male, DZ: blood not typed; ridge counts 199/122, Wendt 62/41, Nixon +9.13; b. 6/33, adm. Letchworth 5/42. Familial. IQ's 71, 77.

Mother hostile, punitive. One of three sibs institutionalized, IQ 62. Birth order, A second; weights 6 lb. 14 oz., 6 lb. (hosp.); B by axis traction and A by breech extraction. Both have rachitic deformities of chest. A, color blind, left strabismus and amblyopia. B not examined. Concordant high-grade.

876, 877. Male-male, MZ: ridge counts 134/123, Wendt 56/52, Nixon —3.07; b. 5/28, adm. Letchworth 8/33. Other forms. IQ's 12, 15.

Parents attended college. One sib. Birth order, A first; weights both 5 lb. Autistic from infancy. Physically normal. Concordant low-grade.

878, 879. Female-female, MZ: ridge counts 158/146, Wendt 52/49, Nixon —3.07; b. 1/26, adm. Letchworth 5/36. Familial. IQ's 32, 33.

Father reportedly had chorea; mother's IQ 73. One of four sibs reportedly subnormal, another had IQ 88 with chorea and rigidity. Birth order, A first; weights both 6 lb. Slight chorea and tremor. A thin, breasts almost juvenile, but estrogenic function judged normal from cervical mucus; metopic suture. Both show fleeting mood swings from hilarity to depression. Concordant low-grade.

881, 882. Female-female, MZ: ridge counts 180/155, Wendt 41/40, Nixon —1.48; b. 6/32, adm. Letchworth 7/37. Undifferentiated. IQ's 19, 19.

Mother sexually promiscuous, possibly psychotic. One sib. Birth order, A first; weights 2600, 2875 Gm. (hosp.). Menarche at age 19, very large breasts. Concordant low-grade.

898. Female-male; b. 2/09, adm. Rome 6/33. Undifferentiated. IQ's 10, 140.

Six sibs mentally normal but one physically "crippled." Meningitis at age 17 months. Increased reflexes, rudimentary speech. Discordant low-grade. History of trauma.

911, 912. Female-female, DZ: blood cells M, D+ C+ E— c+ / N, D+ C+ E+ c+; b. 1/22, adm. Rome 5/35. Familial. IQ's 58, 61.

Parents reportedly subnormal. Two of five sibs institutionalized as subnormal. Physically normal, except for hyperostosis frontalis in B. Concordant high-grade.

948. Female-female, DZ: blood cells MN / M; Nixon +0.98; b. 9/38, adm. Rome 1949. Other forms. IQ's 74, 108.

Huntington's chorea in father and paternal relatives. No sibs. Birth order, A first; weights 3 lb. 14 oz., 4 lb. 2 oz. Pertussis at 7 months, complicated in A by pneumonia and three seizures. A failed second grade, developed motor disturbances between ages 10-13, convulsions at 15, died at 18. B developed chorea while in college. A, at 15, showed spasticity (patellar and ankle clonus), marked intention tremor. Discordant high-grade clinical: cerebral palsy, other major anomalies. History of trauma.

949, 950. Male-female; b. 3/25, adm. Rome 4/40. Familial. IQ's 29, 71.

Mother's IQ 48. Three of four sibs also institutionalized as subnormal. Removed from home as neglected at 11 months. A had a seizure at 18 months. A has depigmentation of rt. iris with (?) cataract; good coordination. Concordant subnormal, discordant low-grade clinical: other major anomaly.

1025, 1802. Male-male, DZ: blood types D+ C— E+ / D+ C+ E—; b. 10/40, A adm. Rome 12/45, B adm. Syracuse 5/51. Familial. IQ's 61, 72.

Father reportedly subnormal. Twin sisters institutionalized as subnormal (see 1349). Three other sibs. Removed from home as neglected at 2 months. Physically normal. Concordant high-grade.

1057, 1058. Male-male, MZ: ridge counts 174/166, Wendt 55/52, Nixon —4.09; b. 10/32, adm. Rome 3/46. Undifferentiated. IQ's 37, 38.

Parents' IQ's 102 and 107. Two sibs, one with IQ 92. Protracted digestive disturbance around 8 months, pertussis at 1 year; B had meningitis at 3. B, strabismus. Concordant low-grade.

1195. Male-male, DZ: blood types D+ C+ E+ / D+ C— E+; Nixon +7.19; b. 1/39, A adm. Rome 10/46, familial; B adm. Syracuse 10/46, familial, but not an index case. IQ's 64, 80.

Mother reported subnormal. Of nine sibs, three are institutionalized as subnormal, one as epileptic, and the status of five is unknown. B spent two 6-month periods in institutions starting at 3 mo. and 3 yrs. Physically normal. Discordant high-grade.

1197. Female-male; b. 7/46, adm. Willowbrook 8/49. Birth trauma. IQ's 20, 111.

Three sibs. Birth order, A second; weights 2800, 2950 Gm. (hosp.), both by breech extraction. A had bilateral acute otitis media at 4½ months, seizures starting at 5 months. Physically normal. Discordant low-grade clinical: convulsive disorder. History of trauma.

1234, 1235. Male-male, DZ: blood groups B / A; b. 5/39, adm. Rome 3/47. Familial. IQ's 65, 69.

Ten sibs. A, healed rickets, head circumference 582 mm. (B, 545 mm), large frontal sinuses and metopic suture. B has ptosis of left eyelid. Evidence of emotional problems, especially in A. Concordant high-grade.

1336. Female-female, DZ: ridge counts 143/95, Wendt 61/44, Nixon +4.85; b. 12/39, adm. Syracuse 6/47. Familial. IQ's 71, 82 at age 7, later 52, 62.

Mother's IQ 58. Two of four sibs institutionalized subnormal. In orphanage from 1940 to 1947. Discordant high-grade.

1343, 1344. Male-male, MZ: ridge counts 194/160, Wendt 55/52, Nixon —.73, Slater —.80, stature 152/152 cm; b. 10/38, adm. Syracuse 7/46. Familial. IQ's 65, 68 at age 7, later under 50.

Mother reported subnormal or psychotic. No full sibs. Physically normal. "Organic" signs on Bender Gestalt test, B shows severe personality disorder. Concordant high-grade.

1349, 1350. Female-female, MZ: ridge counts 74/72, Wendt 40/38, Nixon —3.65; b. 1/38, adm. Syracuse 5/47. Familial. IQ's 54, 64.

Twin brothers institutionalized subnormal (see 1025). Removed at age 2½ as neglected, B has brachyphalangy of left hand. Concordant high-grade.

1379. Male-male, MZ: ridge counts 139/138, Wendt 57/53, Nixon —.78; b. 6/42, adm. Rome 1/47. Cerebral palsy. IQ's 11, 86.

Mother reported subnormal. Seven sibs. A appeared paralyzed at birth. Occasional convulsions from age 3 months. Severe generalized spasticity and atrophy, head circumference 501 mm. B has been institutionalized repeatedly for behavior disorder. Discordant low-grade clinical: cerebral palsy, microcephaly, convulsive disorder.

1410, 1719. Male-male, MZ: ridge counts 183/177, Wendt 51/49, Nixon —3.28; Negro; b. 8/37, adm. Syracuse 2/48 and 7/50. Undifferentiated. IQ's 69, 73.

Parents separated 1945. Four full or half-sibs reported normal. At age 19, testicles were of subnormal size. Behavior disorders; stealing and aggressiveness. Concordant high-grade.

1453, 1454. Female-female, MZ: ridge counts 65/57, Wendt 38/37, Nixon —3.03; b. 10/28, adm. Syracuse 7/48. Familial. IQ's 64, 71.

Mother's IQ 69, father deserted family. One of three sibs blind, institutionalized subnormal. Twins born with cleft palates, repaired between ages 4 and 6. Hearing impairment. Concordant high-grade clinical: other major anomalies.

1471. Female-male; b. 1/40, adm. Syracuse 6/48. Familial. IQ's 67, 85.

Mother's IQ 84, institutionalized in 1949 as psychotic, later as subnormal. No full sibs. Birth weights 4 lb. 9 oz., 5 lb. 7 oz. Raised in institutions and foster homes. Physically normal. B labeled constitutional psychopath. Discordant high-grade.

1495, 1496. Male-male, DZ: blood cells B, Fy (a+) / 0, Fy (a—); b. 9/38, adm. Syracuse 12/48. Familial. IQ's 73, 79.

Mother alcoholic. Father died 1957. Birth weights, both 5 lb. B had cleft palate and lip; repaired. Foster homes from age 6. Both have some hearing loss. Concordant high-grade, discordant clinical: other major anomaly.

1512, 1513. Female-female, MZ: ridge counts 180/179, Wendt 66/65, Nixon —5.07; Negro; b. 11/34, adm. Letchworth 9/54. Familial. IQ's 56, 59.

Two sibs institutionalized with IQ's 46 and 56; six other sibs. Birth order, A second; weights 5 lb., 5½ lb. Hospitalized at age 15 as psychotic, not confirmed. A, slight bilateral ptosis. Concordant high-grade.

1521, 1522. Male-male, DZ: blood cells M / MN, Nixon +3.32; Negro; b. 1/37, adm. Letchworth 8/40. Undifferentiated. IQ's 20, 42.

Mother intermittently hospitalized as schizophrenic. One sib retarded (Case 1523), three normal. Birth order, A second; weights 5 lb., 5 lb. 2 oz; A by version and extraction. Physically normal. IQ of A has fallen, that of B has risen slightly with age. Concordant subnormal, discordant low-grade.

1523. Male-male, DZ: blood types D— C— E— / D+ C+ E—; Negro; b. 6/45, adm. Willowbrook 8/48. Familial. IQ's 19, 108.

Brothers of cases 1521-1522. Birth order, A first; weights 6 lbs. 14 oz., 6 lb. 13 oz. (hosp.); B by breech extraction. Several convulsions since admission; vitreous (?) opacities. Discordant low-grade clinical: convulsive disorder.

1524, 1525, 1526. Male-male-male, two-egg triplets; ridge counts 206/205/140, Wendt 67/67/44, Nixon —4.71 (AB), +10.05 (AC), +9.59 (BC); Negro; b. 2/45, adm. Willowbrook 11/48. Familial. IQ's 24, 24, 32.

Six sibs. Birth order, A first, B second; weights 5 lb. 5 oz., 4 lb. 5 oz., 4 lb.

9 oz. (hosp.). A and B vertex presentations, C, footling breech. All had pertussis at six weeks. High palates; A and B, inguinal hernias; B, right cataract. Concordant low-grade. History of trauma.

1529. Male-male, DZ: blood groups A / O, Nixon +9.88; b. 2/46, adm. Willowbrook 11/48. Undifferentiated. IQ's less than 25, B undetermined.

No sibs. Birth order, A second; weights 2 lb. 10 oz., 3 lb. 6 oz. (hosp.). Both required artificial respiration at birth, A particularly. A's neonatal course complicated by otitis. A's head circumference 454 mm. at age 9; short distal phalanges, external strabismus. B physically and scholastically normal. Discordant low-grade clinical: microcephaly. History of trauma.

1531. Male-male, DZ: blood types D+ C+ E— / D+ C— E—, Nixon —1.52, Slater +0.25; b. 8/44, adm. Willowbrook 2/49. Infection. IQ's 13, 92.

Two normal sibs. Birth order, A second; weights 5 lb. 13 oz., 7 lb. 6 oz.; A, breech extraction. A had encephalitis at 10 months and two convulsions at age 4. Right spastic hemiparesis, head circumference 497 mm. at age 11. Discordant low-grade, clinical: cerebral palsy, microcephaly, convulsive disorder. History of trauma.

1575. Female-male; b. 5/46, adm. Willowbrook 6/49. Undifferentiated. IQ's 21, 101.

One normal sib. Birth order, A first; weights 3 lb. 4 oz., 3 lb. B (normal) hospitalized with meningitis at 4 months; bronchopneumonia at 11 months. Discordant low-grade.

1599. Male-female; b. 5/44, adm. Willowbrook 8/49. Cranial anomaly. IQ's 22, 121.

Mother hemorrhaged at 6 months. Six normal sibs. Birth weights, both 3 lb., kept in incubator 3 months (A), 40 days (B). Head circumference 50 cm.; external strabismus. Discordant low-grade clinical: microcephaly. History of trauma.

1619, 1620. Female-male; b. 12/38, adm. Rome 11/44. Familial. IQ's 62, 66.

Mother institutionalized as subnormal. No sibs. Raised in foster homes until admission. A, undernourished in first year, had rickets and recurrent otitis. A has myopia, high palate and stenosed auditory meatuses. Concordant high-grade.

1699. Male-male, DZ: blood types D+ C+ E+ c+ / D+ C+ E— c—; b. 5/46, adm. Willowbrook 3/50. Birth trauma. IQ's 49, 81.

One normal sib. Birth order, A first; weights 3 lb, 2 lb 14 oz (hosp.). A's head was severely molded; mother thought he was jaundiced later. A's left eye enucleated at 7 months; benign tumor. Numerous pigmented nevi, personality disorder. Discordant high-grade.

1716. Male-female; b. 2/40, adm. Letchworth 4/45. Birth trauma, B institutionalized as epileptic at age 10. IQ's 12, 59.

Mother reported two falls during pregnancy. Birth order, A second; weights 5 lb. 4½ lb. (hosp.). Both footling presentations, easily extracted. A began to have seizures at 4 months and at 8 months bilateral optic atrophy was diagnosed. B has had seizures since age 8 and is emotionally disturbed. A has hyperreflexia, left Babinski, defective vision and a heart murmur. Concordant subnormal clinical: convulsive disorder; discordant low-grade clinical: other major anomalies.

1721. Female-female, MZ: ridge counts 121/121, Wendt 45/43, Nixon -3.68; b. 1/08, adm. Wassaic 7/50. Cerebral palsy. IQ's less than 10, B undetermined.

Six normal sibs. A had convulsions from about 9 months and left hemiplegia following convulsion at age 6. Confined to bed since 1943. Spastic quadriplegia with contractures. Discordant low-grade clinical: cerebral palsy, convulsive disorder.

1732, 1733. Female-female, MZ: ridge counts 72/58, Wendt 42/39, Nixon -2.06; b. 2/47, adm. Willowbrook 8/52. Familial. IQ's 66, 67.

Mother sexually promiscuous. Two normal full or half-sibs. Birth order, A first; weights 5 lb. 7 oz., 5 lb. 6 oz. (hosp.); single amnion. Early growth retardation was later nearly compensated. Concordant high-grade.

1740, 1741. Male-male, DZ: blood groups B / O; Nixon +12.61; b. 1/49, adm. Willowbrook 8/50. Other forms. IQ's 21, 34.

Three normal sibs, one prior stillbirth. Rh antibodies detected during gestation, replacement transfusion given at birth. Birth order, A second; weights 5 lb. 7 oz., 5 lb.

14 oz. Pertussis and pneumonia in infancy. A had cerebral hemorrhage at 7 months. Both have severe choreoathetosis; A, healed skull fracture. Concordant low-grade clinical: cerebral palsy. History of trauma.

1742, 1743. Female-female, MZ: ridge counts 127/118, Wendt 53/47, Nixon —.51; Negro; b. 10/46, adm. Willowbrook 8/50. Familial. IQ's 30, 31.

Mother and only sib reportedly subnormal. Father deserted at twins' birth. Birth order, A second; 5 lb., B unknown; A breech, B vertex. Found severely neglected at 3½. At age 8 active but scarcely able to walk; postural occipital flattening. Electroencephalogram of A showed focal discharge; not recorded for B. Concordant low-grade.

1744. Female-male; b. 6/47, adm. Willowbrook 9/50. Birth trauma. IQ's 18, 115.

No sibs. Labor induced 48 hours after rupture of membranes because of fetal heart signs. Birth order, A first; weight 4 lb. 10 oz., 5 lb. 2 oz. Convulsions from age 3 months. Head circumference at age 7, 474 mm., generalized spasticity. Discordant low-grade clinical: cerebral palsy, convulsive disorder, microcephaly. History of trauma.

1745. Female-male; b. 1/48, adm. Willowbrook 8/50. Undifferentiated. IQ's less than 20, 114.

Birth order, A second; weights 4 lb. 4 oz., 5 lb. 13 oz.; A, breech presentation delivered by high forceps. Respiratory obstruction at 5 weeks requiring tracheotomy. Head circumference 457 mm. at age 7, unable to stand. Discordant low-grade clinical; microcephaly. History of trauma.

1763. Female-male; b. 1/40, adm. Willowbrook 11/50. Undifferentiated. IQ's 26, 80.

Birth order, A first; weight 5 lb. 7 oz., B unknown; mid-forceps deliveries. B had convulsions neonatally. A had at least one convulsion after admission. Discordant low-grade clinical: convulsive disorder.

1764. Female-male; b. 7/44, adm. Willowbrook 11/50. Undifferentiated. IQ's 24, 100.

Two normal sibs. Twins both breech presentations, A first; weight 6 lb., less than 5 lb. Seizures from age 6 months. Facial asymmetry, high palate, funnel chest, neurologically normal. Discordant low-grade clinical: convulsive disorder.

1765, 1766, 1767. Female-male-male, trizygotic: males, blood types D+ C— E+ c+ / D+ C+ E+ c—; b 7/41, adm. Willowbrook 12/50. Familial. IQ's 55, 65, 67.

Family disorganized, nine sibs or half-sibs. Birth order, A first, B third; weights 5 lb. 1 oz., 3 lb. 14 oz., 4 lb. 13 oz. (hosp.); breech extractions. Hospitalized at 2 months with anemia. A, extremely myopic, B has ptosis and internal strabismus. A and B show personality disorders. Concordant high-grade.

1803, 1804. Female-female, MZ: ridge counts 45/40, Wendt 34/31, Nixon —4.04; b. 9/36, adm. Wassaic 12/50. Familial. IQ's 54, 63.

Previously reported as the "M" twins (2). Three normal sibs. Birth order, A first; weights 5 lb. 10 oz., 4 lb. 3 oz. Erythroblastosis fetalis, more prolonged in A. Pertussis at 11 weeks. A, impaired coordination and slight choreoathetosis, B, slightly impaired coordination. Concordant high-grade, discordant clinical: cerebral palsy. History of trauma.

1805, 1806. Female-male, Negro; b. 6/39, adm. Wassaic 4/51. Familial. IQ's 65, 75.

Father alcoholic. Four sibs, one hospitalized as schizophrenic. Physically normal. Concordant high-grade.

1807, 1808. Male-male, DZ: ridge counts 128/107, Wendt 49/37, Nixon +2.92, different eye color; b. 6/36, adm. Syracuse 8/50. Undifferentiated. IQ's 62, 76.

Mother sickly, died of tuberculosis 1945. Slightly impaired coordination; A has impaired stereognosis and B, a right Babinski sign. Concordant high-grade.

1810. Male-male, MZ: ridge counts 135/127, Wendt 51/50, Nixon —2.64; Negro; b. 11/45, adm. Willowbrook 5/51. Undifferentiated. IQ's 27, 74.

One sib. Birth order, A first; weights 3 lb. 12 oz., 5 lb. 4 oz. A cried feebly at birth and was intermittently cyanotic. Bilateral congenital macular degeneration diagnosed at age 1½. B has a small blue sector in the right iris. Discordant low-grade clinical: other major anomalies.

1812, 1826. Female-female, DZ: blood cells O, D+ C+ E— c— / A, D+ C+ E— c+; b. 10/37, adm. Newark 3/53, Syracuse 6/51. Familial. IQ's 48, 64.

Mother's IQ 72, both parents negligent. Six of seven sibs had IQ below 74. A weighed 5½ lb. at birth. Physically normal; emotionally disturbed. Concordant high-grade.

1853. 1854. Male-male, DZ: ridge counts 93/17, Wendt 48/25, Nixon +10.08; b. 3/40, adm. Wassaic 5/45. Familial. IQ's 62, 76.

Both parents previously institutionalized as subnormal. Two normal sibs. Gestation complicated by maternal toxemia. Birth order, A first; weights 5 lb. 2 oz., 4½ lb. Raised in orphanage from 6 months to 2 years. Head circumferences 542, 587 mm. B also has frontal bosses, wide interocular distance (39 mm.). A shows a personality disturbance. Concordant high-grade, discordant clinical: other cranial anomaly.

1855, 1856. Male-male, DZ: blood cells M+ N+ S+ / M+ N+ S—, Nixon +3.699; Negro; b. 12/39, adm. Wassaic 1/51. Familial. IQ's 75, 79.

Rejected by mother and stepfather. No full sibs. Birth order, A second; weights both between 4 and 5 lb. A has slightly abnormal EEG pattern, head circumference 505 mm. (B's head, 520 mm.). Concordant high-grade.

1858. Female-female, DZ: blood cells M+ N—, Fy(a—) / M+ N+ Fy (a+); b. 7/44, adm. Willowbrook 10/51. Birth trauma. IQ's less than 20, 103.

No sibs. Birth order, A first; weights both 4 lb. 13 oz. (hosp.). Hyperreflexia, infantile gait. Discordant low-grade.

1859. Female-male, Negro; b. 2/50, adm. Willowbrook 9/51. Cerebral palsy. IQ's less than 20, 86.

Delivery by Cesarean because of maternal toxemia. Birth order, A first; weights 4 lb. 11 oz., 5 lb. (hosp.). Severe febrile seizure with pneumonia at 2 months. At age 5, opisthotonic, head circumference 443 mm. Discordant low-grade clinical: cerebral palsy, microcephaly. History of trauma.

1877, 1878. Female-female, DZ: blood types D+ C+ E— c— / D+ C+ E— c+, Nixon —.91, ridge counts 153/111; b. 5/45, adm. Syracuse 7/51. Familial. IQ's 62, 64.

Father killed mother and self 1947. Five full sibs, one institutionalized defective, another reported defective. B has impaired vision (20/50). Concordant high-grade.

1944. Male-male, MZ (?): ridge counts 200/163, Wendt 50/46, Nixon —.73, Slater —1.13, ears dissimilar, one has an anterior hair whorl; b. 9/43, adm. Letchworth 12/47. Undifferentiated. IQ's 31, 81.

Illegitimate, raised in orphanage and foster homes. Birth weights 3 lb. 9 oz. (A or B), 3 lb. 5 oz. (hosp.). Both had umbilical hernias at birth, undescended testicles at age 10. Discordant low-grade.

1946. Male-male, MZ (?): ridge counts 126/115, Wendt 43/42, Nixon —5.10, Slater —2.56 (several siblings have similar fingerprints); Negro; b. 12/40, adm. Letchworth 8/52. Epilepsy. IQ's 11, 65.

Three sibs, several half-sibs. Birth order, A second; weights 3 lb. 12 oz., 6 lb. 7 oz. A had convulsions from second day of life and at age 12 was dwarfed and microcephalic (head circumference 474 mm.). B physically normal. Concordant subnormal, discordant low-grade clinical: cerebral palsy, convulsive disorder, microcephaly.

1949, 1950. Male-male, MZ: ridge counts 198/196, Wendt 68/66, Nixon —4.20; b. 3/40, adm. Letchworth 8/47. Familial. IQ's 54, 55.

Mother's IQ 60, father's 86. Father alcoholic. Four or more sibs. Raised mainly in foster homes. Color blind. Personality disorder. Concordant high-grade.

1953, 1954. Male-male, MZ: ridge counts 195/194, Wendt 45/43, Nixon —3.92; b. 6/45, adm. Letchworth 7/50. Down's syndrome (?). IQ's 16, 18.

Mother chronically hypothyroid, 42 at delivery. One normal sib 2 years older than twins. Birth weights 6 lb. 3 oz., 5 lb. 12 oz. Subnormality confirmed at 15 months but type could not be determined at Babies Hospital, New York. Head shape, mineralized nasal bones and dermatoglyphics inconsistent with Down's syndrome. Head circumferences 475 and 472 mm. at age 8. Concordant low-grade clinical: microcephaly.

1957. Male-male, DZ: blood types D+ C+ E+ / D+ C+ E—, Nixon —1.17, Wendt 50/44, Slater —0.35; b. 8/46, adm. Letchworth 2/48. Cerebral palsy. IQ's 11, 93.

Three normal sibs. Birth order, A first; weight 5 lb. 3 oz., 5 lb. 14 oz. (hosp.).
Spontaneous vertex delivery of A, but respiration was not established for 38 minutes.
B had hemorrhagic disease neonatally. Opisthotonic, head circumference 430 mm. at
age 6. Discordant low-grade clinical: cerebral palsy, microcephaly. History of trauma.

1958. Male-male, MZ: blood not typed; ridge counts 203/182, Wendt 57/55, Nixon
—2.57; b. 10/46, adm. Letchworth 11/48. Other forms. IQ's less than 20, 94.

Previously reported as the "R" twins (2). Both hemophilic (PTC deficiency). Birth
order, A second; weights 5 lb. 5½ lb. A had neonatal intracranial hemorrhage. Spastic,
head circumference 486 mm. at age 6 (B, 518 mm.). Discordant low-grade clinical:
cerebral palsy, microcephaly. History of trauma.

1959. Female-female, DZ: blood types D+ C+ E— c— / D+ C+ E— c+, Nixon
+2.71; b. 1/40, adm. Letchworth 1/48. Birth trauma. IQ's 55, 71.

Parents separated, twins raised in foster home first year. One sib. Birth order, A
first; weights 2 lb. 13 oz., 3 lb. 1 oz. (hosp.). A reportedly blue at birth; had bronchopneumonia at 1 year. A has left spastic hemiplegia; B, myopia and a web over the inner
canthus of each eye. Concordant high-grade, discordant clinical: cerebral palsy.

1960. Male-female; b. 12/44, adm. Letchworth 6/52. Familial. IQ's 23, 89.

Three sibs. Birth order, A second; weights 3 lb. 14 oz., 4 lb. 15 oz. (hosp.). B had
several acute illnesses including pertussis at 3 months. At age 10, A had severe spastic
paraparesis, head circumference of 45 cm, hyperacusis, some speech. Discordant low-
grade clinical: cerebral palsy, microcephaly.

1961. Female-female, DZ: blood cells K+ / K—, Nixon +3.79; Puerto Rican; b.
6/37, adm. Letchworth 6/51. Undifferentiated. IQ's 49, 67.

Family disorganized. At least one of two sibs is scholastically retarded. A, sexually
delinquent; B has rheumatic heart disease. Concordant high-grade.

1967. Male-female, Puerto Rican; b. 5/44, adm. Letchworth 7/51. Undifferentiated.
IQ's 59, 62.

Family disorganized, no full sibs. Birth weights 5 lb. 7 oz., 5½ lb. A, belligerent;
has malocclusion. Corcordant high-grade.

1968, 1978. Female-female, DZ (?): ridge counts 153/143, Wendt 55/43, Nixon
+2.37; Negro; b. 4/47, adm. Letchworth 7/52. Familial. IQ's 25, 36.

No full sibs. Birth order, A second; weights 4 lb. 12 oz., 5½ lb. (hosp.); A from
breech presentation. Separate fetal membranes. Each has a right cervical rib, B, bilateral
extensor plantar response. Concordant high-grade.

2013, 2014. Male-male, DZ: blood types D+ C— E+ / D— C— E—; b. 6/36,
adm. Letchworth 6/46. Familial. IQ's 67, 72.

Mother reportedly subnormal, one of two sibs had IQ 60. Father died 1936. Birth
weights 3 lb. 4 oz., 3 lb. (hosp.). A is left-handed, B has pectus carinatum. Concordant high-grade.

2015, 2016. Female-female, MZ: ridge counts 86/74, Wendt 45/41, Nixon —3.56;
Negro; b. 2/34, adm. Letchworth 2/47. Familial. IQ's 75, 79.

Mother and three of six sibs institutionalized as psychotic. Father paranoid with IQ
112. Birth weights 2100 (A or B), 2150 Gm. (hosp.). Physically normal. Concordant
high-grade.

2017, 2018. Male-male, MZ: ridge counts 185/179, Wendt 53/53, Nixon —4.42;
b. 9/42, adm. Letchworth 8/46. Undifferentiated. IQ's less than 20.

Two normal sibs. Delivery uncomplicated; birth weights 4 lb. 3 oz., 4 lb. 2 oz. Development was slow from the start. At age 12, legs thin but not spastic; barely able to
walk; Babinski signs and absent abdominal reflexes; one testicle of each atrophic or undescended. Head circumference 49 cm. in both. Concordant low-grade clinical: microcephaly.

2033. Male-male, DZ: blood cells O, D+ C+ E+ / A, D+ C— E+; b. 9/47, adm.
Letchworth 9/49. Birth trauma. IQ's 49, 110.

Two normal sibs. Birth order, A second; weights 2 lb. 14 oz., 3 lb. 5 oz. (hosp.).
A was intermittently cyanotic in the first few days, fed poorly. At age 5, generalized
spasticity, severe internal strabismus, but progressing well. Discordant high-grade clinical: cerebral palsy.

1971. Male-female; b. 1/06, adm. Letchworth 8/50. Undifferentiated. IQ's 15, 120.
Five normal sibs. Labor prolonged. Retardation not suspected until dismissal after 1 year of school. Concussion with unconsciousness at age 12. High arched palate, enlarged external occipital protuberance, anesthesia to pin–prick. Evidence of regression. Discordant low-grade.

1974. Female-female, zygosity undecided: ridge counts 27/18, Nixon —2.13, Slater +2.40; Negro; b. 10/43, adm. Letchworth 2/49. Infection. IQ's less than 10, 63.
Mother single. Birth order, A second; weights 4 lbs 4 oz., 4 lb. (hosp.). Common chorion reported. Pertussis at age 5, followed in A by encephalitis. At age 10, A had right spastic hemiplegia, no speech. Concordant subnormal, discordant low-grade clinical: cerebral palsy. History of trauma.

1976. Male-female; b. 3/40, adm. Letchworth 8/49. Undifferentiated. IQ's 50, B undetermined.
Three normal sibs. Birth order, A first; weights 3 lb. 11 oz., 2½ lb. (hosp.). Mother says A had ugly instrument marks on head, was not expected to live, and was jaundiced for 2 months. Indirect Coombs test negative 1955. B scholastically normal. A at 14 had constant tachychardia (confirmed on EKG 1958) and anxious mood, slight choreiform movements, tendency toward disuse of left arm, malocclusion. Discordant high-grade clinical: cerebral palsy. History of trauma.

1977. Female-female, MZ: reciprocal skin grafts; b. 11/41, adm. Letchworth 5/45. Cranial anomaly. IQ's less than 10, 96.
Previously reported (17). One sib. Birth order, A second; weights 1220, 2150 Gm. (hosp.). A an arrested breech extraction with two coils of cord around neck. A had unsuccessful cataract operations at 7 and 16 months for what was probably retrolental fibroplasia. Seizures from 8 months. At age 12, A was recumbent, spastic, head circumference 45 cm. Discordant low-grade clinical: cerebral palsy, convulsive disorder, microcephaly. History of trauma.

1980, 1981. Male-male, DZ: blood cells Fy (a—)/Fy (a+), Nixon +7.38; b. 8/39, adm. Letchworth 1/45. Undifferentiated. IQ's 15, 22.
Mother harsh, father alcoholic. Two normal older sibs, one younger, sickly. Birth order, A second; weights 5 lb. 3 oz., 4 lb. 1 oz. (hosp.). Rachitic and anemic neonatally. Repeated hospitalizations from age 4 months, retardation diagnosed at 1 year. This pregnancy was unwanted, and was followed immediately by another. Poor motor coordination; hyperopia in B and extreme myopia in A. Concordant low-grade.

1982, 1983. Male-male-female, MZ male pair: ridge counts 101/114, Wendt 51/44, Nixon +0.84, Slater —0.57; female died neonatally; b. 12/39, adm. Letchworth 3/49. Other forms. IQ's 46, 57.
Two normal sibs, one died at 22 months with convulsions. Cesarean section necessitated by abruptio placentae. In incubators for several weeks. Convulsions in A responded to calcium. Motor development retarded, behavior destructive; given electroshock at age 8. Myopia and vitreous opacities; A had an old right choreoretinal lesion and x-ray evidence of old mastoid disease. Thought content psychotic. Concordant high-grade. History of trauma.

1988, 1989. Male-male, MZ: ridge counts 140/138, Wendt 43/40, Nixon —1.31; b. 8/21, adm. Letchworth 10/47. Familial. IQ's 38, 40.
Three normal sibs. Birth order, A first; weights 6½ lb., 6 lb. Prolonged pertussis at 1 year. Atrophic skin condition. B has noticeable hypsicephaly. Concordant low-grade, discordant clinical: other cranial anomalies. History of trauma.

1991, 1992. Male-male, DZ: blood types D+ C+ E+ c+ / D+ C+ E— c—; b. 1/42, adm. Letchworth 7/47. Familial. IQ's 51, 59.
Mother single, twins raised in orphanage. Birth weights both 4 lb. 2 oz. (hosp.). A has undescended testicles, malocclusion, metopic suture; B has impaired manual coordination. Concordant high-grade.

1993. Male-male, MZ: ridge counts 146/141, Wendt 51/46, Nixon —1.52; b. 11/37, adm. Letchworth 2/52. Familial. IQ's 68, 56.
Mother's IQ 79, two of five sibs required special classes. Birth order, A second; weights

both 1½ lb. according to mother. A institutionalized because of aggressiveness. Concordant high-grade.

2007. Male-male, DZ: blood cells M / MN, Nixon +4.26; b. 4/50, adm. Willowbrook 10/52. Cranial anomaly. IQ's 10, 100.

Two normal sibs. Mother in a mental hospital for 9½ months after delivery. Birth order, A second; weights 4 lb. 14 oz., 5 lb. 15 oz. (hosp.). A's delivery by breech extraction; on third day had fever, cyanosis and hypocalcemic tetany attributed to aspiration pneumonia. Spastic quadriplegia, head circumference 498 mm. Seizures from age 2. Discordant low-grade clinical: cerebral palsy and convulsive disorder. History of trauma.

2008, 2009. Male-male, MZ: ridge counts 59/59, Wendt 41/37, Nixon —2.56; b. 8/43, adm. Letchworth 1/49. Undifferentiated. IQ's less than 10, 12.

Mother hard of hearing. Two normal sibs. Birth order, A second; weights 4 lb. 6 oz., 4½ lb. (hosp.). A had seizures between 10 and 15 months, B, from 8 months to the present. At age 10, both have funnel chest, hyperreflexia, A, possibly choreiform movements. Head circumferences 490 and 493 mm. Concordant low-grade clinical: convulsive disorder and microcephaly.

2010, 2011. Female-female, MZ: ridge counts 226/220, Wendt 58/56, Nixon —0.24; b. 6/41, adm. Letchworth 1/49. Other forms. IQ's 53, 56.

No sibs. Cesarean section at term because of toxemia. Birth order, A first; weights 7 lb. 13 oz., 7 lb. 15 oz. (hosp.). Both had convulsions in first year. Gigantism noted from age 5. Enlarged ventricles, abnormal EEG. At age 11, stature 169 and 167 cm., head circumferences 590 and 599 mm. Digital deformity and ptosis. Concordant high-grade clinical: other cranial anomaly and other major anomalies.

2012. Female-female, DZ: blood cells MN / M; Nixon +8.28; b. 5/36, adm. Letchworth 12/51. Endocrine. IQ's 32, 117.

One normal sib. Birth order, A second; weights both 4 lb. 5 oz. Blood cholesterol elevated at age 13, skin dry and insensitive, metabolic rate *elevated*. Menses delayed and irregular, stature 137 cm. at age 17. Myopia, heavy freckling, simian crease in palms. Discordant low-grade clinical: other major anomalies.

2037, 2028. Male-male, MZ: ridge counts 89/84, Wendt 33/32, Nixon —3.87; White Puerto Rican; b. 7/42, adm. Letchworth 12/51. Familial. IQ's 45, 46.

One of two sibs institutionalized, IQ 70. Birth weights 4 lb. 12 oz., 4 lb. B had two convulsions around age 4. Concordant high-grade.

2065. Male-male, DZ: blood types D+ C+ E— c+ / D+ C+ E— c—, Nixon +1.03; b. 11/38, adm. Wassaic 9/41. Familial. IQ's 67, 96.

Most of children removed from home as neglected while infants. Two sibs in mental hospitals, one institutionalized with IQ 80 or less. Birth weights 6 lb. 14 oz., 6 lb. 9 oz. (hosp.). B hospitalized from age 11 to 17 as schizophrenic. Discordant high-grade.

2071. Male-male, DZ: blood groups O / B, Nixon +10.76; half Philippino, b. 6/40, adm. Letchworth 2/53. Undifferentiated. IQ's 59, 63.

Mother unstable, indecisive, parents divorced. One brother, vagrant, attended special classes. Birth order, A second; weights both 7 lb. A sadistic, thievish. B had a duodenal ulcer at age 5. Both stammer, A more than B. Head circumferences 563, 592 mm. Concordant high-grade, index case undifferentiated (partner has macrocephaly).

2091, 2092. Male-male, DZ: blood types D+ C+ E— / D+ C+ E+, Nixon + 1.26; b. 2/38, adm. Syracuse 3/53. Familial. IQ's 69, 74.

Father deserted; mother considered an improper guardian in 1941. Twins raised in a foster home. Physically normal. Concordant high-grade.

2093, 2094. Female-female, MZ: ridge counts 81/74, Wendt 39/39, Nixon —2.06; b. 6/42, adm. Syracuse 3/53. Familial. IQ's both 60.

Mother neglected children. One of two sibs reportedly retarded, the other, IQ 87. Half-sib died at age 4 with idiocy and microgyria. Birth weights just over 3 lb. One has 20/50 vision and strabismus, the other has normal vision. Psychomotor tests indicate organic disease. Concordant high-grade.

2112, 2113. Female-female, DZ: blood cells O, D+ C+ E— c+ / A, D+ C+ E— c—; b. 11/31, adm. Letchworth 5/48. Familial. IQ's 58, 60.

Father alcoholic, mother reportedly borderline. Two of seven sibs institutionalized as subnormal. Birth weights between 5 and 6 lb. A shows a personality disorder. Concordant high-grade.

2127, 2128. Male-male, DZ: blood cells MN, Fy(a+) / M, Fy(a—); b. 1/40, adm. Letchworth 4/53 and 2/53. Familial. IQ's 68, 70.

Mother hospitalized since late 1940 as schizophrenic. Nine sibs. Twins raised in five foster homes. Always poorly adjusted, B destructive. A has heart murmur and herniorrhaphy scar, B, malocclusion and slight scoliosis. Concordant high-grade.

2129. Male-female; b. 3/44, adm. Letchworth 2/53. Familial. IQ's 79, 75.

Mother institutionalized age 14-16 with IQ 57. No full sibs; one of three half-sibs institutionalized as defective delinquent. Birth order, A second; weights 7 lb., 6½ lb. A destructive and uncontrollable; borderline hypertelorism (Romanus' index 321), malocclusion. Concordant high-grade.

2130. Female-male; b. 1/39, adm. Newark 11/47. Birth trauma. IQ's 10, 81.

Two normal sibs; one younger sib died at age 4 with chronic convulsive disorder. Birth order, A second; weight 8½ lb., B not known. A's birth delayed an hour, airway obstructed. A has had convulsions since birth. At age 16, spastic, scissors-gait, dorsal kyphosis, head circumference 509 mm. Discordant low-grade clinical: cerebral palsy, convulsive disorder. History of trauma.

2134. Female-male; b. 5/44, adm. Newark 12/48. Birth trauma. IQ's 30, 61.

Seven sibs, nearly all scholastically retarded. Birth order, A second; weights 4½ lb., 5½ lb. Delivery difficult, A by breech extraction. Twice hospitalized for malnutrition. A had convulsions between 8 months and 6 years. At age 10, stature 120 cm., head circumference 494 mm., left spastic hemiparesis. Concordant subnormal, discordant low-grade clinical: cerebral palsy, microcephaly, convulsive disorder.

2138. Male-male, DZ: blood types D+ C— E+ / D+ C— E—, Nixon —1.26, Slater +1.93; Negro, b. 1/44, adm. 11/50. Familial. IQ's 33, 64.

Mother subnormal, father deserted. Three sibs. Birth weights 6 lb., 7 lb. Twins removed as neglected at age 1. Both twins and at least two sibs had unilateral polydactyly. B, like mother, has impaired vision; A, bilateral cataracts from about age 8. Concordant subnormal, discordant low-grade clinical: other major anomalies.

2143. Female-female, DZ: blood cells Fy (a+) / Fy (a—), Nixon +0.22, ridge counts 244/158; b. 10/45, adm. Newark 10/52. Birth trauma. IQ's 60, 107.

Three normal sibs. Birth order, A second; weight 7 lb. 2 oz., B not known (hosp.). Severe neonatal respiratory problems ("atelectasis"). Frequent convulsions starting neonatally. Discordant high-grade clinical: convulsive disorder. History of trauma.

2146. Male-female. Negro; b. 11/39, adm. Newark 10/48. Familial. IQ's 35, 83.

Three normal sibs, one apparently retarded with ptosis and rheumatic heart disease. Birth reportedly normal. Physically normal except for severe acne, not sebaceous adenoma. Discordant low-grade.

2147, 2148. Female-female, MZ: ridge counts 167/150, Wendt 50/48, Nixon—1.55; b. 9/28, adm. Newark 9/44. Familial. IQ's 49, 53.

Family disorganized. One sib, institutionalized, IQ 42. Twins institutionalized because of sexual delinquency. One had unilateral polydactyly at birth, both physically normal now. Concordant high-grade.

2151. Male-female, Negro; b. 9/35, adm. Wassaic 5/47. Undifferentiated. IQ's 70, 68.

Nine sibs, none apparently subnormal. When A had a high fever at 6 months, doctor warned that he would have behavior problems. Head always appeared large. Both twins attended special classes, but A was enuretic and aggressive. At age 20, A's head circumference was 580 mm., cephalic index 65.4. B's head was 516 mm., index 78.2. A had schizoid and paranoid traits. Concordant high-grade.

2152. Female-female, DZ: blood types D+ C+ E— c+ / D+ C+ E— c—, Nixon +4.24; b. 8/24, adm. Wassaic 10/49. Familial. IQ's 42, 75.

Twelve sibs, one hospitalized two years as schizophrenic. Birth order, A second; weights both over 9 lb. B completed high school. A resented special class placement and became delinquent. On examination, A is strikingly muscular, with facies and body build suggestive of chondrodystrophy, but stature is 150 cm. (B, 160 cm.) and long bones are normal. Concordant high-grade.

2154, 2155. Male-female; b. 8/40, adm. Wassaic 6/49. Familial. IQ's 35, 36.

Mother's IQ 52, children removed as neglected. Of two elder sibs, one is reportedly dull. Twins were in an institution from 6 to 18 months, thereafter with elderly foster parents. Physically normal. Concordant low-grade.

2157, 2158. Female-female, DZ: blood groups, B / O, Nixon +2.78; b. 6/39, adm. Wassaic 5/48 and 8/47. Familial. IQ's 24, 28.

Mother twice admitted to mental hospitals. No sibs. Intense fear responses from early childhood. A uses speech in meaningful protest, B only in parrot-like singing. Concordant low-grade.

2159. Female-male; b. 4/43, adm. Wassaic 6/48. Birth trauma. IQ's less than 10, 132.

No sibs. Mother 44 years old at delivery, died 10 days later. Birth order, A first; weights 7 lb. 3 oz., 6½ lb. A's delivery was from ROP position by mid-forceps after 15 hours of labor and secondary uterine inertia. B's delivery normal. A could not feed neonatally, had convulsions from age 5 or earlier. At age 10, could walk but showed spasticity, athetosis and external strabismus. Head circumference 485 mm. No speech. Discordant low-grade clinical: cerebral palsy, microcephaly, convulsive disorder. History of trauma.

2160, 2161. Female-female, DZ: blood groups O / A, Nixon +11.39; b. 8/46, adm. Newark 7/53. Familial. IQ's 17, 26.

Eight sibs are apparently normal. Birth weights 3 lb. 6 oz., 3 lb. 12 oz. Retarded in growth as in motor development, stature 104, 107 cm. at age 6½. Both had metopic sutures and, at age 14, head circumferences were 498 and 525 mm. Concordant low-grade, discordant clinical: microcephaly.

2178. Male-male, MZ: ridge counts 111/109, Wendt 48/47, Nixon —4.01; b. 9/45, adm. Wassaic 4/47. Cranial anomaly. IQ's less than 10, 106.

Father once institutionalized as defective. Two younger sibs. Birth order, A first, both by breech extraction; weights 3 lb. 4 oz., 6 lb. 4 oz. (hosp.). At age 1½; A's head was enlarged, but at age 9, the circumference was only 45 cm. Spastic quadriplegia, undescended testicles. Discordant low-grade clinical: cerebral palsy, microcephaly.

2185, 2186. Female-male; b. 3/40, adm. Wassaic 8/48. Familial. IQ's 71, 79.

Mother reportedly of borderline intelligence, family broken since 1942. Birth order, A first; weights 2½ lb. (A or B), 3 lb. Sickly and rachitic as infants. A has strabismus, B, hyperreflexia. Concordant high-grade.

2192. Male-female; b. 2/40, adm. Wassaic 7/45. Undifferentiated. IQ's 52, 87.

One normal sib. Birth weights 4 lb. 3 oz., 4 lb. A's head circumference measures 57 cm., gait shuffling, muscles spastic or manifesting cogwheel rigidity. Discordant low-grade clinical: cerebral palsy.

2197, 2479. Male-female; b. 9/47, adm. Willowbrook 9/49 and 6/55. Cranial anomaly (A), Familial (B). IQ's 43, 67.

Three of seven sibs subnormal, IQ's below 20 in two and 55 in the third. Another sib has cleft palate. Birth order, A second; weights 3½ lb., 4 lb. A had bronchopneumonia neonatally. Hydrocephaly diagnosed at 3 months in A, was not evident after age 2. At age 8, A had left internal strabismus, undescended testicles, head circumference 518 mm; B, slight ptosis of left eyelid. Concordant high-grade. History of trauma.

2211, 2212. Female-female, MZ: ridge counts 286/281, Wendt 70/70, Nixon —4.88; b. 5/13, adm. Letchworth 5/30. Undifferentiated. IQ's 28, 34.

Father alcoholic, mother institutionalized as subnormal. A had duodenal ulcers, seizures; B, Bell's palsy. Concordant low-grade, discordant clinical: convulsive disorder.

2250. Male-male, MZ: blood cells B, D+ C+ E— c— / D+ C+ E— c+; Negro; b. 3/48, adm. Letchworth 5/53. Postnatal trauma. IQ's 6, 100.

Two sibs. Birth order, A first, breech; weights 2590, 2650 Gm. A operated on 12/52 for strabismus; after cardiac arrest, never regained consciousness. Generalized atrophy and spasticity. Discordant low-grade clinical: cerebral palsy. History of trauma.

2257. Female-male; b. 11/37, adm. Willowbrook 11/53. Undifferentiated. IQ's 74, 72.

Paternity uncertain. Two normal half- (?) sibs. Birth order, A second; weights 6 lb, 10 oz., 6 lb. 11 oz. A had pneumonia at 1½ years. Both attended school, A aggressive. Concordant high-grade.

2259. Male-female; b. 8/47, adm. Letchworth 6/53. Cerebral palsy. IQ's less than 20, 114.

One younger sib. Birth order, A first; weights 2200, 1800 gm. Neonatally, both had intermittent cyanosis and moderate jaundice; on the third day A was edematous. Both were Rh +, mother Rh —. On 5th day, A's incubator overheated. Generalized muscular atrophy, opisthotonus. Discordant low-grade clinical: cerebral palsy. History of trauma.

2262. Female-male, Negro; b. 11/36, adm. Letchworth 10/53. Undifferentiated. IQ's 67, 65.

Family disorganized. Two normal sibs. Birth order, A second; weights 3 lb. 9 oz., 3 lb. 6 oz. A had pneumonia neonatally. A has WISC verbal IQ of 80; sexually delinquent. Concordant high-grade. History of trauma.

2263, 2264. Male-male, MZ: ridge counts 131/114, Wendt 47/44, Nixon —2.77; Negro; b. 12/46, adm. Letchworth 7/53. Familial. IQ's 57, 68.

Mother single, hospitalized as schizophrenic in 1951. A but not B once diagnosed as childhood schizophrenia. Electroencephalograms diffusely abnormal. Myopia of 15 and 20 diopters. Concordant high-grade.

2270. Male-female; b. 12/42, adm. Rome 5/48. Cerebral palsy. IQ's less than 10, 94.

One sib. Birth order, A first; weights 2 lb. 4 oz., and 4 lb. (hosp.), both breech presentations. Left microphthalmia and hydrocephaly diagnosed neonatally. Pertussis before age 1. At present, left microphthalmia, right optic atrophy, spastic paraparesis, head circumference 480 mm. Discordant low-grade clinical: cerebral palsy, microcephaly, other major anomalies. History of trauma.

2281. Female-female, DZ: ridge counts 73/54, Wendt 38/32, Nixon +2.5 (prints-male, unsatisfactory), hair colors different; b. 5/23, adm. Willowbrook 2/54. Birth trauma. IQ's 13, 126.

One normal sib. Membranes ruptured one week before delivery. Birth order, A second; weights 3 lb. 1 oz., 2 lb. 11 oz.; A presented as breech. Both Rh +, mother Rh —, A more jaundiced and given more oxygen. A had retrolental fibroplasia and transient hydrocephaly. Head circumference at 2½, 508 mm. Discordant low-grade clinical: other cranial anomalies. History of trauma.

2301. Female-female-male, trizygotic: females' blood cells M/MN, Nixon +6.91; Puerto Rican; b. 5/48, adm. Letchworth 12/53. Infection. IQ's less than 20, 89, 91.

Three sibs, at least two normal. Birth order, A last. A, reportedly had an acute illness with CNS involvement before age 1. Frequent seizures from infancy. At age 7, right spastic hemiplegia, head circumference 45 cm. Discordant low-grade clinical: cerebral palsy, convulsive disorder, microcephaly. History of trauma.

2302. Male-male-male, dizygotic or trizygotic: blood types D+ C+ E+ c+ / D+ C+ E— c— / D+ C+ E— c—, Nixon (AB) +.75, (AC) + 5.13, (BC) —.15, stature 101, 110, 112 cm; Puerto Rican; b. 8/48, adm. Letchworth 11/53. Undifferentiated. IQ's 20, 50, 60 (language barrier).

Two younger sibs, at least one normal. Birth order, A last; weights 3 lb., 3½ lb., 3½ lb. Internal strabismus, growth retardation (101 cm. at 6½ years). Concordant subnormal, discordant low-grade.

2303, 2304. Male-male, MZ: ridge counts 201/188, Wendt 64, 61, Nixon —2.75; b. 1/45, adm. Letchworth 3/54. Familial. IQ's 45, 48.

One of three sibs died neonatally with visceral anomaly, one institutionalized with findings as in the twins. Birth order, A first; weights 4 lb. 12 oz., 5 lb. 2 oz. Heads small and round: at age 9, circumferences 492, 495 mm., indexes 86.3, 87. Hands short with dermatoglyphic features of Down's syndrome but ears large. B had internal strabismus and undescended testicles. Bizarre mannerisms. Concordant high-grade clinical: microcephaly.

2305. Male-female; b. 8/48, adm. Letchworth 11/53. Undifferentiated. IQ's 74, 77.

Family broken, twins orphaned at 3½ years. Three sibs. Birth order, A second. A slower in development, spoiled by mother, disturbed after her death. Concordant high-grade.

2311, 2312. Female-male, Negro; b. 4/52, adm. Willowbrook 4/54. Birth trauma. IQ's 18, 18.

Nine normal sibs. Birth order, A first; weights 2 lb. 5 oz., 2 lb. 11 oz. Retrolental fibroplasia recognized neonatally. At 3½ A is blind and unable to stand; B, some vision, stands with support. Head circumferences 479 and 484 mm. Concordant low-grade. History of trauma.

2320, 2321. Female-female, DZ: blood cells A, D+ C+ E— c— / O, D+ C+ E+ c+; b. 10/50, adm. Rome 11/53. Undifferentiated. IQ's 31, 36.

Three normal sibs, one younger than the twins. Birth order, A second; weights 2120, 2160 Gm. (hosp.). Retarded in motor and speech development; physically normal according to institution's examination. Concordant low-grade.

2322, 2323. Male-male, DZ: blood groups O / B, Nixon +7.44; b. 8/44, adm. Rome 10/51. Familial. IQ's 61, 61.

Parents and two of five sibs reportedly subnormal, two others institutionalized (2341-2342). A's arm broken at birth. Kept in a crib usually, until age 3. Institutionalized two years earlier than their older and equally retarded sisters. Impaired manual coordination. Psychomotor tests indicated organic pathology. Concordant high-grade.

2324, 2325. Male-male, MZ: ridge counts 55/52, Wendt 25/23, Nixon —5.49; Negro; b. 12/45, adm. Rome 8/52. Familial. IQ's 65, 68.

Mother unstable, father unknown. No full sibs. Excluded from school because of behavior problems. Visual acuity approximately 15/40 in both. Rorschach tests revealed neurotic personality disturbance. Concordant high-grade.

2328, 2329. Male-male, MZ: ridge counts 155/146, Wendt 56/55, Nixon —1.58; b. 4/41, adm. Rome 9/48. Familial. IQ's 44, 47.

Mother reportedly subnormal, two of seven sibs institutionalized as subnormal. Both have internal strabismus, but no other abnormality noted in the institution's examination. Concordant high-grade.

2341, 2342. Female-female, DZ: blood groups A / B; b. 9/43, adm. Rome 4/53. Familial. IQ's 48, 54.

Sisters of cases 2322, 2323. Stayed in kindergarten until age 9. Enuretic. At age 10½ A had hypertelorism (interocular distance 36 mm., Romanus' index 297), unusually thick and firm subcutaneous tissue, and very low manual strength (dynamometer). B had Hoffman and Babinski signs on the left. Coordination normal. Concordant high-grade, discordant clinical: cranial anomaly.

2344. Female-male; b. 4/46, adm. Rome 2/48. Undifferentiated. IQ's 28, 150.

One sib. Gestation complicated by toxemia. Birth order, A first; weights both 5 lb 4 oz; A vertex, B breech. Tooth eruption delayed to 11 months in A. At age 1 year, air studies revealed internal and external hydrocephalus with cortical atrophy. At age 9, head circumference 51 cm, slight funnel deformity of chest, scattered purpuric spots; muscle stretch reflexes could not be elicited. Discordant low-grade.

2347. Male-male, MZ (?): ridge counts 101/98, Wendt 42/38, Nixon —.29, Slater —1.44, iris color dissimilar; b. 9/44, adm. Rome 1/48. Cerebral palsy. IQ's unmeasurable in A, 121 in B.

One normal sib. Birth order, A first; weights 5 lb. 7 oz., 5 lb. 9 oz. Prolapse of umbilical cord before delivery. At age 10, head circumference 497 mm., spastic quadriplegia, undescended testicles. Socially responsive but without speech. Discordant low-grade clinical: cerebral palsy, microcephaly. History of trauma.

2348. Male-female. b. 3/44, adm. Rome 12/47. Cranial anomaly. IQ's 11, 106.

Three normal sibs. Birth order, A second; weights 3 lb 5 oz., 5 lb. 14 oz.; both breech. Mental defect diagnosed at 3 months. At age 11, stature 108 cm., head circumference 457 mm.; flat occiput, bilateral simian creases, loud diastolic heart murmur. Umbilical hernia, scrotal hypospadias, granular conjunctivitis. Facies not suggestive of Down's syndrome. Discordant low-grade clinical: microcephaly, other major anomalies.

2351. Male-male, zygosity undetermined: ridge counts 80/60, Wendt 45/39, Nixon

—.23, Slater +.38, palmar main lines dissimilar; Negro; b. 4/47, adm. Willowbrook 5/54. Cerebral palsy. IQ's 30, 75.

Nine normal sibs. Birth order, A first; weights 3 lb. 14 oz., 3 lb. (hosp.). A has had several convulsions, B, one with fever at age 4½. Both boys have blue sectors in both eyes, internal strabismus, hyperopia. A has spastic quadriplegia but is socially responsive. Concordant subnormal clinical: convulsive disorder; discordant low-grade clinical: cerebral palsy.

2352, 2353. Female-male, Puerto Rican; b. 4/44, adm. Letchworth 12/53. Familial. IQ's 19, 53.

One sib. Birth order, A first by several hours; A premature and B normal in size. At age nearly 12 years, A was 111 cm. tall, head circumference 470 mm.; B, 133 cm. and 515 mm. Concordant subnormal, discordant low-grade clinical: microcephaly.

2355. Female-female, DZ: blood cells Fy (a—) / Fy (a+), Nixon + 3.62; b. 1/43, adm. Letchworth 3/54. Cerebral palsy. IQ's 32, 107.

Mother is unsteady of gait, has an intention tremor; her mother had a tremor that diminished with age. One sib of normal intelligence was diagnosed by a neurologist as having disease of the basal ganglia with pyramidal and extrapyramidal signs. Birth order, A first; weights 4 lb. 5 oz., 5 lb. (hosp.). At age 11½ had spastic paraplegia with bilateral Babinski; menarche had occurred at age 10 and breasts were extremely large. B normal despite recent concussion and brain surgery. Discordant low-grade clinical: cerebral palsy.

2368. Female-female, MZ: ridge counts 30/26, Wendt 29/27, Nixon —2.26; b. 5/53, adm. Willowbrook 8/54. Birth trauma. IQ's 20, B undetermined (scholastically normal at age 7).

One younger sib. Maternal preeclampsia. Birth order, A second; weights 4 lb. 4 oz., 6 lb. (hosp.); A from breech, B from vertex presentation. At 9 months A was found to have cerebral palsy and primary optic atrophy. At 3 years, spastic quadriplegia, head circumference 418 mm. Discordant low-grade clinical: cerebral palsy, microcephaly, other major anomaly.

2395. Male-male, MZ: ridge counts 153/139, Wendt 55/48, Nixon —1.99; b. 6/49, adm. Willowbrook 7/54. Familial. IQ's 18, less than 33.

No sibs, no prior pregnancies. Birth order, A first, breech; weights 3 lb. 4 oz., 4 lb. 3 oz. (hosp.). A became jaundiced at 4 weeks with diagnosis of probable intermittent biliary obstruction. Both institutionalized before age 1 because of psychosis in mother. At 6½ years, A had reduced muscle strength and tonus, toddling gait; B physically normal. Concordant low-grade. History of trauma.

2406, 2407. Female-female, MZ: ridge counts 118/105, Wendt 40/40, Nixon —4.58; Negro; b. 7/48, adm. Willowbrook 12/54. Familial. IQ's 42, 52.

Two normal sibs. Birth weights 4 lb. 10 oz., 4 lb. 14 oz. A, thought to have congenital heart disease. Growth difference: at age 6½, A was 114 cm. tall, B, 126 cm.; head circumference of A 527 mm., of B, 538 mm. Otherwise normal. Concordant high-grade.

2412, 2413. Male-female, Puerto Rican; b. 12/45, adm. Letchworth 12/54. Familial. IQ's 60, 62.

Mother single, no full sibs. Birth order, A second; weights 3 lb. 2 oz., 4 lb. Physically normal. Concordant high-grade.

2426. Male-female; b. 2/50, adm. Willowbrook 2/55. Epilepsy. IQ's, less than 10, B undetermined.

One normal sib. Birth order, A first; weights 6 lb. 11 oz., 5 lb. 13 oz. (hosp.). Labor was protracted and A's delivery an instrumental breech extraction. Convulsions began at 5 months. Cerebral palsy diagnosed at age 2. At age 9, he had spastic paraplegia, head circumference of 48 cm., left retinal lesion of the macula. B reportedly normal. Discordant low-grade clinical: cerebral palsy, microcephaly, convulsive disorder. History of trauma.

2435. Female-female, MZ: ridge counts 163/160, Wendt 52/51, Nixon —2.18; b. 2/52, adm. Willowbrook 3/55. Undifferentiated. IQ's 27, B undetermined.

No sibs. Birth order, A second; weights 3 lb. 1 oz., 3 lb. 11 oz. (hosp.); both breech presentations. Retrolental fibroplasia severe in A, slight in B. A also thought to have congenital heart disease. B at least normal in development. Discordant low-grade.

2441, 2442. Female-female, zygosity undetermined: ridge counts 131/107, Wendt 48/40, Nixon +0.35, Slater —0.37, physically similar; b. 12/51, adm. Willowbrook 3/55. Birth trauma. IQ's 17, 18.

Two normal sibs; one malformed sib died on first day. Mother bled for two months before delivery. Birth order, A first; weights 1295, 1410 Gm. (hosp.). Retrolental fibroplasia diagnosed before hospital discharge. Brief right-sided convulsion observed in B at age 1½, electroencephalogram abnormal. At 3½ years, A had some vision and was active, B had no vision. Concordant low-grade. History of trauma.

2446, 2447. Female-female, DZ: blood cells MN / M, Nixon —.54, Slater —1.69, but physically very dissimilar; Puerto Rican; b. 4/39, adm. Letchworth 1/55 and 2/55. Familial. IQ's 31, 42 (language barrier).

Mother died 1942. One of two elder sibs reportedly subnormal. A remained in Puerto Rico until 1953; B, only until 1948. IQ's discounted in this analysis. Examinations by the state school revealed no relevant pathology. Concordant high-grade.

2454. Male-male, MZ: ridge counts 136/120, Wendt 41/40, Nixon —4.50; b. 7/41, adm. Newark 8/55. Birth trauma. IQ's 53, 70.

Mother died of rheumatic heart disease in 1946. No full sibs. Birth order, A first; weights 4 lb. 7 oz., 3 lb. 6 oz. (hosp.). Placenta dichorionic. B had grand mal seizures from age 9, institutionalized in 1953. Both had myopia and undescended right testicle. Concordant high-grade, discordant clinical: convulsive disorder—index case unaffected.

2466. Male-male, MZ: bloods not obtained; ridge counts 150/126, Wendt 47/43, Nixon —2.24; hair, iris and ears closely similar; b. 5/54, adm. Newark 3/55. Cranial anomaly. IQ's undetermined.

Two normal sibs. Mother received pelvic radiation treatment about time of conception; confined to bed in the fifth month because of bleeding and cramps. Birth order, A first; weights 5½ lb., 5 lb. 3 oz. (hosp.). A presented as LOP., labor was prolonged, and he had extensive ecchymoses at birth. Both had jaundice till the fourth week. Hydrocephalus noted at 3 months, progressing until death at 1 year. B, normal. Discordant low-grade clinical: other cranial anomaly. History of trauma.

2591, 2592. Male-male, MZ: ridge counts 131/104, Wendt 45/42, Nixon —1.018; b. 2/41, adm. Letchworth 11/55. Familial. IQ's 54, 58.

Father hospitalized as schizophrenic since 1942. One of three sibs scholastically retarded. Birth order, A first; weights 6 lb. 14 oz., 6 lb. 11 oz. (hosp.); B's delivery, breech. At age 15, B was 9 cm taller. Concordant high-grade.

TABLE 1. DISPOSITION OF THE 592 PLURAL BIRTH SETS
ORIGINALLY ASCERTAINED

	Sets	Index Cases
Total	592	739
Omitted (not in state schools)	61	71
Omitted (not mentally defective)	11	12
Verified subjects	520	656
One or both dead	143	156
Defined twin population	376	500
Sample	177	261

TABLE 2. DESIGNATIONS OF ADMISSION DIAGNOSES AS GIVEN
IN THIS REPORT AND CORRESPONDING OFFICIAL DIAGNOSES
IN MOST OF THE STATE SCHOOL RECORDS

Abridged Admission Diagnosis	Official Diagnosis
Familial	Familial
Undifferentiated	Undifferentiated
Down's syndrome	Mongolism
Birth trauma	Due to trauma during birth
Cranial anomaly	With developmental cranial anomaly
Cerebral palsy	With congenital cerebral spastic infantile paralysis
Epilepsy	Due to epilepsy
Infection*	Due to infection
Postnatal trauma*	Due to trauma after birth
Endocrine*	With glandular disorder
	With familial amaurosis
Other forms	With other organic nervous diseases
	Other forms

*Combined with "Other forms" in some tables.

TABLE 3. VERIFIED INDEX CASES BY NEW YORK STATE FISCAL YEAR
OF ADMISSION, BY NUMBER OF INDEX CASES PER SET, AND BY OCCURRENCE
OR NONOCCURRENCE OF DEATH BEFORE JULY, 1952

		Before 1940	1940-1944	1945-1949	1950-1955	1956	Total
Members of intact pairs	Double-index	74	30	54	81	7	246
	Single-index	42	35	78	95	4	254
	Total	116	65	132	176	11	500
One or both dead	Double-index	10	5	5	6		26
	Single-index	23	24	29	52	2	130
	Total	33	29	34	58	2	156
All cases		149	94	166	234	13	656

TABLE 4. VERIFIED INDEX CASES BY ADMISSION DIAGNOSIS, BY NUMBER
OF INDEX CASES PER SET (TRIPLE-INDEX TRIPLETS COUNTED AS
"DOUBLE"), BY SEX CONCORDANCE, AND BY DISPOSITION

| | | Disposition | | | | | | |
| | | Studied | | Not Studied | | Excluded by death | | |
		Double-index	Single-index	Double-index	Single-index	Double-index	Single-index	Total
Familial	Same-sex	96	8	44	28	6	16	198
	Opposite-sex	17	10	14	18	2	11	72
Undifferentiated	Same-sex	32	7	12	36	5	19	111
	Opposite-sex	0	14	4	31	0	18	67
Down's syndrome	Same-sex	4	6	0	2	6	1	19
	Opposite-sex	0	8	0	3	0	3	14
Birth trauma	Same-sex	2	8	0	14	0	10	34
	Opposite-sex	2	6	0	8	0	4	20
Cranial anomaly	Same-sex	2	5	0	3	2	4	16
	Opposite-sex	1	3	0	3	0	9	16
Cerebral palsy	Same-sex	2	6	2	3	3	6	22
	Opposite-sex	0	4	0	2	0	13	19
Epilepsy	Same-sex	0	1	1	0	2	2	6
	Opposite-sex	0	1	0	3	0	4	8
Infection	Same-sex	0	4	0	0	0	1	5
	Opposite-sex	0	0	0	0	0	2	2
Other forms	Same-sex	8	4	3	4	0	4	23
	Opposite-sex	0	0	0	1	0	3	4
Total		166	95	80	159	26	130	656

TABLE 5. COMPARISON OF SAMPLE WITH REMAINDER OF THE DEFINED
TWIN POPULATION WITH RESPECT TO FISCAL YEAR OF ADMISSION,
NUMBER OF INDEX CASES PER SET, AND SEX-CONCORDANCE

			Before 1940	1940-1944	1945-1949	1950-1955	1956	Total All Years
Sample	Single-index	Same-sex	1	3	16	28	1	49
		Opposite-sex	6	2	16	22		46
		Total	7	5	32	50	1	95
	Double-index	Same-sex	30	10	47	56	2	145
		Opposite-sex	2	2	4	12	1	21
		Total	32	12	51	68	3	166
Remainder	Single-index	Same-sex	19	21	27	22	1	90
		Opposite-sex	16	9	19	23	2	69
		Total	35	30	46	45	3	159
	Double-index	Same-sex	34	16	2	8	2	62
		Opposite-sex	8	2	1	5	2	18
		Total	42	18	3	13	4	80

TABLE 6. COMPARISON OF SAMPLE WITH REMAINDER OF THE DEFINED
TWIN POPULATION WITH RESPECT TO AGE ON ADMISSION, NUMBER OF
INDEX CASES PER SET, SEX-CONCORDANCE, AND SEX OF
INDEX CASES

			Age on First Admission					
			Under 5	5-9	10-14	15-19	20	Total
Sample	Double-index	Same-sex, M	15	43	26	4	2	90
		Same-sex, F	6	24	12	12	2	56
		Opposite-sex	4	14	2	0	0	20
		Total	25	81	40	16	4	166
	Single-index	Same-sex, M	18	8	4	0	0	30
		Same-sex, F	6	6	3	2	2	19
		Opposite-sex, M	4	15	2	1	1	23
		Opposite-sex, F	9	7	3	3	1	23
		Total	37	36	12	6	4	95
Remainder	Double-index	Same-sex, M	0	10	10	10	0	30
		Same-sex, F	4	8	8	10	2	32
		Opposite-sex	4	4	10	0	0	18
		Total	8	22	28	20	2	80
	Single-index	Same-sex, M	7	4	24	9	2	46
		Same-sex, F	6	13	7	10	8	44
		Opposite-sex, M	8	7	12	3	1	31
		Opposite-sex, F	5	9	9	9	6	38
		Total	26	33	52	31	17	159

SECTION IV: FUNCTION OF A MEDICAL GENETICS DEPARTMENT IN THE FIELD OF MENTAL HEALTH

23

Introduction

WILLIAM MALAMUD, M.D.

THE PRIVILEGE OF INTRODUCING the contributors to the fourth section of these proceedings is a particularly distinctive and gratifying one for a number of reasons. It may have come to me, I guess, on account of my peculiar ability to wear *three hats* at one time. Although by no means being among my regular habits, this slightly immodest faculty apparently lent more than ordinary weight to my long-planned and rather single-minded participation in this splendid program — a rare opportunity which I would not have missed even without a hat.

As it was, I not only happened to be incoming president of the Eastern Psychiatric Research Association when this memorable symposium was held, but I had also been asked by Dr. Walter Barton, the present president of the American Psychiatric Association, to convey the most cordial greetings of our esteemed mother organization to Dr. Kallmann's group. The third hat denoted my presence as the current field director of the Scottish Rite Committee on Research in Schizophrenia. This is the usually rather hard-boiled committee which wants to put its limited funds to the best possible use. In almost 25 years, however, it never hesitated to renew its support of Dr. Kallmann's genetic studies, the soundness of which was clearly recognized by our first field director, Dr. Nolan D. C. Lewis.

May I state here on behalf of our entire committee that we are as proud of the fact that Dr. Kallmann, the organizer of this symposium and the concluding speaker in this section, was among the earliest recipients of a Scottish Rite Committee grant, as we are of his solid contributions to the growth of *mental health genetics* in this country during the past quarter of a century. This joint report on the function of a medical genetics department in the field of mental health, prepared by distinguished experts from three different continents, is so distinctly along the lines pursued by Dr. Kallmann for many years that it amounts to a veritable tribute to his own work.

Viewed from the standpoint of American psychiatry, another reason for our particular interest in the reports presented in this section may be seen in the varied national and professional backgrounds of its contributors. In a symposium that deals with the relevance of *basic genetic variations,* but is amply interspersed with somewhat embarrassed references to the ghost of the old nature-nurture controversy, every attempt to evaluate *cross-cultural differences* is bound to be helpful in appreciating the effect of universal genetic factors. In order to bring about a real rapprochement in regard to the outdated heredity versus environment dispute, more recently identified with the innate and the experiential components of human existence, an important step forward is what our distinguished participants from abroad have successfully done in their reports; namely, to give us a clear over-all picture of *different genetic research trends* in their countries.

In this *international panel,* Great Britain is represented by two prominent geneticists, Dr. John A. F. Roberts and Dr. Eliot Slater. Both are full-fledged Londoners, and capitalizing on many years of experience as teachers and researchers, have authored widely used textbooks of medical genetics and clinical psychiatry, respectively. Having been frequent visitors to our shores, they count many of their American colleagues among their personal friends.

Scandinavia's equally well accredited representative is Dr. Erik Strömgren, and that of South Africa, Dr. Lewis A. Hurst. The former is professor of psychiatry at the Danish University of Aarhus, while the latter, a previous associate of Dr. Kallmann, holds a similar position at the University of the Witwatersrand in Johannesburg. Both are no strangers and always welcome here.

The geneticist assaying the development of medical genetics in the United States, Dr. C. Nash Herndon of the Bowman Gray School of Medicine in Winston-Salem, is even less in need of a formal introduction. He is a professor of preventive medicine rather than psychiatry, but he is well known to us through his extensive family studies and counseling work in disorders of the central nervous system, in inborn errors of metabolism, and in genetically determined forms of drug idiosyncrasy. Like Dr. Kallmann, he is a former president of the American Society of Human Genetics, and he currently serves as the editor of its Journal of Human Genetics.

It is a real privilege to introduce this provocative account of the function of a *modern genetics department* to our fellow workers in the field of mental health.

24

Genetics in the Medical School Curriculum

J. A. FRASER ROBERTS, M.D., D.Sc., F.R.C.P.

GENETICS OCCUPIES such a central place in general biology that an adequate grounding in its principles and relations to other subjects is evidently essential in all branches of biological science, including medicine.

In the specific field of medicine there are many practical applications which are now assuming an ever growing importance. Indeed, today it is no longer so much a matter of geneticists attempting to interest their colleagues, working in other specialties, in the value and usefulness of the subject, as of receiving from those colleagues increasing demands for exposition, cooperation in researches, and instruction for their students.

It is easy to give a selection of practical applications of interest to many medical men. Beyond doubt, the most important is the provision of genetic advice for those people who need it. The proportion of the population that really needs genetic advice in regard to the chances of defect in children, or further children, may not be very large. However, there are few medical practitioners, apart from those in some of the nonclinical specialisms, who will not at intervals be specifically asked for genetic advice. Obviously, it is their duty to provide it to the extent that knowledge permits, and that is to a very considerable extent.

Medical men may rest assured that if they do not give the answers, or are vague or noncommittal, the inquirers will get them in abundance from other, and very ill informed, sources. It is well known that the subject of the future of the unborn child has gathered around itself a wealth of foolish superstitions and old wives' tales, often of the most gloomy and alarming character. The odds can often be specified precisely, and it may prove to be fortunate that this is usually so if the risks are bad, for then one particularly needs to know where one is. In other instances, though the genetics may be obscure, the results of large-scale surveys provide over-all empirical risks of the defect's recurrence in a further child. Luckily, these empirical risks are often good.

Experience shows that the great majority of risks fall into two groups. First, there are the bad ones, say, worse than 1 in 10. Secondly, there are the good ones, say, better than 1 in 20. It is seldom that the estimate of risk falls into the region in between. It would be reasonable to call 1 in 20 or better a relatively good risk. After all, the chance that any random pregnancy will end with some serious malformation or other, or that some serious developmental error will manifest itself in early life, is probably not less than 1 in 40.

Of course, *genetic counseling* involves more than the mere calculation

214

of odds. Feelings of guilt, overt or not, may have to be dispelled. Parents may need to be encouraged to see that they are not different from other people. They will have to realize that they have suffered a misfortune which might have been the lot of any one of us. In many instances, they can be helped to face their bad luck realistically; perhaps, if the risk is altogether too big, they may adopt a child. On the other hand, if, as so often happens, the outlook is good, they can go ahead with confidence.

Genetic knowledge can on occasion be useful in making an *early diagnosis* when this is important in the matter of treatment. A few examples may be quoted. In nephrogenic diabetes insipidus, which is due to a sex-linked gene, diagnosis is not easy. If the child is not given adequate fluids, it may well die, or be left with serious cerebral damage. [2] Knowledge that the risk is 1 in 2 for any subsequent boy will ensure an early diagnosis, so that harmful consequences may be averted. Moreover, nearly all, if not all, of the female carriers can be identified by their failure to produce a normally concentrated urine. Hence, it can be determined which female relatives run the 1 in 2 risk of having an affected boy.

Galactosemia, which is due to a recessive gene, falls into much the same category. [7] Here, too, it is vital to make an early diagnosis if lactose is to be withheld in time. Toward the end of the first week signs of damage appear, going on to severe malnutrition, gross liver damage, cataracts and severe cerebral impairment. Only prompt avoidance of lactose may secure relatively normal development.

In congenital pyloric stenosis, early diagnosis is also important, and the results of treatment are very good indeed. Although the genetics are rather obscure, it is useful to know what a mother who was herself affected runs a risk of 1 in 4 or 5 that any son will also be affected. [1]

More generally, the number of known *inborn errors of metabolism* is now large, certainly exceeding 50. The rapidly advancing subject of biochemical genetics, with all the light it throws on the pathways of intermediary metabolism, is of prime importance to every student. Incidentally, it may be mentioned that although so many inherited conditions are rare or very rare, they are very numerous. In the aggregate, therefore, they are of appreciable practical significance.

The subject of *drug-induced disease* has also become of increasing practical importance in recent times. Here we are dealing with genes which under natural conditions apparently do little or no appreciable harm; but the administration of certain drugs may produce serious or sometimes disastrous results. Some of these genes are common, at least in certain populations. For example, there is the porphyria variegata of South Africa, due to a dominant gene possessed by no less than one person in 100 in parts of that country. [4] Barbiturates, or especially a barbiturate anaesthetic, may produce very serious effects, and many fatalities have been reported.

Pseudocholinesterase deficiency, due to a recessive gene, came to light through the use of suxamethonium as a muscle relaxant during anaesthesia. [6] Those persons carrying the gene may suffer from a prolonged and dangerous apnoea. Primaquine sensitivity, a sex-linked condition, is of course very common in

Negroes and in some other peoples, and a variety of drugs may induce a haemolytic anaemia. [3] Serious risks of this kind raise important questions in relation to the protection of the health of susceptible individuals.

The vast subject of *serology,* with all its ramifications in blood transfusion, in haemolytic disease of the newborn, and in legal medicine, is to a considerable extent an exercise in applied genetics. There is the current interest in the genetic effects of *radiation,* not only in connection with fears of the use of atomic energy in warfare, but also in relation to the medical and industrial uses of x-ray. The recent discoveries, dating from the beginning of 1959, of *abnormalities of chromosome behavior* have established a new branch of medical genetics. In relation to Down's syndrome, and to intersex states of various kinds, there are useful practical applications of the new techniques for the counting and examination of chromosomes.

It is unnecessary to multiply examples further. It is clear that the medical student must be taught genetics, first as a *basic scientific discipline,* and secondly, because of its *practical applications.* Moreover, it is evident that practical applications are rapidly becoming more numerous. There are many that were almost unknown, or quite unknown, ten years ago.

Instruction in genetics can be given at three stages before or during the medical curriculum. It must be given during premedical training in biology. It can be given during the preclinical course. It can be given during the clinical part of the course. Ideally, it should be given at all three levels.

Having no experience in premedical teaching, I will only say that we trust that our students will come to us with a thorough grounding in general genetics. Just one point may be made in this connection. When I was a student of biology (long before I had thought of turning to medicine), one of my favorite textbooks was Graham Kerr's Zoology for Medical Students. [5] I should like to quote a rather extensive passage from the preface.

(The author) . . . has kept before him three objects which he believes to be of pre-eminent importance.

1. To awaken and develop, so far as the animal kingdom is concerned, interest in biological science. Medical students are training themselves to be efficient practitioners of a particular department of applied biology. It is of vital importance that they should become inspired at the earliest possible stage in their curriculum with a living interest in the study of the animal body. One of the first endeavors then of the teacher of Zoology should be to cast over the minds of his pupils some of the fascination of the most fascinating of sciences, so that they may pass on their way quickened and inspired by the stimulus of its interest.

2. To lay an adequate foundation for the superstructure of detailed knowledge of the animal body imparted in the course of Anatomy, Physiology, and Pathology, with their clinical applications in the later parts of the curriculum.

3. To provide a reasonably up-to-date account of the more important animal parasites, more especially of the pathogenic microbes of animal nature, and the ways in which they are carried or harboured by members of the animal kingdom other than man.

Of these objects the last mentioned, though seeming at first sight to be very important, is actually of far less importance than the first two; for specialized knowledge of the type indicated can readily be added at a later stage, provided always that a sound foundation of general zoological knowledge has been laid. Many teachers indeed favour its relegation to a special course at a later stage of the medical curriculum. The present writer is on the whole in favour of retaining it in the general course in Zoology: 1) because the later parts of the curriculum are already much complicated by the multiplicity of subjects, and tend to become more and more so with increase of specialization; 2) because various parasitic forms of life are best studied along with their free-living allies; and 3) because many of the animal organisms that would naturally come into such a specialized course can quite well be made use of in the general course.

The analogy is, I think, a good one. Kerr's book accomplished all he aimed at. There is no doubt that it stimulated the interest of many medical students at a very early stage of their careers. Although the book stressed human applications, it was none the worse as an excellent general text of zoology. Indeed, as has been mentioned, it was one of my favorite books, although I had no thought at that time of ever taking up medicine. Those who are teaching genetics to premedical students could usefully adopt the same approach. Where a human example will serve as well as any other, and this is often so, the interest of students will be especially quickened, and a useful basis laid for application later in the course.

In contrasting the advantages of instruction at the preclinical and clinical levels, we encounter a basic difficulty. At the preclinical level, the student is not familiar with the abnormalities used as examples, or indeed with the principles of pathology. As one teacher of renown remarked, "A knowledge of pathology is what distinguishes the doctor from the layman." On the other hand, if medical instruction in genetics is postponed until late in the course, when a knowledge of pathology and the main characteristics of various disease conditions has been acquired, the student will have missed the illumination which instruction in genetics, general and applied, could have given him throughout his clinical years.

If a choice between the two alternatives must be made, my own preference is for a course in medical genetics *as late as possible* in the clinical years. This statement is made although many, probably the majority, of teachers will disagree with me. Most probably, the best plan is to avoid this disagreement by giving genetic instruction at both stages.

A course towards the end of the preclinical years should include *general genetics* with as much in the way of human application as is reasonably practicable. Thus, gene transmission in man should be stressed, and extended reference made to the manner in which inherited anomalies appear in human populations. This task requires some instruction in the methods of *population genetics*. The methods of *cytogenetics* should be demonstrated, and in these days the elements of *microbial genetics* should also be taught.

An accompanying *practical course* is of much value. Provided that an adequate foundation has been laid in premedical days, perhaps 12 hours might be regarded as a reasonable minimum time, although more could be profitably utilized.

If such an extensive course has been completed, instruction in the clinical years could be quite brief. The emphasis may then be placed on the demonstration of patients with inherited and partly inherited conditions, combined with the working out of family histories and a discussion of the principles of genetic prognosis. Provided that facilities are available, clinical lectures and instruction in the wards could largely replace formal systematic lectures.

The situation is different if the first teaching of genetics in the medical course proper is during the clinical years. In order to bridge the gap between clinical training and the general biology of the premedical course, systematic lectures will be essential. The student must be reminded of the principles he once learned, and be directed to their applications in the human field. It will probably be impossible in this case to cover much more than strictly human and medical genetics, but even such a limited course would be useful. A conservative estimate would be, say, seven to nine lectures, together with some clinical lectures or demonstrations. If necessary, it may be possible to accomplish quite a lot in four or five hours provided that this is all the time that can be spared.

In actuality, it has to be recognized that many students of the present day qualify without any instruction in genetics which is remotely adequate. At a number of schools no such course as the one briefly outlined is being given during the preclinical years. Consequently, there are several generations of students who would definitely benefit by a systematic course during their clinical years. It is to be hoped, however, that the time is not far distant when this schedule will become unnecessary. If the foundations have been securely laid, *instruction late in the course* can be concentrated on practical human applications, making the demands on these busy years relatively modest. Indeed, it may be possible to give a considerable proportion of this genetic curriculum incidentally during general clinical training. What is no longer possible, however, is to ignore genetics in the medical school curriculum altogether.

REFERENCES

1. Carter, C. O.: The inheritance of congenital pyloric stenosis. Brit. Med. Bull. 17: 251, 1961.
2. Carter, C., and Simpkiss, M.: The "carrier" state in nephrogenic diabetes insipidus. Lancet 2: 1069, 1956.
3. Childs, B., et al.: A genetic study of a defect in glutathione metabolism of the erythrocyte. Bull. Johns Hopkins Hosp. 102: 21, 1958.
4. Dean, G., and Barnes, H. D.: The inheritance of porphyria. Brit. M. J. 2: 89, 1955.
5. Kerr, J. G.: Zoology for Medical Students. London, Macmillan, 1921.
6. Lehmann, H., and Ryan, E.: The familial incidence of low pseudocholinesterase level. Lancet 2: 124, 1956.
7. Schwarz, V., et al.: A study of the genetics of galactosaemia. Ann. Human Genet. 25: 179, 1961.

25

Trends in Psychiatric Genetics in England

ELIOT SLATER, M.D.

Since early in 1960, reports of original observations on human chromosomes have been appearing in the British medical journal, *The Lancet,* at an average rate of nearly one a week. There have, in fact, been so many new studies of this kind that a number of the reports, although presenting significant scientific information, have been confined to the span of a letter to the editor. In addition, there have been reviews, annotations, letters of comment or criticism, similar publications in other British journals and, of course, two important specialized symposia.[5,18]

Since Britain is only one of a number of countries where *chromosomal investigations* have been pursued, the growth of this particular aspect of medical genetics may at the present time be regarded as almost explosive in its rapidity. Not only is it the case that established centers of research into human genetics have turned over part of their resources to work of this kind, but we also find that men whose background has not been in genetics proper — for instance, clinical pathologists in some of our great hospitals — have turned to cytogenetics as a field of extraordinary promise. While these developments have brought genetics into the center of the picture in the broad field of general medicine, they have also done much to bring psychiatry into closer view for many workers in the general field. Actually, there is not one of the chromosomal anomalies so far discovered which is not likely to be associated with psychiatric abnormality.

The effects have not been less impressive in the psychiatric world itself. Mental deficiency, so long an area of relative neglect, now assumes a role of central importance. It is here rather than in the pathological processes of later life, that the biggest contribution to our understanding of etiology is likely to be made.

It is as yet quite impossible to say how far and how fast further developments along this line will take us. However, we may confidently look forward to a rapid accumulation of items of new information, which, bit by bit, will sum up to constitute a map of the territory we have now begun to explore. We have already seen the adumbration of hitherto unrecognized syndromes, associating anomalies of particular chromosomes with recognizable clinical patterns, to add to the one certainly known case of Down's syndrome. We shall be able to estimate their individual frequencies, to begin with, in such special classes of the population as the mentally defective or the infertile, and finally in the general population as a whole. Rapid improvements in technology will

219

presumably enable us to implicate more and more chromosomes in the line of advance. There is definite hope, too, that regularities will be discovered in the mode of expression of the anomalies of each of them, in the frequencies of chromosomal mutations, in the relation of these frequencies to maternal and paternal age, and so forth. Finally, it may be expected that work of this kind will lead to the beginnings of an understanding of the mode of development of the pathological processes set in motion by the abnormal chromosomal constitution.

Two pathways can be thought of as appropriate and promising. One might, for instance, adopt one of the techniques of *animal genetics*. A systematic study of early human embryos might end in the discovery that specified chromosomal abnormalities resulted in a perversion of the normal processes of development taking place at a particular stage in the life of the embryo and affecting particular tissues. In this manner, the chain of cause and effect might be followed through all its ramifications. Grüneberg's brilliant elucidation of the developmental process in the case of the lethal cartilage anomaly in the rat provides a master-example of this approach. [9]

Another pathway would be to apply to chromosomal anomalies the techniques of *enzyme chemistry*. In our own unit, some work of this kind has been done. In a study of the mothers of patients with Down's syndrome, Coppen and Cowie [3] were unable to confirm the observation by Ek [7] that there were indications of thyroid abnormality in a raised level of protein-bound iodine in the serum. They did find, however, that women who had borne a mongoloid child at the age of 27 years or younger distinguished themselves from the older mothers by a raised androgyny score. An increase in the androgyny score was also shown by mothers who had had multiple miscarriages.

This observation led to investigation [15] of steroid excretion in the mothers of mongoloid children, which confirmed the existence of a chemical difference between mothers with earlier and with later maternities of this kind. Mothers who had borne a mongoloid child early in life showed a remarkable increase in the ratio of output of dehydroepiandrosterone to total output of 17-ketosteroids. The mean level was about twice that of the other mothers, and there was no overlap.

There are a number of possible explanations for this finding. One of them would be that the older mothers are constitutionally normal, while many of the younger mothers may be carriers of a balanced translocation, a chromosomal deviation from normality insufficient to cause any pathological appearance, but sufficient to lead to a difference in steroid metabolism. Hamerton and co-workers [10] have found that an increased incidence of mongolism in the sibships of mongols is practically confined to the families of the younger mothers.

In this brilliant future, are there any considerations which should act as a warning or as a caution? It would certainly be disastrous if all effort in human genetics were confined to chromosomal studies. In such well-investigated species as the fruit-fly and the mouse, it is known that of all observed variance which can be put down to hereditary constitution, only a small fraction can be allocated to gross chromosomal deviations. By far the larger part of the observed variation is associated with *microgenetics,* with single gene effects, the effects of combinations of genes, position effects, genetic-environmental interactions, and so forth. In man, too, we can estimate that at the end of the story a similar relationship will hold. If expansion in chromosomal genetics were to lead to the neglect of, let us say, biochemical genetics, we should be making a grave error.

I doubt that such a mistake will be made. The main development which has taken place so far has led to the influx into genetics of workers, money and laboratory resources from outside the genetic field. Among workers within that field, no great diversion has so far occurred. Furthermore, the psychiatrist can point to the fact that people mainly want to do and actually do the kind of research work for which they are fitted by temperament and special gifts. For instance, mathematicians are not likely to start looking down microscopes. One of the great advantages of chromosomal work is that the techniques of cell culture and histology rely on the gifts with which humankind is best endowed, the ability to manipulate and the ability to see, and hardly at all on our more stunted capacities, such as that for abstract conceptual thinking. If men of a practical turn of mind are enabled to play a larger part in the development of our science, it will be greatly to our advantage. There will always be plenty of tasks for the others.

These reflections might perhaps be interpreted as motivated by the need to console ourselves, for those of us who clearly are going to play no personal part in the exciting world which is opening up. If so, we surely have stronger grounds for hope. No major development occurs in science with its effects being shown in a single field. Work in frontier territories is always beneficially affected, and ideas and techniques which penetrate across the border are rapidly adopted. An illustration can be given from work in my own unit.[17]

Many years ago, Theo Lang suggested that *human homosexuality* might represent, in part or in toto, a form of intersexuality. The idea was supported by the finding of an elevated sex ratio, with an excess of males, among the sibs of male homosexuals. Only in recent years has a more critical test of this hypothesis been provided by the technique of nuclear sexing, and the result was negative. Pare[13] reported that male homosexuals were chromatin-negative, corresponding in their lack of Barr bodies with the normal male. However, this finding alone was not sufficient to dispose of the idea altogether that some anomaly at the chromosomal level may play a part in the causation of homosexuality.

It is well established that there is a very marked shift in both birth order and maternal age in the case of Down's syndrome, and there are suggestions of heterogeneity in the increased variance of maternal age in Turner's and Klinefelter's syndromes.[14] Hence, an investigation of the given background factors seemed indicated in homosexuals, and such a study was made in a series of male homosexuals admitted to the Bethlem and Maudsley Hospitals between January 1, 1949, and December 31, 1960.[17]

In this study, the *maternal age* associated with 355 out of the 401 homosexuals admitted was found to have a mean value of 31.3 years, as compared with 28.5 years for the general population, and 36.7 years for Penrose's material of patients with Down's syndrome.[14] In the homosexuals, the distribution of maternal ages was such that it might have been practically duplicated by a mixture of one mongoloid person to two members of the general population, and the variance of 50.8 was actually higher than that observed with mongoloid cases.

Maternal age is not a very convenient statistic with which to work, since it is subject to a variety of influences affecting marriage and procreative patterns in the population. *Position in birth* order is much easier to study and is closely related to maternal age. With respect to birth order, adventitious influences such as affect the statistics of maternal age are compensated for, with the birth order of the sibs constituting control material. If an individual comes mth in order in a sibship of n individuals, then the ratio $(m - 1)/(n - 1)$ can readily be calculated, together with its mean, variance and standard error. The limits of the ratio are 0 and 1, and the expected mean is 0.5. In terms of this statistic, the birth order of 389 male homosexuals was 0.58, a figure which differed from the expected mean of 0.5 by more than three times its standard error. In other words, homosexuals tend to come late in birth order, and this finding suggests that there may be a certain proportion of bearers of chromosomal anomalies among them.

This investigation may have been rather limited in scope, but it illustrates the fructifying influence of advances along one line on research along other lines. It is also mentioned here for the purpose of drawing attention to a tool of research which might be more widely used by way of a sieve, to sort out syndromes worth special genetic attention.

The knowledge which we may hope to gain from the study of chromosomal anomalies represents a breakthrough, by which psychiatric material will for the first time be used to provide the basis of a fundamental advance in human genetics. In psychiatric genetics, the debt is usually in the opposite direction, and the advances which are made are contributions to psychiatry rather than to genetics. Such nosology as there is in psychiatry depends as much on genetic work as on any other basic scientific discipline. It is the genetic findings in schizophrenia which provide the main justification for the present interest in the *biochemistry* of the psychoses.

The immediate prospects in *schizophrenia* are not entirely encouraging. With a lot of work done, nothing very distinctive has been discovered so far. We are up against the difficulty that any anomalies are as likely to be secondary to the total disturbance of normal life caused by the psychosis, as primary to the psychotic process itself. The outlook is probably better with the *affective disorders,* where investigations of water and electrolyte chemistry offer hopes of getting to an understanding of the basic pathology. When the time comes for the chemists to lay their hands on a good working hypothesis, we must hopefully look forward to the acuity of clinical research workers who will try it out on genetically defined groups. If there is a definable anomaly in the chemistry of the cyclothymic, it becomes of the highest importance to see whether the same or related anomaly is to be found in his sibs.

The vexing question of the heterogeneity of schizophrenia remains a live issue. Personally, I belong to the school which regards the bulk of schizophrenics as being related to a single genetic and pathological syndrome. This hypothesis would not exclude the existence of a twilight area of heterogeneity surrounding the nuclear group. In clinical work in a neurological hospital, I have been greatly struck by the occurrence in long-standing epileptics of *paranoid psychoses* very closely resembling paranoid schizophrenia.

With my colleagues at the National Hospital,[2] we investigated the histories of 69 such patients. It was found that the bulk of them were temporal lobe epileptics, with some degree of cortical atrophy being a very common feature. There were, however, some clinical symptoms which seemed to differ from those of the common schizophrenic picture, especially the relatively satisfactory preservation of capacities of affective response. On follow-up, the course of illness also tended to differ from that seen in schizophrenia. Deterioration of personality occurred with great frequency, but generally towards an organic type of personality defect, rather than a schizophrenic one.

The genetic findings in this study were even more distinctive. While the incidence of schizophrenia was not increased in the parents and sibs of "schizophrenia-like" epileptics, the incidence of epilepsy in their families approximated the rate generally observed in the families of what used to be called "symptomatic" epileptics. Apparently, there is considerable justification for the view reached by Gruhle[7] many years ago. According to this view, it may be assumed that the psychotic illness of epileptics, despite its close resemblance to schizophrenia, is not schizophrenic at all.

A different conclusion was reached by Kay and Roth,[1] who recently studied 99 paraphrenic patients over the age of 60 (42 patients from a British hospital and 57 patients from Stockholm) and compared these probands with matched cases of affective and organic illness. Among social and environmental factors which were reported as having been prominent in causation, deafness and social isolation were found to be particularly common. By contrast, evidence of a genetic predisposition seemed correspondingly attenuated. For instance, there was only a 3.4 per cent incidence of schizophrenia among the sibs and children of the 57 Stockholm probands.

Although this figure might have been due to heterogeneity of the clinical material, the investigators rejected this explanation. They claimed that all the cardinal symptoms of schizophrenia were shown by their cases, and the indications of hereditary loading were thought to have been more evenly spread than, say, in Stenstedt's study of involutional depression.[20]

In line with this pattern of reasoning, Kay and Roth regarded their genetic findings as most easily explained on a multifactorial hypothesis. In the predisposed personalities of paraphrenics, they say, we are probably dealing with extreme variants of the normal rather than with a rare and specific constitution. Monohybrid theories have to be buttressed by ad hoc hypotheses of reduced manifestation, influence of polygenes on age of onset, etc., and no theory of this kind is entirely satisfactory to the investigators. Instead, they propose that in the light of the new evidence which is now being accumulated about the importance of environmental factors, the simpler hypothesis that the predisposition to schizophrenia may be a graded character, depending on quantitative variation, merits more consideration than it has yet received. The all-or-none phenomenon, by which the predisposed individual is transmuted into someone recognizably suffering from schizophrenia, could be explained by threshold effects. Transitional stages between the schizophrenic and the normal are to be found in the formes frustes, paranoid psychopathy, and so forth. Conditions known to be due to single genes are probably less influenced by the environment than schizophrenia appears to be. The social circumstances, which have been found to be associated with schizophrenia in early life, are likely to prove to be causes of the illness, and not just effects, although their contribution may be less than it is in paraphrenia.

Since this is an interesting line of thought, it would be possible to find further support for it. According to Edwards,[6] it appears that the familial relationships of conditions showing quasi-continuous variation may closely resemble those seen in single-factor inheritance with reduced penetrance. He writes: "If we consider the simple cases of multifactorial inheritance, and of an abrupt threshold such that a proportion p of the population lies beyond it, then the intensity of familial aggregation shows a simple approximate relationship to p" (page 65). With a correlation coefficient of 0.5, over a wide range of values of p, the incidence in first-degree relatives approximates the square root of p. Edwards continues: "It is interesting to note that in the range of incidence between 0.1 per cent and 1.0 per cent, within which lie epilepsy, schizophrenia, diabetes, spina bifida, anencephaly, pyloric stenosis and mental deficiency of unknown cause, the incidence in first-degree relations expected on a multifactorial hypothesis is very similar to that found" (page 67).

In the proceedings of a special symposium of the kind we have the pleasure of attending here, one cannot possibly think of genetic contributions to psychiatry without touching on the vast field of *twin research*. None of us questions the value of the contributions which have been made through twin studies in the past. We are gathered at this institute to honor the work carried on by Dr. Kallmann and his school and to acknowledge the increasingly general recognition among psychiatrists that genetic work, and particularly work with twins, has done much to clarify fundamental psychiatric problems. Of course, we may ask the question whether there should be the same level of scientific investment in work on twins in the future as in the past. My own opinion is that the work should go on, but should be extended to cover new territory, rather than go over old ground.

In our twin research unit at the Maudsley Hospital, one of the two main groups of twins presently investigated by my colleague James Shields [16] is a series of twins from the general population, ascertained through a television program. This study was organized in such a manner that twins, who were willing to subject themselves to inquiry as volunteers, sent their names to the British Broadcasting Corporation. Among them were 42 members of MZ pairs who upon separation in early life had been brought up apart. Matched with an equal number of nonseparated MZ twins who served as controls, the given pairs were further compared with a series of 28 DZ pairs of the same sex, who had been separated early in life. On the whole, the design of the study has been such as to show up those environmentally determined differences in personality and life story which might be rooted in early childhood life. Despite some degree of repetition, this study is distinguished from the well-known investigations of Newman, Freeman and Holzinger[12] in that the number of cases is larger, comparable controls are available, and the line of investigation has been rather different.

In general, our samples showed almost equal similarity between members of pairs in both the MZ groups, whether separated or control, while members of the DZ pairs differed from one another to a much greater extent. This finding holds for all data on which correlation coefficients could be calculated, including height, tests of verbal and non-verbal intelligence, and tests of extraversion and neuroticism on Eysenck's Maudsley Personality Inventory. The only exception was the correlation coefficient in respect to body weight in females, which was much smaller in the separated MZ pairs than in either of the other groups.

With a more subjective rating of personality, environmental effects were more clearly discernible. As a rule, the MZ control twins were found to be more alike, though not significantly so, than the separated pairs. An attempt to identify the nature of this environmental factor led to the discarding of a number of plausible possibilities, but did provide a suggestion that the kind of home made some difference. The twin brought up in the psychologically less favorable home tended to have the poorer mental health rating.

Both separated and control pairs in the MZ category disclosed substantial evidence of similarity in mannerisms, voice, temperament, tastes and other aspects of personality, including sexual behavior. Personalities verging on the extreme with respect to quick temper, anxiety, emotional lability, rigidity and cyclothymic tendencies were no less concordant in the one group (separated) than in the other (controls). The variables which produced personality differences — some of which were quite noteworthy — were usually found to be multiple. Since physical and social influences arising at different times in life seemed to interact with one another, the effect of the original home background as a differentiating factor tended to be obscured. In some pairs, twin partners remained obstinately alike, in spite of relatively large environmental differences.

The other main series of twins on whom we have recently been working consists of nearly 200 pairs, in whom the twin index case had been given a diagnosis of neurosis or psychopathy by the admission service of the Bethlem-Maudsley Hospital. A few months ago, a detailed report [18] was presented on those cases of the series diagnosed as "hysteria."

Our main finding may be seen in the inability to confirm the status of hysteria as a genetic syndrome. At least, the data were of a very different order from what one would have expected if the disorder had been not hysteria but, let us say, schizophrenia. As you know, twin studies have been criticized on the ground that high concordances must appear every time, whatever the group investigated, and hence have little meaning. Obviously, this view is quite unrealistic.

In our series of neurotic twins, data are presently available on 52 twin index cases (from 39 pairs), admitted to the Children's Department of the Maudsley Hospital between January 1, 1949, and December 12, 1958. Varying in age from two to 15 years when first seen, all twins have been followed up for a period of two to 11 years, except for four patients whom we have not yet been able to contact. It is unfortunate, however, that the given observation period has not been long enough to take more than a few cases beyond adolescence into adult life.

Some problems arise here in deciding the method of calculating concordance. In eight of the 25 MZ pairs and in two of the 27 DZ pairs, the twin partners were referred together. Clearly, therefore, their referrals were not independent, so that the ordinary method of counting doubly ascertained pairs twice would not be justifiable. The alternative method proposed by Allen [1] would seem to be preferable. In this manner, we have found a concordance in MZ twins of 61 per cent, and in DZ pairs of 29 per cent. Clinically, the children constitute a heterogeneous material. Diagnosis in child psychiatry is usually allowed little importance. However, a rough and ready classification indicates that in seven pairs the principal problem was associated with mental deficiency, and in eight with an organic syndrome. The other cases were behavior disorders; 19 of the aggressive type, and 18 of the nonaggressive type. Differences in concordance between MZ and DZ pairs were more striking in the first two categories than in the others.

The previously mentioned study of separated twins may serve as an example of the use of genetic methods, designed not only to elucidate the existence of conformities which might be attributed to genetic causes, but even more to discover dissimilarities which might be confidently attributed to the environment. This has always seemed a very promising line of investigation, and it is a pity that when it is followed, the results are so often negative. It would be most welcome if the proponents of environmental etiology in psychiatry could provide us with some other controlled method of bringing out the psychological and social causes of illness and maladaptation. Such methods as have been used in the epidemiological and ecological approaches do indeed turn up interesting data, but always of a kind which lack critical value. For instance, the finding that schizophrenia is more common in the poorest social classes than it is at higher levels is somehow suggestive of environmental causation. However, the suggested environmental factors remain totally obscure, and the participation of genetic factors has by no means been excluded.

The difficulties encountered in family studies of this kind are demonstrated by the still unpublished results of another study of our unit, [4] which dealt with the psychiatric history of the children of psychotic patients. According to environmentalist views, these children should be more than normally liable to the neurotic disturbances of childhood, and also to psychiatric disorder of any and every kind later in life. However, the data obtained have not confirmed this expectation. Whether one dealt in terms of historical events or in terms of psychological test results, the children of psychotic patients showed no greater tendency to neurotic disorders than did the children of a matched group of subjects from medical and surgical hospital patients. Nevertheless, the findings were not entirely negative. Those neurotic disturbances which were observed seemed to occur preferentially during the two years following the onset of the psychosis in the parent.

Our original plan had been to match this study with a completely different type of investigation. The subjects for investigation were to be girls admitted over a calendar year into a so-called "classifying school," while the analysis was to be concerned with psychosis in the parents of patients with behavior disorder, rather than with neurosis in the children of psychotics. Unfortunately, however, administrative technicalities interfered with bringing this study to a satisfactory conclusion.

In closing, let me say that this brief survey may not have portrayed a full picture of present trends in psychiatric genetics in our country. I do hope, however, that my report has given you a fair idea of what those workers in the field have been doing in recent years, with whom I have been in personal contact.

REFERENCES

1. ALLEN, G.: Comments on the analysis of twin samples. A. Ge. Me. Ge. 4: 143, 1955.
2. BEARD, A. W., AND SLATER, E.: The schizophrenic-like psychoses of epilepsy. Proc. Roy. Soc. Med. 55: 311, 1962.
3. COPPEN, A., AND COWIE, V.: Maternal health and mongolism. Brit. M. J. 1: 1843, 1960.
4. COWIE, V.: Children of psychotics. Acta psychiat. scandinav. 37: 37, 1961.
5. DAVIDSON, W. M., AND SMITH, D. R. (Eds.): Human Chromosomal Abnormalities: Proceedings of a Conference Held at King's College Hospital Medical School. London, Staples Press, 1961.
6. EDWARDS, J. H.: The simulation of mendelism. Acta genet. 10: 63, 1960.
7. EK, J. I.: Thyroid function in mothers of mongoloid infants. Acta Paediat. 48: 33, 1959.
8. GRUHLE, H. W.: Über den Wahn bei Epilepsie. Ztschr. ges. Neurol. Psychiat. 154: 395, 1936.
9. GRÜNEBERG, H.: Animal Genetics and Medicine. New York, Hoeber, 1947.
10. HAMERTON, J. L., et al.: Chromosome studies in detection of parents with high risk of second child with Down's syndrome. Lancet 2: 788, 1961.
11. KAY, D. W. K., AND ROTH, M.: Environmental and hereditary factors in the schizophrenias of old age ("late paraphrenia") and their bearing on the general problem of causation in schizophrenia. J. Ment. Sc. 107: 649, 1961.
12. NEWMAN, H. H., FREEMAN, F. N., AND HOLZINGER, K. J.: Twins: A Study of Heredity and Environment. Chicago, Univ. Chicago Press, 1937.
13. PARE, C. M. B.: Homosexuality and chromosomal sex. J. Psychosomat. Res. 1: 247, 1956.
14. PENROSE, L. S.: Parental age and non-disjunction. In Davidson, W. M., and Smith, D. R., Eds.: Human Chromosomal Abnormalities: Proceedings of a Conference Held at King's College Hospital Medical School. London, Staples Press, 1961.
15. RUNDLE, A., COPPEN, A., AND COWIE, V.: Steroid excretion in the mothers of mongols. Lancet 2: 846, 1961.
16. SHIELDS, J.: Monozygotic Twins Brought Up Apart and Brought Up Together. Oxford, Oxford Univ. Press, in press.
17. SLATER, E.: Birth order and maternal age of homosexuals. Lancet 1: 69, 1962.
18. ——: The Thirty-Fifth Maudsley Lecture: "Hysteria 311." J. Ment. Sc. 107: 359, 1961.
19. SMITH, D. R., AND DAVIDSON, W. M. (Eds.): Symposium on Nuclear Sex. London, Heinemann, 1958.
20. STENSTEDT, A.: Involutional melancholia. Acta Psychiat. (suppl. 127), 1959.

26

Trends in Psychiatric Genetics in Scandinavia

ERIK STRÖMGREN, M.D.

IT IS DIFFICULT to express in words how much the opportunity to participate in the program of this anniversary symposium has meant to me. Throughout these 25 years, I followed Dr. Kallmann's work with great admiration, first from a distance and later through close personal contact.

Although my homeland, where our own studies in psychiatric genetics have been carried on, is Denmark, my report here will cover recent trends in this field in all Scandinavian countries. This extension is justified not only by a desire to do justice to the fine research which is being conducted in such other Scandinavian countries as, for instance, Sweden, but also by the marked similarities in our investigative procedures and the range of our population problems.

There are some obvious reasons for the longstanding interest of Scandinavian psychiatrists in genetic studies. The Scandinavian countries are distinguished not only by relatively stable and fully registered populations which are readily accessible to genetic investigations, but also by remarkable homogeneity in their social and economic structure. Whatever environmental differences do exist are limited in scope and usually so well known that they are easily appraised by the investigator. With environmental constellations being so stable and statistically assessable, it would seem to be a fair assumption that the majority of observable differences among individuals are due to *genetic* factors.

The expected interplay of nature and nurture is more difficult to evaluate in populations which are less stable and homogeneous than those in Scandinavia. Where an extreme degree of environmental variability is the rule in regard to both space and time, a greater proportion of individual differences may be explainable on *environmental* grounds. By the same token, genetically determined variations are more difficult to assess in a population that is known to be heterogeneous in its genetic backgrounds. Hence, Scandinavian psychiatrists have had definite advantages in attacking intricate problems of this kind.

As to the *methods* and *objectives* of psychiatric-genetic research, it is not surprising that they are closely related to those of demographic or "epidemiologic" investigations. Whenever a geographical variation is observed either in the prevalence or in the incidence of mental disorder, we must ask whether such a variation may be due mainly to differences in environment or to differences in hereditary background factors. In the latter case, it may be assumed that the observed variation is probably a consequence of *migration*.

In studying the mechanisms and effects of migration, preferably of migration *within* a country, it is important to bear in mind that most environmental differences encountered within a relatively homogeneous population are apt to be much smaller than those between two different countries. The implications of internal migration in a Scandinavian population have recently been investigated by Astrup and Ødegaard.[4]

In this study of first admissions to Norwegian mental hospitals, the rates of first admission were found to be significantly lower for migrants than for nonmigrants. The latter category was defined as consisting of persons who resided in their native communities at the time of first admission. Particularly low rates were connected either with short-distance migration or with migration from rural districts to cities. Migrants from cities tended to have higher rates, probably because of the atypical reasons for this type of migration. The city of Oslo formed an exception in that migrants to the city had higher admission rates than the city-born. On the whole, *selective migration* was regarded as the most likely explanation for the observed differences.

In the *prevalence* of hospitalized psychiatric patients, there are striking geographical differences even within a small country like Denmark. When we studied this problem in collaboration with Dr. Kaj Arentsen a few years ago,[3] the prevalence differences between counties were found to be inconsiderable, except for some geographical areas with a highly mobile population. While the prevalence was generally high in those parts of the country where the population size was stable or decreasing, it was comparatively lower in areas with an increasing population. Such differences seem to indicate that populations which decrease in size tend to acquire the character of "residual populations." One may hypothesize that persons leaving the area are usually in good health, while those who are ill, and especially those who require hospitalization for a long time, are likely to remain in the area. Even those persons who become ill within a few years after their departure may be expected to return to their place of origin where they will sooner or later become hospital patients. It is advisable, therefore, that we exercise extreme caution before we attribute the immediate cause of morbidity differences between population groups to special environmental differences between the areas compared.

In our current investigation of *migration phenomena* (University of Aarhus), the ascertainment of psychiatric subjects is limited to the County of Aarhus with a population of 220,000. It is planned not only to synchronize the rates obtained for different social, economic and geographical groups, but also to compare them at regular intervals. In order to relate these differential rates to the movements of the population within the county, a reporting system has been established which will provide us with information about almost all psychiatric cases. This registration center will receive reports from all hospitals and other institutions admitting psychiatric patients from the county, as well as from all medical practitioners in the district and from a great number of social and other official agencies. In this manner, we hope to accumulate comprehensive data on some of the essential factors responsible for psychiatric morbidity variations in different population groups.

For obvious reasons, *longitudinal studies* designed to follow a certain patient for a long time are also facilitated by the relative stability of the Danish population. The results of such a study were reported by Fremming,[9] whose population sample consisted of 5,500 individuals born in a Danish county in the years 1883-1887. This investigator succeeded in finding over 92 per cent of the given individuals at the time when they were 55-60 years old. Of course, his morbidity risk figures for psychiatric and other pathological conditions had a definite "age limit." In particular, little or nothing could be said with respect to the disorders of old age. It may be mentioned, therefore, that another psychiatric follow-up study of Fremming's index cases, who are now 74-78 years old, has recently been undertaken by Dr. Myschetzky.

The same *catamnestic* method, originally employed by Klemperer in Germany in 1933, [14] has been used by Professor Tomas Helgason of Reykjavik, a member of the staff of the Aarhus Institute during the last two years. His sample consists of 5,400 individuals born in Iceland between 1895 and 1897. That conditions for such studies are especially favorable in Iceland is demonstrated by the fact that Helgason succeeded in tracing 99.8 per cent of the total sample. He obtained direct information bearing on the subjects' mental health in 99.4 per cent. In general, it was found that the expectancy rates for psychiatric disorders in Iceland tended to be very similar to those computed by Fremming in his Danish material. The results of Helgason's study will soon be published as a monograph.

With respect to the much disputed clinical classification of *paranoid psychoses* in old age, one of the basic questions is whether they are late cases of schizophrenia or have an entirely different etiology. Since the studies of Kay and Roth, [13] Knoll [15] and Schulz [17] have been inconclusive, further studies are called for. Hence, a member of our staff, Dr. Thorkild Funding, is engaged in a still unpublished* study of the relatives of 152 index cases with paranoid psychoses which developed after the age of 50. According to his preliminary observations, the expectancy of schizophrenia seems to be higher in these families than in the general population, but significantly lower than among the relatives of schizophrenics. However, the total psychosis risk is practically the same as in the families of schizophrenics, although the psychoses observed appear to be non-schizophrenic in nature and evidently include many reactive cases and senile dementias. From a psychiatric-genetic standpoint, this seems to be an extremely heterogeneous category which requires further investigation.

In another recent study, Hallgren and Sjögren[10] paid particular attention to possible relations between *schizophrenia* and mental deficiency. They found, as Brugger[6] and Kallmann[12] reported before them, no statistical evidence for a genetic relationship between these two types of mental abnormality. However, one unexplained finding was an increased mental deficiency risk of 10.5 per cent for schizophrenic index cases as compared with a risk of 3 per cent in the corresponding general population. Although no adequate explanation could be given for this increase, the investigators rejected the possibility of a genetic causation.

In Finland, Alanen[1] studied the personalities and mother-child relationships of 100 mothers of schizophrenic patients, taking a special interest in the possible significance of these relationships in the etiology of schizophrenia. The

---

*Since this writing, Funding's study has been published in Acta psychiat. scandinav. 37: 267, 1962.

psychosis risk was found to be very high among parents of schizophrenics, and even higher among the mothers than among the fathers. Therefore, the disturbed mother-child relationship in these cases was regarded as an important factor in the etiology of schizophrenia in the children. This conclusion has been widely criticized, especially by Essen-Möller[8] who pointed out that the fertility of psychotic persons, and particularly of schizophrenics, tends to be lower than it is in the general population, and that the decrease in fertility is more pronounced in male than in female patients. This factor would suffice to explain the observed excess of mothers among the psychotic parents of schizophrenics, calling at the same time for a reappraisal of Alanen's conclusions which seem to have been accepted rather uncritically.

In the area of *twin studies,* Professor Kemp's staff at the Institute of Human Genetics in Copenhagen continues to collect extensive data on all twins born in Denmark during the period 1870-1910. At present, about 6,000 of these twin pairs have been traced, but the psychiatric evaluation of this material is only in its early stages. In Sweden, where Essen-Möller's department at the University of Lund is also engaged in twin studies, Dencker[7] reported on a series of 128 twins with head injuries, using co-twins as controls. There can be no doubt that this is likewise an excellent method of studying the effect of well-defined extrinsic factors, and it is a pleasure to state here that similar problems are being studied in Lund. For instance, Kaij's[11] investigation of chronic alcoholic deterioration in a series of 174 twin pairs yielded interesting information about the etiology of overindulgence in alcohol. Strangely enough, so-called alcoholic deterioration was not found to be significantly correlated with the degree of alcohol consumed. According to Kaij, the deterioration which may occur in some cases is not an effect of alcohol, but an etiological factor in its abuse.

At our institute in Aarhus, Drs. Juel-Nielsen and Mogensen carried out psychiatric-psychological studies in 12 one-egg pairs of twins who were 22 to 77 years old and had been reared apart. In view of the relatively small size of our series, elaborate plans were made to examine the twins intensively over a long period and to collect material from as many sources as possible. This type of data is especially important in such studies, because an adequate statistical treatment is impossible for many of the given factors. All twin partners were separated during early childhood and, despite some contacts later in life, have continued to live apart from each other. In many instances, the environments of the twins had been very different. The investigative methods included detailed psychiatric interviews (Dr. Juel-Nielsen), psychometric tests, electroencephalographic, electrocardiographic and other special examinations, as well as the usual tests for zygosity. The psychological tests were administered by Dr. Mogensen and included the Wechsler-Bellevue Intelligence Scale, Raven's progressive matrices, the Rorschach test and a few more specialized tests. Estimates of reliability were obtained by a retest which was given at least six months after the original testing.

I shall briefly review here some preliminary results of this twin study, the detailed results of which will be published as a monograph sometime in 1962. On the Wechsler-Bellevue Intelligence Scale, the correlation coefficients between the twin partners were 0.62 for the total I.Q., 0.78 for the verbal score and 0.49 for the performance score. The reliability coefficients measured by test-retest varied from 0.84 to 0.98 and were in agreement with those reported by Wechsler. The similarity between twin partners on the various subtests, expressed as correlation coefficients, ranged from 0.19 to 0.84, apparently in close relation to the reliability of the subtest with a range from 0.32 to 0.94. The correlation coefficient between the twins on Raven's test was 0.73 for the I.Q., and 0.79 for the raw scores. Thus it was found that the two members of a twin pair tend to have more similar scores than do people selected at random, and probably more similar ones than siblings in general. However, they did not resemble each other as closely as each twin resembled himself within a short-term interval on retesting. An analysis of the twins' intelligence profiles revealed that their high degree of resemblance was unlikely to be the result of chance. When environmental variations in formal school training were rated, a significant relationship between differences in training and test results was seen in the verbal tests, but not in the performance tests or Raven's progressive matrices. These findings confirm the data of Shields[18] on his series of separated twins studied at the Maudsley Hospital.

Statistical analysis of the personality tests was considered inadvisable. Instead, the personality description and psychological classification assigned on the first and second testings, together with a "double-blind" evaluation by another psychologist, were clinically appraised and then compared with the psychiatrist's descriptive categories. These independent assessments show a close agreement in the majority of cases, so that the testing added little to the information gathered through interviews.

In the few pairs of twins with psychiatric disorders, a close resemblance between the partners was observed in respect to their type of reaction, regardless of whether it was psychotic, neurotic, psychopathic, or psychosomatic in nature. In all cases, however, there were differences in degree and symptomatology which could be attributed with reasonable certainty to differences in the partners' life experiences in childhood or in later life. Similar tendencies were found in those pairs, who had no psychiatric history or showed evidence of only moderate psychoneurotic or psychosomatic symptoms. On the other hand, some of the twin pairs were strikingly similar in their personality developments or varied only slightly in their phenotypes, even though they apparently lived in very different childhood environments. The twins' electroencephalograms were practically identical in all cases and in both normal and pathological features. Extensive longitudinal observations undoubtedly reduced the problem of attaching undue importance to dissimilarities arising from temporary discordances or from the use of different systems of reference.

Another Danish twin study may be mentioned here, that of Norrie[16] on *congenital dyslexia,* not only because of its merits, but also because it has been published only in Danish. In a series of 39 pairs, all nine one-egg pairs were found to be concordant as to dyslexia, while 20 of the 30 two-egg pairs were classified as discordant.

In a Swedish study of 50 monozygotic pairs of twins and their families, Alström[2] re-examined the question of genetic factors in *intelligence.* Various intelligence tests were used to determine the correlations among family members, and their results were found to conform to theoretical expectations under the hypothesis of a multifactorial mode of inheritance. Like other investigators, Alström stressed the confusing fact that the given correlations may be higher as a consequence of assortative mating in these families, but he was unable to disentangle the ensuing complexities, thus confirming the need for additional studies of intrafamily correlations with regard to intelligence. Considering the vast number of intelligence tests which have been administered everywhere, it is indeed amazing that there have been so few careful analyses of intrafamily correlations.

In the *cytological* branch of genetic research, it is well known that laboratory activity has been especially lively in Sweden. It may be noted, for instance, that it was at the Institute of Genetics in Lund that Tjio and Levan[19] finally determined the exact number of human chromosomes. Much cytogenetic work is now going on in this institute as well as in the Institute of Medical Genetics in Uppsala where several new types of chromosomal abnormality, some of them associated with mental deficiency, have been described under Böök's direction.[5]

The exciting achievements which have been recorded in that particular field should not, however, draw the attention from the serious technical problems encountered in this new research area. Although various medical specialties are asking cytologists for immediate help through chromosome studies in relation to a great number of pathological conditions, genetic departments are still reluctant to take up large-scale studies because of the intricacy and laboriousness of the cytological work required. Lack of sufficient human control material adds to their cautiousness in accepting clinical specimens.

Therefore, one of the principal goals of contemporary medical genetics should be the establishment of close cooperation among the various centers engaged in cytological work. Immediate objectives should be to obtain sufficient control materials and to simplify techniques in such a way that mass investigations become possible. Such a cooperative organization is currently being developed in Scandinavia.

One might ask whether further advances in cytological genetics may be expected in the near future to make obsolete our traditional methods of *clinical genetics*. Most definitely, the answer will have to be in the negative. It is improbable that a substantially increased proportion of inherited abnormalities will soon be traced to specific chromosomal disarrangements. Even in the case of gross chromosomal aberrations, the result obtained by means of traditional methods and those obtained by cytology will have to supplement each other fruitfully.

REFERENCES

1. ALANEN, Y. O.: The mothers of schizophrenic patients. Acta psychiat. scandinav. (suppl. 124) 1958.
2. ALSTRÖM, C. H.: A study of inheritance of human intelligence. Acta psychiat. scandinav. 36: 175, 1961.
3. ARENTSEN, K., AND STRÖMGREN, E.: Patients in Danish psychiatric hospitals. Results of a census in 1957. Acta Jutlandica 31, 1959.

4. ASTRUP, C., AND ØDEGAARD, Ø.: Internal migration and disease in Norway. Psychiat. Quart. (suppl. 34) 116, 1960.

5. BÖÖK, J. A.: Clinical cytogenetics. In Gedda, L., Ed.: De Genetica Medica. Rome, Istituto Gregorio Mendel, 1961, Vol. 3.

6. BRUGGER, C.: Die erbbiologische Stellung der Pfropfschizophrenie. Ztschr. ges. Neurol. Psychiat. 113: 348, 1928.

7. DENCKER, S. J.: A follow-up study of 128 closed head injuries in twins using co-twins as controls. Acta psychiat. scandinav. (suppl. 123) 1958.

8. ESSEN-MÖLLER, E.: Mating and fertility patterns in families with schizophrenia. Eugenics Quart. 6: 142, 1959.

9. FREMMING, K.: The Expectation of Mental Infirmity in a Sample of the Danish Population. London, Eugen. Soc. Publ., 1951.

10. HALLGREN, B. AND SJÖGREN, T.: A clinical and genetico-statistical study of schizophrenia and low-grade mental deficiency in a large Swedish rural population. Acta psychiat. scandinav. (suppl. 140) 1959.

11. KAIJ, H. L. Alcoholism in Twins; Studies on the Etiology and Sequels of Abuse of Alcohol. Stockholm. Almqvist & Wiksell, 1960.

12. KALLMANN, F. J., et al.: The role of mental deficiency in the incidence of schizophrenia. Am. J. Ment. Deficiency 45: 514, 1941.

13. KAY, D. W. K., AND ROTH, M.: Environmental and hereditary factors in the schizophrenias of old age ("late paraphrenia") and their bearing on the general problem of causation in schizophrenia. J. Ment. Sc. 107: 649, 1961.

14. KLEMPERER, J.: Zur Belastungsstatistik der Durchschnittsbevölkerung: Psychosenhäufigkeit unter 1000 stichprobenmässig aus den Geburtsregistern der Stadt München (Jahrgang 1881-1890) ausgelesenen Probanden. Ztschr. ges. Neurol. Psychiat. 146: 277, 1933.

15. KNOLL, H.: Wahnbildende Psychosen der Zeit des Klimakteriums und der Involution in klinischer und genealogischer Betrachtung. Arch. Psychiat. Nervenkr. 189: 59, 1952.

16. NORRIE, E.: Ordblindhedens (dyslexiens) arvegang. Laesepaedagogen, June 1954.

17. SCHULZ, B.: Über die hereditären Beziehungen paranoid gefärbter Alterspsychosen. Ztschr. ges. Neurol. Psychiat. 129: 147, 1930.

18. SHIELDS, J.: Twins brought up apart. Eugenics Rev. 50: 115, 1958.

19. TJIO, J. H., AND LEVAN, A.: The chromosome number of man. Hereditas 42: 1, 1956.

27

Trends in Psychiatric Genetics in South Africa

LEWIS A. HURST, M.D., Ph.D.

Hailing as I do from the land of the Taungs skull and living within a stone's throw of the Sterkfontein Caves which house the fossil lady "Mrs. Ples" (the Sterkfontein Ape Man Plesianthropus), and working in a country noted for such eminent scholars and teachers as Lancelot Hogben, Robert Broom, Raymond Dart and M. R. Drennan, I should perhaps preface my remarks about South African trends in psychiatric genetics by some sort of picture of the more general genetic matrix in which these trends were cradled.

HISTORY OF HUMAN GENETICS IN SOUTH AFRICA

The *anthropological* aspects of human development spring to mind first, especially when we think of the diverse ethnic groups in South Africa, the Bushman, the Hottentot and the Bantu, in addition to the White population with its varied countries of origin in Europe. Our Departments of Anatomy and Physical Anthropology in Johannesburg and Capetown are fortunate in having such outstanding genetic workers as Professor Phillip V. Tobias and Dr. R. Singer. The former has done excellent work in basic and cytological genetics[35-37] apart from having been concerned with the application of the data of physical anthropology to evolutionary theory,[34,38] with the question of local evolution in South Africa versus hybridizing migrations, and with racial theory.[32] His investigations of Bushman-European hybrids[39] yielded the first recorded descriptions of hybrids between two such extreme human physical types as Caucasoids and Bushmen. One of his main findings was the lack of evidence of physical disharmony or infertility in the hybrids. It may also be of interest to note here that in extending the earlier work of Pijper[30] on the blood groups of the Hottentots, Singer and Weiner[31] observed very low frequencies of group O and high frequencies of blood groups A and B.

The liaison between *genetics* and *anthropology* was successfully fostered by the Institute for the Study of Man in Africa, founded in 1958 in honor of Professor Raymond A. Dart on his retirement from the University of the Witwatersrand. Since the principal objective of this institute was to study the medical and cultural aspects of the living peoples in Africa, as well as the life of their predecessors, a museum was established to enshrine and perpetuate the vanishing Africana. Within the broad over-all program of the institute, educational activities and information services in relation to man in Africa have been combined with the organization of research which covers anthropological as well as genetic subjects.

Other *genetic research units* have been developed by the Institute of Agriculture at the Universities of Bloemfontein (G. Eloff), Pretoria (I. D. Hofmeyr) and Stellenbosch (B. E. Eisenberg and F. X. Laubscher) as well as by the Veterinary Institute Onderstepoort near Pretoria. While Eisenberg[9] is probably best known for his biometric analysis of anthropological characters, Eloff[10] has been engaged in a genetic study of apperception. At the University of the Witwatersrand, Nolte's work on eye pigments and polymorphism in Drosophila, on swarm formation in the locust, and on genetic drift in sand mussel populations have aroused particular interest.[28,29]

Within the province of the *medical sciences,* it may be said in retrospect that human genetics was introduced to South Africa by Dr. J. G. Davel[6] in 1944. Subsequent studies of note which fell into the area of medical genetics were those of Griffiths[11] on the distribution in South Africa of the sickle cell trait; of Anderson and Leonsins[2] on the familial aspects of gastrointestinal polyposis (Peutz-Jeghers' syndrome usually following the dominant mode of inheritance); of Tobias[33] on an Indian family with almost 60 members showing an association of deafness with blue sclerae, arachnodactyly and fragility of the bones; and of Klintworth and Anderson[22,23] on a family which in five generations presented a combination of clinodactyly with marked hyperkeratosis (referred to as tylosis palmaris et plantaris). Particularly active in the cytogenetic field has been Dr. S. Klempman[21] of the University of the Witwatersrand.

It has already been mentioned that one of the advantages which we have in South Africa for studies in human genetics is the diversity of ethnic groups. Another advantage is the tendency within the White population to marry early and to have large families. Also, there is the fortunate circumstance that, in 1820, de Villiers published a monograph in which the pedigrees of all the original Cape Settlers were recorded. Thus it is possible not only to trace the ancestry of many South Africans through three centuries back to the original immigrants, but also to demonstrate consanguinity where it would otherwise be missed.

Equally helpful in South African investigations in human genetics is the manner in which Afrikaner families name their children. Until recently, all such families christened their offspring according to an accepted convention. The eldest son was always named after the father's father, the second eldest after the mother's father, and the third eldest after the father. Similarly, the eldest daughter was given the name of the mother's mother, the second the name of the father's mother, and the third the name of the mother. Therefore, if one knows the name of the eldest uncle, one also knows the name of the paternal greatgrandfather ("oupa grootjie"). Likewise, if the birth order of the father's and mother's siblings is known, it is easy to determine the names of their ancestors. Finally, invaluable aid in our family studies is often rendered by the Family Bible of Afrikaner families, in which it is customary to inscribe the names and dates of birth of parents and their children.

Retrospectively, it would seem justified to say that human genetics in South Africa came of age in 1956 with the foundation of the South African Genetics Society, which meets monthly in Pretoria. When the First National Congress of Genetics was held in July 1958, there were some 70 members in the attendance.

HIGHLIGHTS OF PSYCHIATRIC GENETICS IN SOUTH AFRICA

South African interest in mental health genetics is traceable to *the work* and *personal leadership* of Franz J. Kallmann of the Department of Medical Genetics of the New York State Psychiatric Institute, where we convened a few months ago to celebrate the mighty achievements of a quarter of a century.

In looking through the literature for this report, I happened—quite by chance — upon an article of my own, which was written in 1940.[14] The article commenced in the following way: "When the history of psychiatry comes to be written a century hence, F. J. Kallmann's demonstration, once and for all, of the hereditary basis of schizophrenia, together with the constitutional factors modifying the manifestation of this genetic predisposition, will overshadow the contribution of most other investigators." Even today I vividly recall how the editor had to tone down the more enthusiastic original version of my opening paragraph to the "restrained" statement just quoted. The given article appeared in the year of my return from a two-year apprenticeship in Dr. Kallmann's department. Since that time, I have attempted to keep in close contact with significant developments in his department and, to the best of my ability, have relayed them to my South African colleagues and students through my writings [13-19] as well as through my courses of instruction at the Universities of Capetown, Pretoria and Johannesburg (Witwatersrand).

For an appraisal of *original work* in psychiatric genetics which has been carried on in South Africa, the following selection of topics may be of particular interest here:

a.   Through the painstaking investigations of Dr. Geoffrey Dean of the Provincial Hospital in Port Elizabeth[7,8] and of Dr. H. D. Barnes of the Institute for Medical Research in Johannesburg,[3] *porphyria* has been shown to be a genetically determined disorder which causes severe disturbances in the metabolism of pyrrole pigments. The condition is relatively common in South Africa and occurs in both Whites and non-Whites. In the acute phase, the urine is reddish brown and darkens on standing, due to the great excess of porphyrin and porphobilinogen. In the stools, coproporphyrin and protoporphyrin are increased.

Psychiatrically, the condition calls for general attention, because approximately one-third of the South African cases tend to display marked emotional disturbances. In line with my own observations and those described in the literature, the psychiatric changes may be divided into the following main categories: paresthesias associated with psychoneurotic and hypochondrical symptoms, depressive reactions and other signs of emotional instability; delirious states; and an array of imperious, demanding, querulous and paranoid attitudes. Because of the prominence of psychiatric features, proper urine tests have been made a routine procedure for all new admissions to psychiatric services in South Africa.

According to Dean's genetic studies,[7] it is certain that in the common, adult form of porphyria nearly all White cases in South Africa are of old Afrikaner stock and are descendants of one forebear who came to the country 300 years ago. It has been possible to trace the genealogies of 32 porphyric families, in which a total of 324 persons (168 males and 156 females) showed clinical manifestations.

In one of the typical family groups, careful field studies revealed that of the 478 descendants of the forebear (who was born in 1814), 434 were still alive and traceable to Germany, France, England, the United States and the Rhodesias. Urine tests in all living family members showed that in the four generations descended from the original porphyric forebear, 48 per cent of the offspring of affected individuals were in turn porphyrics, with the rate varying from 41 to 54 per cent in the different generations. There never was more than one affected parent, with the over-all distribution clearly supporting the hypothesis of an autosomal dominant mode of inheritance. It was also indicated by the data that acute porphyria may be less frequent in men than in women.

In Barnes' porphyria studies among the Bantu,[3] the excretion of porphyrins and porphyrin precursors in 15 Bantu cases of cutaneous porphyria was compared with that observed in Whites with variegate porphyria who resided in South Africa and in a series of Swedish patients with intermittent acute porphyria.[8] Important etiological clues emerged from the finding of significant differences among the three groups.

b. According to observations made by Dr. Gordon K. Klintworth of Johannesburg Hospital (personal communication, 1961), the presence of *Huntington's chorea* has been established in 16 South African families. In the White population, the condition seems to be most common among the Afrikaners where it has been ascertained in at least five families. However, further pedigree studies may prove that all the Afrikaner cases belong to one large family. In addition, there are four English families, some pedigrees of Austrian and German descent, and two affected Jewish families in which the possibility of a non-Jewish ancestor could not be excluded.

"Colored" cases of Huntington's chorea (White-Negro hybrids) are known, but a reliable family history is lacking in most instances. In one Bantu family, the "purity" of which has not been fully established, the typical clinical features of the condition have been seen by Dr. H. Reef (Baragwanath Hospital, Johannesburg) in two siblings who had a similarly affected parent.

Klintworth's investigation confirmed the importance of a known family history of Huntington's chorea. While in some hospitalized cases the diagnosis may be suspected without a definite family history, it is often clinched only when it becomes known that the patient is a member of a recognized family. It is not uncommon, however, that a family history is reported as negative, although many other members of the family are similarly afflicted.

Another source of diagnostic difficulties is the fact that the children of clinically recognized patients may have been given for adoption. This possibility must especially be taken into consideration in unmarried women who had illegitimate children prior to the onset of their disease. In two cases of this kind in our material, it has not been possible to trace the children. Should they develop the condition later on, their cases would almost certainly be classified as "sporadic."

The attitudes toward Huntington's chorea in affected South African families are highly diversified. In some instances the majority of people know that their family was afflicted with this illness, but they do not think that they themselves have anything to fear, just because some ancestors had been affected by the discase. Such families rarely see any necessity for limiting their reproductive quota and not uncommonly have as many as 10 children. They simply refuse to believe in the hereditary nature of the condition, even though they are familiar with the histories of numerous affected relatives.

In at least two families, the spouses of patients were fully aware of the hereditability of the disease, but they kept this information from their children in order to avoid upsetting them unnecessarily. Such an attitude may account for the fact that, in certain instances, newly admitted patients seem to be truly unfamiliar with the existence of the disease in their families.

In a few families, younger people decide to disassociate themselves from the others when they discover the family history. While some of them have not married, at least one person is known to have produced several children in his marriage after he had legally changed his name.

It may also be noted that following the discovery of their long-concealed family history, several persons committed suicide. This observation confirmed the need of tactful family counseling services which were already advocated by Huntington[12] and Bell.[4] In the latter's report on suicides, 13 cases occurred in affected, and 7 cases in unaffected members of Huntington's chorea families.

In a limited number of South African families, there is a tendency either to reduce marital fertility in view of the family trait or to resort to complete childlessness through rigidly applied birth control measures. Some couples insist on having at least two to four children of their own, although they recognize that a certain proportion of their offspring may develop symptoms of Huntington's chorea later in life.

c. In a recent survey of neuropsychiatric conditions in the Bantu at the Meadowlands Clinic in Johannesburg,[20] *epilepsy* was found to be the sole category of sufficient dimensions to warrant reporting. Meadowlands is a residential district of the Bantu with a population of nearly 60,000 people. The district is divided into administrative zones of separate ethnic-group demarcation (Nguni, Sotho and Venda-Shangaan), representing a descending scale of socio-economic development and degrees of urbanization. It is planned to conduct a five-year house-to-house study of 10,000 households from each of the following four levels of Bantu civilization: (a) middle class (Dube and Diepkloof); (b) industrialized and partly urbanized (southwestern townships of Johannesburg); (c) rural (Pfokeng Location, Rustenburg); and (d) primitive (Sekekuniland). In our preliminary study, only clinic cases were used.

In this not yet fully investigated series of epileptic Bantu patients, particular attention was paid by the author to the *genetic aspects* of convulsive disease, while the clinical, social and demographic data were studied by the two other collaborators (Drs. Reef and Sachs). New light on the genetic background factors of epilepsy is urgently needed, since the opinions expressed by previous investigators conflict radically.[27] The importance of a hereditary predisposition has been stressed by Conrad[5] in Germany and by Lennox, Gibbs and Gibbs[25,26] in the United States. According to Alström's Scandinavian study, however, the role of an inherited vulnerability would seem to be negligible.[1]

Because of the large size of our Bantu families, the Meadowlands study holds out the prospect of making a substantial contribution to our understanding of the etiology of epilepsy. The average sibship size in the 46 index families studied is 5.8, with the number of sibs ranging from one to 16. As to the ages of the various groups of relatives under investigation, cultural limitations will make it necessary to be content with estimates falling within a defined age range rather than with precisely ascertained ages as used in other morbidity risk studies.

At this stage of our analysis it can be reported only that of the 46 epileptic index families investigated, over one-quarter (28.3 per cent) yielded at least one additional case of epilepsy besides the index case. This morbidity rate is higher than the one obtained by Alström[1] in his Scandinavian sample (8 per cent), but the meaning and validity of this discrepancy need further investigation. The mode of inheritance observed in the 13 families with more than one epileptic member does not seem to be consistent.

d. In the light of recent cytogenetic discoveries, Kluge's findings of changes in the polymorphonuclear leukocytes of patients with *Down's syndrome* were of considerable interest.[24] When the blood films of 60 mongoloids (and of some of their parents) were compared with those of 35 normal adults and of 60 mental defectives without mongoloid symptoms (matched for sex, age, and intelligence quotient), a high proportion of leukocytes with unsegmented nuclei was noted in the mongoloid series, revealing a leukocytic shift to the left on the Arneth scale. During the course of acute infections, however, mongoloids showed a normal regenerative type of shift.

e. Valuable *pedigree studies* included Wolpowitz' observations on a family with *Friedreich's ataxia,* in which the children and grandchildren from the three marriages of an overtly unaffected male were traced, [40] and a family with *spinocerebellar degeneration* in association with mental defect and convulsions, which was presented by Katz, Sandig and myself at the 1960 meeting of the Medical Association of South Africa. In the latter family, 6 out of 10 children displayed the entire syndrome (two without convulsions), while their parents were of low average intelligence and free of neurological symptoms. Certain variations in the clinical features observed in this family gave rise to a lively discussion of the question of pleiotropy.

GENETIC FAMILY COUNSELING

The demonstration of the need for well planned genetic counseling services as advocated by such distinguished workers as Dice, Kallmann, Kemp and Sheldon Reed was initiated almost immediately upon my return to South Africa in 1940, but assumed more organized form only in recent years; after my appointment at the University of the Witwatersrand in 1959, to be exact. Since that time, we have conducted free and entirely voluntary hereditary counseling services in psychiatry as well as in other branches of medicine. Most recently, all counseling problems in general medicine and surgery were taken over by Dr. Ingram Anderson.

To acquaint the medical profession and the general public with the scope of the services offered in our newly developed clinic, we have explained them through the press, suitable periodicals, and lectures to the various groups concerned with the treatment and care of mental defect, epilepsy and cerebral palsy. Also, the purposes and techniques of genetic family counseling have been dealt with in numerous lectures to medical students, graduate nurses, social workers, students of occupational therapy, and postgraduate students in psychiatry, preventive medicine and industrial health.

In geographical terms, it would have been impractical to limit our counseling services to case referrals from the Johannesburg area. Actually, many of our cases have come from Pretoria and other parts of the Transvaal, from the Orange Free State, the Cape Province, Natal and even the Rhodesias, thus reflecting a felt need for such services throughout the country and beyond it in Southern Africa.

While the volume of cases is not very great at present — some three to four cases per month — we have recently taken an important step forward in the expansion of our unit. Owing to the good offices of Dr. K. F. Mills, Medical Superintendent of the Johannesburg Hospital, our accommodations have been considerably increased so that the counseling service of our Medical Genetics Unit can now be considered as firmly established. Hence, we anticipate a much greater volume of referrals in the future.

EPILOGUE AND PROSPECT

As we look back at the past 25 years of genetics in South Africa in its various aspects, we may see some fitful and patchy developments, but at the same time, substantial and significant contributions. In the course of this development, we have noted the emergence of departments and organizations which promise to remain the stable centers of assured advance, inspiration and mutual stimulation. We have observed the coming of age of medical genetics and the sustained development of mental health genetics, deriving its concepts and main impetus from the work of Franz J. Kallmann and his associates at the Department of Medical Genetics of the New York State Psychiatric Institute.

During the year, a special vitality in our field has been apparent in several ways. Together with the contributions of South African geneticists at the Second International Conference of Human Genetics in Rome and with the scheduling of the Second National Conference of the South African Genetics Society in September, 1962, I would like to mention the acquisition of an electron microscope at the University of the Witwatersrand and the planned development of a cytogenetic unit at our Medical School, and, last but not least, the selection of the theme "Heredity and Disease" for the coming Annual Conference of the Students Medical Council (1962).

It is no exaggeration to state that genetics is in the air in South Africa. With our special and rich facilities, I venture to predict dynamic developments in the quarter century that lies ahead, in all branches of the discipline including our own.

REFERENCES

1. ALSTRÖM, C. H.: A study of epilepsy in its clinical, social and genetic aspects. Acta psychiat. neurol. (suppl. 63) 1950.
2. ANDERSON, I. F., AND LEONSINS, A. J.: The syndrome of Peutz-Jeghers. South African M. J. 35: 637, 1961.
3. BARNES, H. D.: The excretion of porphyrins and porphyrin precursors by Bantu cases of porphyria. South African M. J. 33: 274, 1959.

4. BELL, J.: Huntington's chorea. In Pearson, K., Ed.: Treasury of Human Inheritance. Cambridge, Mass., Cambridge Univ. Press, 1934, vol. 4.

5. CONRAD, C.: Die erbliche Fallsucht. In Guett, A., Ed.: Handbuch der Erbkrankheiten. Leipzig, Thieme, 1940, vol. 3, pt. 2.

6. DAVEL, J. G. A.: Some aspects of medical genetics. South African M. J. 18: 93, 1944.

7. DEAN, G.: Porphyria, a familial disease: its diagnosis and treatment. South African M. J. 30: 377, 1956.

8. ———, AND BARNES, H. D.: Porphyria in Sweden and South Africa. South African M. J. 33: 246, 1959.

9. EISENBERG, B. E.: A biometrical analysis of some anthropological characters in Bush-Bantu hybrids. South African J. M. Sc. 57: 8, 1961.

10. ELOFF, G.: Apperception in White and Bantu children. First Congr. S. Afr. Genet. Soc. (1958). Pretoria, Univ. Pretoria, 1958.

11. GRIFFITHS, S. B.: The distribution of the sickle cell trait in Africa. South African J. M. Sc. 19: 56, 1954.

12. HUNTINGTON, G.: On chorea. Med. Surg. Reptr. 26: 317, 1872.

13. HURST, L. A.: Seventh International Congress of Genetics. Ment. Hyg. 23: 677, 1939.

14. ———: Heredito-constitutional research in psychiatry. South African M. J. 14: 384, 1940.

15. ———: Research in genetics and psychiatry. New York State Psychiatric Institute, Columbia University. Eugen. News 37: 86, 1952.

16. ———: Applications of genetics in psychiatry and neurology. South African J. Lab. Clin. Med. 4: 169, 1958.

17. ———: Applications of genetics in psychiatry and neurology. Eugen. Quart. 8: 61, 1961.

18. ———: Classification of psychiatric disorders from a genetic point of view. Second Internat. Conf. Hum. Genet. (Rome 1961). Amsterdam, Excerpta Medica, 1961.

19. ———: Research implications of converging advances in psychiatric genetics and the pharmacology of psychotropic drugs. Third World Congr. Psychiat. (Montreal 1961). Montreal, Dunbar, 1961.

20. ———, REEF, H. E., AND SACHS, S. B.: Neuro-psychiatric disorders in the Bantu. 1. Convulsive disorders. A pilot study with special reference to genetic factors. South African M. J. 35: 751, 1961.

21. KLEMPMAN, S.: Sex chromosomes and abnormal sex development. South African M. J. 35: 701, 1961.

22. KLINTWORTH, G. J., AND ANDERSON, I. F.: Hypovitaminosis-A in a family with tylosis and clinodactyly. Brit. M. J. 1: 1293, 1961.

23. ———, AND ———: Tylosis palmaris et plantaris familiaris associated with clinodactyly. South African M. J. 35: 170, 1961.

24. KLUGE, W.: Leucocytic shift to the left in mongolism, with some observations on segmentation inhibition and the Pelger-Huët anomaly. J. Ment. Defic. Res. 3: Part 1, 1959.

25. LENNOX, W. G., GIBBS, F. A., AND GIBBS, E. L.: Inheritance of cerebral disrhythmia and epilepsy. Arch. Neurol. & Psychiat. 44: 1155, 1940.

26. ———, ———, AND ———: The brain wave pattern, an hereditary trait. J. Hered. 36: 233, 1945.

27. METRAKOS, J.: The centrencephalic EEG in epilepsy. Second Internat. Conf. Hum. Genet. (Rome 1961). Amsterdam, Excerpta Medica, 1961.

28. NOLTE, D. J.: Genetic drift in populations of a sand mussel. First Congr. S. Afr. Genet. Soc. (1958). Pretoria, Univ. Pretoria, 1958.

29. ———: Polygenic polymorphism in South African populations of Drosophila melanogaster. First Congr. S. Afr. Genet. Soc. (1958). Pretoria, Univ. Pretoria, 1958.

30. PIJPER, A.: Blood groups in Hottentots. South African M. J. 9: 192, 1935.

31. SINGER, R., AND WEINER, J. S.: Blood groups of Hottentots. Second Internat. Conf. Hum. Genet. (Rome 1961). Amsterdam, Excerpta Medica, 1961.

32. TOBIAS, P. V.: The problem of race determination. J. Foren. Med. 1: 113, 1953.
33. ———: Blue sclerae, fragilitas ossium, arachnodactyly and deafness in an Indian family. Am. J. Human Genet. 6: 270, 1954.
34. ———: Teeth, jaws and genes. J. Dent. A. South Africa 10: 88, 1955.
35. ———: The origin and behavior of the nucleolus in mammalian cells. Anat. Rec. 124: 372, 1956.
36. ———: Premeiotic mitosis: A new type of cell-division in mammals. J. Anat. 90: 570, 1956.
37. ———: Sexing tests and sex chromosomes. Leech. Johannesb. 28: 7, 1958.
38. ———: Embryos, fossils, genes and anatomy. Inaugural lecture. Johannesburg, Witwatersrand Univ. Press, 1960.
39. ———: Studies on Bushman-European hybrids. Second Internat. Conf. Hum. Genet. (Rome 1961). Amsterdam, Excerpta Medica, 1961.
40. WOLPOWITZ, B.: Friedreich's ataxia with an interesting family tree. South African M. J. 30: 846, 1956.

28

Medical Genetics in the United States

C. NASH HERNDON, M.D.

MY ASSIGNMENT is so broad and all-inclusive that one hardly knows where to grasp it. Of course, many other speakers have found themselves in the same situation. Three weeks ago I had the pleasure of attending a symposium at Duke University with the title, "The Commonwealth of Children." The keynote address was given by Dr. Grayson Kirk, the President of Columbia University. Dr. Kirk remarked that he had experienced some misgivings because of the broad scope of the title, and had requested some guidance as to choice of subject. He was told, "You may talk on any subject you like, as long as it is pertinent to the theme." Dr. Kallmann was equally helpful in writing to me recently that I might discuss "medical genetics as it developed here in the last 25 years, as it functions at present, and as it should function in the future." Dr. Kallmann must be laboring under the misapprehension that I possess the powers of succinct summary that were attributed to President Calvin Coolidge. It is said that after church one Sunday, Coolidge was asked what the minister had discussed. He replied, "Sin." The questioner persisted, "Well, what did he say about sin?" Coolidge answered, "He was against it."

So I can say that I am "for" medical genetics, but it would be beyond my abilities as historian, observer or prophet to paint a panorama of this subject in the scope and color that it so richly deserves. Within recent years, medical genetics has infiltrated and become woven into the fabric of each specialty of medical practice. Each of the sciences basic to medicine has found that genetics can contribute concepts and tools capable of opening new and exciting vistas in fundamental research. Medical genetics has become recognized in its own right as a subject essential to a well balanced medical school curriculum. Ample documentation for these statements has been provided by the interesting papers presented in this symposium. In 25 years the field of medical genetics has expanded and matured so much that a brief summary would fail to do justice, and a comprehensive summary would be impractical.

Rather than attempt to paint so broad a canvas, I would prefer to direct attention to certain events of a more personal nature that have been significant in shaping the course of development of medical genetics in the United States. Certainly, the event that this symposium commemorates, the establishment of the Department of Medical Genetics of the New York State Psychiatric Institute, was an event of major significance. I doubt if the announcement of the establishment of this department pushed much news off the front pages of the local newspapers in 1936, but it was news of much more significance for the future of the nation than many of the stories that drew banner headlines.

population genetics, and both groups may be startled by the reports of biochemists studying gene control of enzyme synthesis. Fortunately, this fragmentation is more apparent than real, and deals with details of subject matter rather than with basic principles of genetics. The genetic hematologist may become lost in the biochemical details of the enzymologist's work, but he can follow the essential genetic reasoning and see a clear relationship to his own work. For this reason, medical genetics continues to exert a unifying influence among the various specialties of modern medical science.

My crystal ball has been a bit cloudy recently, and I would certainly venture no specific predictions concerning future developments in medical genetics. As long as there exist research-oriented groups that emphasize the positive health aspects of heredity, progress will be continuous, logical and orderly. In my opinion, the future of medical genetics would be fully ensured if we could hope to have one scientist like Franz Kallmann in each generation.

REFERENCES

1. HERNDON, C. N.: Basic contributions to medicine by research in genetics. J.A.M.A. 177: 695, 1961.
2. KALLMANN, F. J.: Human genetics as a science, as a profession, and as a social-minded trend of orientation. Am. J. Human Genet. 4: 237, 1952.
3. ———: Heredity in Health and Mental Disorder. New York, Norton, 1953.
4. ———: Genetic factors in aging: Comparative and longitudinal observations on a senescent twin population. In Hoch, P. H., and Zubin, Jr., Eds.: Psychopathology of Aging. New York, Grune & Stratton, 1961.
5. Snyder, L. H.: Old and new pathways in human genetics. Am. J. Human Genet. 3: 1, 1951.

29

Genetic Research and Counseling in the Mental Health Field, Present and Future

FRANZ J. KALLMANN, M.D.

Now THAT ALL THE PERTINENT TOPICS have been expertly reviewed and the main editorial functions duly discharged, this veteran chronicler and senior beneficiary of our special anniversary symposium finds himself in a curiously unruffled frame of mind. His singular feeling of ease may be compared with that of a homeward bound seafarer who has just caught a glimpse of the familiar church steeples of his home port. True, the exact landing time remains to be entered in the logbook, and all the customs regulations will still have to be complied with. But when the harbor's lights are in view, no self-respecting sailor is likely to be bothered by the thought that his long voyage home was not always smooth.

So it is comforting to know that this concluding summary of current and future functions of a *genetic research and counseling unit* in the mental health field can be brief and to the point. It would be useless to anticipate a host of rhetorical questions that are no longer raised by seasoned mental health workers. In particular, few people will still express doubts as to whether the concepts and techniques of psychiatric genetics are now far enough advanced to augur productive work in that once dimly-lit territory forming the microcosmic matrix of man's precisely coded life processes. Instead, the most frequent question now posed is what to do about recruiting skilled manpower for special genetics units so that they can keep up with their expanding goals and responsibilities.

Here, cynics may interpolate, with a nod to the history of medicine and some of the social sciences, that provisional answers to this crucial question will depend not so much on the potential merits of the markers which mental health genetics would like to insert in programs of family guidance and the treatment or prevention of mental illness, as on the momentum of ingrained attitudes of unilaterally trained rank and file workers in the other mental health professions. More tolerantly, one may say that when it comes to accepting the modalities of new techniques in the behavioral sciences, there will always be some unavoidable lag. It may also be inevitable that unfamiliarity with refined tools developed by another discipline should breed boldness and contempt. At present, *cytogenetic tools* may fall into this category, regardless of how useful they will prove to be in family counseling, in the search for ionizing radiation damage to human chromosomes and genes, and in a multitude of other investigative pursuits within the province of psychiatry.

A. General Aims of Mental Health Genetics

Be that as it may, students of human genetics have long been mindful of the fact that this is "a world of changes and chances" (Pericles). Obviously, then, mental health programs, too, should be readily adaptable to the ever-changing pressures on a trembling world seeking peaceful solutions to such threats as grossly disproportionate population growth, creeping social unrest, and haphazard transmutation of cultural values.[7a,7b,8] Bush league practices in the management of crucial health issues only reflect self-deceit and are bound to hasten decline. By the same token, since "health is more than the condition people are in between acute illnesses and accidents," even the most irreverent professionals in the health services will not deny that such services "should be more than a commodity which is offered for sale or donated according to circumstances" (Le Roy, 1962).

In this generally stressful atmosphere, medical geneticists will most certainly be called upon to make real contributions to one of their *primary objectives,* that of guiding man as he struggles to survive in an expanding universe. Hence, every geneticist should be trained to act as expert guardian of all that is solid and good in mankind's genetic code. In discharging these professional responsibilities, he will be expected to protect diligently and with foresight born of knowledge and a genuine humanitarian outlook that which is capable of further improvement through intelligent use of modern technical and scientific principles.

Concerning the practicality of sound mental health programs for the control of intractable deficiencies of genetic origin, it is beyond dispute that there is no simple solution to the task of *guiding human evolution* toward unimpaired health potentials. Certainly, in the conquest of many severe pathological conditions traceable to disarrangements in the gene material, prevention through "biological education" will, for a time, be less difficult to achieve than a complete cure.[2] The general principle here is that each genetic condition has to be evaluated separately, with different solutions for each. Inevitably, "some defects are to be endured, others to be managed environmentally, and still others eugenically".[2] At any rate, while promoting a culture in which one can survive without being fit, we should give at least some thought to a safe method of repopulating the earth.

As to the direction in which man might conceivably learn to influence *his own evolution,* it has been emphasized by some of our finest scholars that selection can be employed with foresight.[1,4,10] In their opinion, with the deleterious effects of most mutant genes "diluted and postponed by an improved environment rather than obliterated," satisfactory population policies call for "birth selection, not death selection . . . for criteria of health, intelligence or happiness, not just survival and fertility."[1]

In line with this general objective, well planned research programs and adequate family counseling procedures become equally important functions of genetics in the mental health field.

B. Research in Mental Health Genetics

As to the goals of our *future research programs,* it is clearly the consensus of all participants in this symposium that thorough investigations at the molecular and chromosomal levels of personality organization cannot fail to enhance our understanding of the genetic aspects of variable health potentials and of a wide spectrum of human behavior disorders. It follows that neither the general nor the mental health geneticist can properly fulfill his functions without well equipped laboratories and appropriately trained research personnel.

In order to meet these two prerequisites for productive genetic research with a minimum of friction and delay, it has been deemed advisable in various countries to establish *self-propelling genetics departments* at every major medical center. Whether such departments specialize in the mental health field or cover all medical specialties would depend on the various factors that go into the local equation of supply and demand; or, to put it another way, on the local climate as determined by available facilities and resources and the preferential interests of the homegrown manpower.

Regarding *the optimum size and composition* of a mental health genetics team and its future research programs, it would seem prudent to heed Slater's warning against the mistaken idea that most of the traditional and necessarily time-consuming methods of genetic studies on human populations may soon be rendered obsolete by the increasing precision of micromanipulative and other cytogenetic techniques (see Chapter 25). Rooted in the complexities of experimental, statistical and biochemical genetics, our particular branch of genetics has grown into a subspecialty which permeates every mental health profession and gives coherence to all the medical and social sciences concerned with mental health and its major imperfections.

Hence, there will always be a need in our field for specially trained experimental scientists as well as for various other groups of workers who are *two- or three-letter men* with respect to their qualifications. The latter are necessary for exploring the quantitative and qualitative aspects of genetically salient mating patterns, or for the task of locating the most suitable subjects for cyto-chemical studies, or that of finding schizophrenics in a deaf population. For such comprehensive programs, we shall remain in need of the sampling expert as well as the twin researcher, the medical specialist as well as the psychometrically competent interviewer, the dogged foot-soldier as well as the daring astronaut willing to test the resilience of chromosomal structures from a long state of weightlessness.

In planning research at *the family and population levels,* neither human genetics in general nor mental health genetics in particular can afford to be an ivory tower science confined to the laboratory and restricted to theoretical deduction and impersonal extrapolation. Through concerted action they form a science of genetics *applied to people,* to benefit people, and to be understood by people for their own good and that of their progeny.[6,7b] The "disciplined imagination" of lofty theoreticians notwithstanding, most biologists are inclined to believe that "creativity and originality are good if they lead to something"[3] —something constructive, that is.

To illustrate the range and complexity of legitimate research and guidance functions which fall into the province of psychiatric genetics, our recently completed pilot study of family and mental health problems in a *deaf com-*

munity such as that of New York State may serve as a case in point.[11] Originally conceived as a fact-finding inquiry into the size, adjustive norms, vocational propensities and reproductive trends of an ostensibly well sheltered population group, the project began in something of a clinical and statistical vacuum. By cumbersome means beyond the comprehension of lofty theoreticians, it gradually proceeded to the documentation of a minimum action program for an aggregate of clearly frustrated but nonvociferous people who in an enlightened society would seem to need family guidance services with as much justification as any of their hearing counterparts.

Obviously, one cannot guide troubled families without knowing something about them, nor is much accomplished in the management of their problems by sweeping them under the carpet. On the other hand, if those textbook inferences were correct in crediting a deaf community with freedom from schizophrenia, suicide and delinquency, one might seriously consider remodeling our genetic and mental health services for the hearing along similar lines.

C. Training in Mental Health Genetics

In accord with the observations made in deaf and similarly afflicted population groups, family counseling facilities assume parity with the work of genetic research teams in the mental health field. However, they also require *trained personnel,* the supply of which depends on the availability of *special training programs.* In the execution of these programs, selected trainees, willing to work full time, should be taught how to shift their frame of reference from strictly clinical or experimental concerns to the health problems of families and whole populations. It is no secret, to be sure, and bears repetition here that a scarcity of both qualified personnel and training centers continues to be one of the major bottlenecks in mental health genetics.

This unwholesome state of affairs is known to our professional and academic authorities. It will have to be remedied before lasting benefits can be derived from those many tangible contributions that psychiatric genetics is able to make to our scientific schemes and preventive programs.

D. Genetic Family Counseling

Among our multiple family guidance functions, one particularly exacting task is that of providing scientifically valid yet psychologically undamaging advice in matters of *marriage* and *parenthood* where there is a pathological condition in one or both of the families concerned. Since there are no more momentous decisions in a man's life than the one to marry and the one to assume parenthood, a truly democratic society owes it to its citizens that anyone who is beset by doubts, whether well founded or not, should have access to competent guidance.[5,9]

This obligation is indisputable, even if one cannot possibly enlighten, comfort, or cure those who, for one reason or another, stay away from clinics where well intentioned advice is available. Fortunately, *an increasing number of people* are asking for and are grateful for frank information regarding possible genetic implications of their family problems, or the advisability of marrying and having children in the presence of a known familial disorder.[6]

The conscientious and soundly trained counselor will be guided by the *general objective* of the geneticist to encourage a person's feeling of responsibility for his own self, without negating the all important concept that a well-planned family is indispensable as a biological, social and cultural unit from society's standpoint, and as a source of strength and stability for the individual. When confronted with a calculable health risk in a predictably unstable home, the counselor will be sufficiently detached to consider that every child born "should be given a fair chance in life."[12]

It is also understood that in order to be of constructive help to unknowing or perplexed people, a good counselor is expected not only to elicit and discreetly evaluate the essential facts bearing on a family's decision, but to attempt to understand the given persons' fears and hopes, defenses and rationalizations. Since the majority of people come to such a clinic session with both *reasonable and unreasonable expectations,* they cannot be assumed to be capable of making important decisions in family matters without clear instruction and reassuring guidance. It is a common observation that even highly intelligent persons, when frightened either by some factual morbidity risk information supposed to dispel their state of perplexity and lack of technical information or by the need to be evaluated in their roles as actual or prospective mates and potential parents, may regress to immature levels of emotion and thought.

It follows, therefore, that information of this nature should neither be given in an impersonal way (for instance, in the form of cold statistics or through third parties) nor without sufficient understanding of the motives and capacities of the persons who come for help. Although the required interviewing sessions need not be categorized as a formal program of psychotherapy, they will greatly gain in effectiveness if conducted along the lines of *short-term psychotherapy,* aimed at reducing anxiety and tension.[9]

Another requirement of genetic counseling is that when the stage is reached where a program of action can be formulated without psychological harm to the person or persons involved, each step should be tailored to their *individual needs and resources,* both as to contents and manner of presentation. In many cases, of course, the decision to marry and the decision to have children will have to be dealt with as *two separate problems.* If one or the other question raises serious doubts, it will be advisable to act in accordance with the truism that healthy children (healthy in terms of genetic endowment, developmental circumstances, and emotional climate in the home) are both the product and the source of health in the parents.

While illustrative examples of such explanatory or manipulative forms of genetic counseling sessions have been included in some earlier reports,[7b,9,11] it should still be noted here that familiarity with *current adoption procedures* is another facet of a genetic counselor's responsibilities. When a preference for a couple's childlessness is indicated on genetic grounds, there emerges the need for a frank discussion of the modes of operation and potential risks of these procedures. Certainly, the hazards of unwittingly adopting the natural child of two schizophrenics overshadow the risks of harelip or diabetes in a child of one's own.

Justifiable fears of this kind cannot be allayed by the glib assertion that the effect of heredity in man is negligible.

E. Conclusions

In conclusion, it may again be stressed that as a member of a *health service team,* a professional geneticist is called upon to empathize with persons in need of guidance and to follow the age-old medical principle of *nil nocere.* It is just as inappropriate for him to create anxiety in a research subject as it is to withhold tension-relieving support from perplexed individuals when it lies within his power to provide such help in a counseling situation. At the same time, it is no less improper for any medical or other specialist in the mental health field to offer advice in genetically rooted family problems without being familiar at least with the simple facts of human genetics.

By giving sufficient emphasis to each of these three important functions of a genetics department in the mental health field, *research, training* and *counseling,* we shall be able to discharge our responsibilities to best advantage and take our rightful place alongside the other health professions.

If our anniversary symposium has helped to further this objective, it has been truly successful. Once again, may I thank all the participants, and express my personal gratitude by saluting their thought-provoking contributions with one of Lincoln's prophetic messages fully suited to our era of scientific upheaval:

"The dogmas of the quiet past are inadequate to the stormy present . . .as our case is new, so we must think anew and act anew."

REFERENCES

1. Crow, J. F.: Mechanisms and trends in human evolution. Daedalus 90: 416, 1961.
2. Dobzhansky, T.: Man and natural selection. Am. Scientist 48: 285, 1961.
3. Eiduson, B. T.: Scientists: Their Psychological World. New York, Basic Books, 1962.
4. Herndon, C. N.: Basic contributions to medicine by research in genetics. J.A.M.A. 177: 695, 1961
5. ———, and Nash, E. M.: Premarriage and marriage counseling. J.A.M.A. 180: 395, 1962.
6. Kallmann, F. J.: Heredity in Health and Mental Disorder. New York, Norton, 1953.
7a. ———: Heredity in the etiology of disordered behavior. In Hoch, P. H. and Zubin, J., Eds.: Comparative Epidemiology of the Mental Disorders. New York, Grune & Stratton, 1961.
7b. ———: New goals and perspectives in human genetics. A. Ge. Me. Ge. 10: 377, 1961.
8. ———: The future of psychiatry in the perspective of genetics. In Hoch, P. H., and Zubin, J., Eds.: The Future of Psychiatry. New York, Grune & Stratton, 1962.
9. ———, and Rainer, J. D.: Psychotherapeutically oriented counseling techniques in the setting of a medical genetics department. In Stokvis, B., Ed.: Topical Problems of Psychotherapy. Basel, Karger, Vol. 4, in press.
10. Muller, H. J.: Survival. A.I.B.S. Bull. 40: 15, 1961.
11. Rainer, J. D., Altshuler, K. Z., and Kallmann, F. J. (Eds.): Family and Mental Health Problems in a Deaf Population. In press.
12. Slater, E.: Galton's heritage. Eugen. Rev. 52: 91, 1960.

30

Discussion

Dr. Baroff

In discussing the genetic aspects of Down's syndrome, Dr. Jervis suggested that the risk of having another affected child may not be the same in cases of a trisomy 21-anomaly and in those involving a chromosomal translocation. This difference would seem to be an important point to be taken into consideration in genetic family counseling.

Dr. Jervis

This problem has been dealt with in a recent article by Hamerton et al. (Lancet 2: 956, 1961). Apparently, if the defect is due to a translocation, the chances of having a second affected child is greater for female than for male carriers.

Dr. Impastato

In using anectine to relax the muscles during electroshock therapy, we have encountered a number of patients who violently react even to such small doses as 5 mg. I understand that this unusual reaction has been ascribed to a genetically determined low titer of pseudocholinesterase. It would be of interest to know whether geneticists have made some progress in studying this problem.

Dr. Rond

I should like to know whether there are some genetic data on the psychoneuroses. It appears that at least the hysterical reaction syndrome and the mixed type of psychoneurosis have some constitutional basis.

Dr. Slater

It has been emphasized by Dr. Jarvik that the various specific forms of drug idiosyncrasy, including susceptibility to the effect of anectine, are extremely important from a genetic as well as from a clinical standpoint. In England, I believe, it is Dr. A. C. Stevenson who has taken a particular interest in this complex field. I have also been told by Dr. Roberts that according to Dr. Lehmann's data, the incidence of pseudocholinesterase deficiency in the population seems to be as high as one in 1000 persons for the homozygous recessive condition.

As to the genetic aspects of the psychoneuroses may I say that at the Bethlem and Maudsley Hospitals in London, we have collected extensive data on a consecutive series of neurotic patients who are twins. While our total series consists at present of approximately 200 same-sex pairs in the adult range, only our study of hysteria in twins has been completed. The results have been presented in a recent paper entitled "Hysteria 311" (J. Ment. Sc. 107: 359, 1961), since the international code number of hysteria is 311.

According to our findings, the category of hysteria cases seems to be a heterogeneous one. In other words, the classification "hysteria 311" is really a code number rather than a syndrome. With approximately equal concordance rates for monozygotic and dizygotic twin pairs, there appears to be no sound basis for considering hysteria a unified genetic syndrome.

As to other types of psychoneurosis, however, it is unlikely that our data will yield evidence of a similar degree of heterogeneity. In obsessive-compulsive states, for example, we expect to find a relatively homogeneous syndrome with a genetic basis. The same seems to be true for certain anxiety and tension states. On the other hand, psychopathic personality will probably prove to be a heterogeneous classification. Like hysteria, it may have to be regarded as a clinical category comprising diverse conditions rather than as a specific syndrome.

Dr. Kalinowsky

I would like Dr. Strömgren to say a few words about sterilization laws in the Scandinavian countries and the practical effectiveness of these laws.

Dr. Malamud

Would Dr. Strömgren be good enough to elaborate on those conditions facilitating genetic and demographic studies in Scandinavian countries?

Dr. Strömgren

The given laws are different in each country. In Denmark we have two laws which date back to the 1930's: one concerning mental defectives and the second concerning other categories of mentally disturbed persons who may need sterilization. In theory, involuntary sterilization is possible, but it has never been used. In actual practice, sterilization is limited to those cases of severe mental deficiency where there is a definite eugenic risk, and to cases where childlessness is important from the standpoint of the individual's health or social adaption. The eugenic consequences of severe mental disorders, such as schizophrenia, may not have been very great because of the reduced fertility of these patients. With regard to mental deficiency, however, Professor Tage Kemp has estimated that the number of new mental deficiency cases is now half the figure that it would have been if our sterilization law had not been in effect for the last 25 years. The adjustment problems after sterilization have been explored by Martin Ekblad in a follow-up study of 225 Swedish women(Acta psychiat. scandinav. [suppl. 161] 37, 1961).

As to Dr. Malamud's question, may I re-emphasize that Scandinavian countries are particularly suitable for family and population studies because of our registration systems and the homogeneous social structure of the population. We have virtually no difficulty in locating all our research subjects, even if we know only where they lived 25 years ago.

Dr. Holt

It is well known that many members of the clergy function in the role of marriage counselors, advising prospective couples about their degree of fitness to marry and to have children. Although some of us believe that this is primarily a medical problem in many instances, I would like to know Dr. Kallmann's attitude toward the advisability of holding educational courses for interested members of the clergy to prepare them for their marriage counseling responsibilities.

Dr. Kallmann

In my opinion, everything that has been said regarding the social responsibilities of professional mental health workers would seem to be valid for various clergymen, too. Whenever they are called upon to act as family counselors in the presence of a clearly recognizable case of mental disorder or mental defect of possibly hereditary origin, it would be most helpful for them to be familiar with the simple facts of human genetics. A similar statement may be made with respect to the professional personnel of adoption agencies.

SECTION V: TESTIMONIALS AND AWARDS

31

Anniversary Banquet

LAWRENCE C. KOLB, M.D.

TASTEFULLY ATTUNED to the serene setting of Columbia University's Faculty Club, the banquet session in honor of the 25th anniversary of our Medical Genetics Department was a most congenial affair. A flair of academic dignity was added to the decorum of a convivial family dinner by the presence of many distinguished guests, who joined the symposium participants and a score of other friends of Dr. Kallmann's group to celebrate this important milestone in the growth and recognition of their solidly established research organization in the field of psychiatric genetics. Fittingly, full shares of the tribute which the speakers of the session paid to the department's work during the past 25 years went to Helly Kallmann as one of the most loyal and widely traveled members of its research staff; to Dr. Nolan D. C. Lewis; Dr. Paul Klemperer, Dr. David Levy and General Frederick Osborn as the earliest supporters of its research program present at the banquet; and to all the former and current members of the departmental staff, both those who were present and those who were not.

Of the co-sponsoring societies, the American Psychopathological Association was represented by Dr. Lauretta Bender; the American Eugenics Society by Dr. Harry Shapiro; the American Society of Human Genetics by Dr. C. Nash Herndon; the National Association for Mental Health by Dr. William Malamud; and the Eastern Psychiatric Research Association by Dr. Charles Buckman. The congratulations of the Governor and the Department of Mental Hygiene of the State of New York were expressed by Commissioner Paul H. Hoch, and those of Columbia University by its Vice President in charge of medical affairs, Dean H. Houston Merritt. Both speakers pointed to the impressive advances of genetics into every branch of the basic as well as the clinical sciences and acclaimed Dr. Kallmann's leadership in traversing the no man's land between human genetics and clinical psychiatry.

Other congratulants were Dr. Bentley Glass for the participants in the symposium, Dr. William Horwitz for the clinical services of the Psychiatric Institute, Dr. Sandor Rado for the New York School of Psychiatry, and the Nobel Prize laureate and neurospora expert, Dr. Edward L. Tatum, for the basic sciences. Each of them added some intriguing background material for a biographical sketch of Dr. Kallmann's career as may be exemplified by a few brief excerpts.

258

Dr. Glass

In a recent UNESCO report, convincing evidence was presented to substantiate the estimate that the amount of significant scientific knowledge in the twentieth century is doubling about every 10 years. At this rate of advance, it is safe to predict that teachers of human biology will soon have to spend one year out of three as learners. We have entered an era in which even the average tenth-grade student wants to know about DNA and RNA as well as the structure and control of enzymes. In other words, the real problem in our current generation is not concerned with the students but with the teachers.

At this juncture, I appreciate the opportunity to pay tribute to my good friend, Franz Kallmann. Not only has he made great contributions to our present volume of significant scientific knowledge in one important area of human genetics, but he has always remained a learner himself. At a very early stage, he clearly saw the crucial relationship of one scientific field to another, and he was the first president of the American Society of Human Genetics who succeeded in bringing the disciplines of medicine and genetics together. I hope that none of us will ever forget this achievement.

Dr. Rado

Earlier this evening, our chairman identified several guests as witnesses of the birth of Dr. Kallmann's department. This reference places my report into the position of an authentic account of the prenatal period of this department or, at least, of its chief worker. In 1926-27 and 1927-28, when Dr. Kallmann was an assistant of Prof. Karl Bonhoeffer, the noted chairman of the department of psychiatry and neurology at the University of Berlin, he was advised by his chief to become a student at the Berlin Psychoanalytic Institute where I was one of the teachers. Some years later, when we began to teach psychoanalysis at the New York State Psychiatric Institute where he had meanwhile established his own department, we decided to ask him to teach genetics in our basic science course.

Needless to say, our psychoanalytic graduate students were somewhat bewildered at this decision, and a similar degree of reluctance was observed when we included Dr. Kallmann's lectures on genetics in our present psychoanalytic training course for state hospital residents. The position of genetics in medicine was still very shaky in those years, and our students had to be requested "to be a little patient" when they wanted to know what genetics had to do with psychoanalysis. I told them that both genetics and psychoanalysis would gradually change, and that their common features would become obvious with further advances in scientific knowledge.

As we are now standing at the threshhold of an era in which the entire proud edifice of medicine — including psychiatry as a whole as well as psychoanalysis — will rest on genetics, all our students are pleased to have the necessary foundations in this rapidly advancing science. I am glad to have this opportunity, therefore, to express on my own behalf and that of the New York School of Psychiatry our deep appreciation to Dr. Kallmann from whom we have learned so much. We are proud to have him as one of our teachers, while my personal impression is that he had a unique pleasure in his life when he began to work in genetics.

Dr. Tatum

Although I am not a psychiatrist, I consider it a great privilege to add my voice to the well deserved tribute which has been paid to Dr. Kallmann for his leadership and inspiration in firmly establishing genetics in the medical sciences. He is widely admired as a man who was far ahead of his time in recognizing the significance of our genetic heritage and that of the science of genetics in medicine and human biology in general and in the areas of mental health and mental disorder in particular. In acknowledging our esteem for a resourceful research worker of his stature, we owe it to ourselves to look forward, with the same clarity of thinking as has been shown by Dr. Kallmann during the past 25 years, to the ever growing scope of genetics in the public health field. It is obvious, too, that future medical generations cannot fulfill their obligations to humanity, unless they are adequately trained in genetics.

The need of well balanced medical school courses in genetics, so emphatically alluded to by Dr. Tatum, was fully endorsed by the principal speaker of the session, Dr. John A. Fraser Roberts of the famous Hospital for Sick Children in London. The informative address of this experienced geneticist, printed in full in another section of the proceedings (Chapter 24), was a veritable masterpiece of scientific objectivity and fair understatement.

The evening session came to a close with the presentation of the EPRA Gold Medal to Dr. Kallmann (Chapter 33 and frontispiece), his modest speech of thanks for the many honors and congratulations received by him, and a hilarious talk by the ladies' committee representative, Mrs. J. A. F. Roberts. Although the report of this well-known English actress was less concerned with chromosomes and genes than with certain evolutionary aspects of human anatomy, it was wildly applauded.

Altogether, it was a most enjoyable evening.

32

Presentation of R. Thornton Wilson Awards in Genetic and Preventive Psychiatry (1961)

ALEXANDER G. BEARN, M.D.

AS THIS EXCELLENT SYMPOSIUM comes to a close, ending a truly memorable event influenced so much by the work and the name of Dr. Kallmann, it is my proud privilege to present the R. Thornton Wilson Awards for the year 1961. As you know, these two awards are given to contributors of scientific reports within the broad areas of genetic and preventive psychiatry, one award going to a research worker in the basic sciences, the other for research at the clinical level.

On behalf of the Awards Committee, consisting of Dr. William L. Holt, Jr., Dr. William Malamud and myself, may I say that we deliberated long and hard to select the two contributions. It is no ordinary platitude to state that this was a formidable task, in view of the high scientific quality of all papers and the excellence of their presentations.

In selecting a contribution to the *basic aspects* of psychiatric genetics, we have been mindful of the fact that despite occasional fears to the contrary, basic research often sheds light on the clinical problems of the day. In no field has this truism been more self evident than in *human cytogenetics*. Tjio and Levan's discovery that the chromosomal complement of man is formed by 46 and not by 48 chromosomes, and Lejeune's finding that the usual form of Down's syndrome (mongolism) tends to be associated with a complement of 47 chromosomes, precipitated what has been appropriately referred to as a *chromosomal explosion*. In these days when explosions are so frequently to the detriment of mankind, it is good to be able to recognize an explosion aimed at a better understanding of human problems.

One of the chief architects of this noninjurious explosion has been Dr. Ferguson-Smith. On account of his original research, his mature scholarship and the brilliance of his presentation in this symposium, he is deemed a particularly worthy recipient of the Wilson Award in the basic sciences.

In the area of research at *the clinical level,* it is the opinion of the committee that the contribution made by the team of Dr. Kenneth Z. Altshuler and Dr. Bruce Sarlin is especially outstanding by its scholarly approach and the clarity of its conclusions. Their investigation into the interrelation of communication stress (deafness), maturation lag and schizophrenia risk has elucidated the relationship of stress to schizophrenia. It is with great pleasure that I ask Dr. Altshuler and Dr. Sarlin on behalf of the committee to share the second Wilson Award.

33

Presentation of the Eastern Psychiatric Research Association Gold Medal for Special Scientific Achievement

DAVID J. IMPASTATO, M.D.

Secretary-Treasurer, Eastern Psychiatric Research Association

ON BEHALF of the Eastern Psychiatric Research Association (EPRA), I am honored to present a deserving scholar with our Gold Medal which is awarded now and then for *special scientific achievement*. The medal, artfully designed by Mr. Leon Mednikow of New York City, has been awarded only once. The first recipient was Dr. Ugo Cerletti, the noted Italian psychiatrist who recently received an honorary M.D. degree from the University of Montreal.

The second recipient is known to every member of our society and to many scientists throughout the world. Some of us have come to know him only through his writings or those of his colleagues. Others, much more fortunate, have come to know him as students or associates. Beginning with what at first appeared to be a side interest, his achievements have been very imposing. With the selfless and unending help of his wife, Helly, and that of a few devoted associates, he nurtured this apparent side interest into one of the major trends in contemporary psychiatry; namely, *psychiatric genetics*.

It would seem to be appropriate here to give you a brief account of the professional background of this tireless research worker: Franz J. Kallmann, presently Professor of Psychiatry at Columbia University, received his M.D. degree in 1919 from the University of Breslau (Silesia), the same university where his public-spirited father was trained to be a surgeon. In 1928, following his training in psychiatry, criminology, psychoanalysis and neuropathology, he became director of the neuropathological laboratories of two mental hospitals in Berlin and, at the same time, was given a fellowship at the celebrated Max Planck Institute of Psychiatry in Munich where he was associated with such well known geneticists as Rüdin, Lange, Luxenburger, Bruno Schulz, and others. Under this influence, with his interest in genetic family investigations fully aroused, he immediately set out on his first major research project in psychiatric genetics, a study of the incidence of schizophrenia among the siblings and descendants of 1,087 schizophrenic hospital patients. The data collected in this extensive study formed the basis for his first book, The Genetics of Schizophrenia (1938).

Luckily for us, before this book was published here, Dr. Kallmann had come to the New York State Psychiatric Institute (1936) where he organized the

---

For illustration of Gold Medal, see frontispiece.

first research department in psychiatric genetics. Through his painstaking work, his foresight, his persistence, his teaching, his inspiration, his meticulousness in organization and his multidisciplinary approach to medical research, he gradually developed the discipline of psychiatric genetics to that level where we may truly say today that it has come to flower. Current interest in medical genetics is widespread as is indicated by the eagerness with which chairs of genetics are being established throughout the country, as well as by the ever increasing number of scientific papers, symposia and textbooks on this subject. Our own symposium marks 25 years of psychiatric genetics in the United States, made possible only through Dr. Kallmann's thinking, planning, working and organizing.

It has already been mentioned in this symposium that Dr. Kallmann gave the Salmon Memorial Lectures in 1952 and the Hamilton Memorial Lecture in 1960. The former lectures were published under the title of "Heredity in Health and Mental Disorder" (1953). He also helped to organize the American Society of Human Genetics as well as the International Congresses of Human Genetics in Copenhagen (1956) and Rome (1961). For these many accomplishments, the University of Torino bestowed on him an honorary M.D. degree in 1957.

These are but few of the honors and achievements of Franz J. Kallmann. He himself seems especially proud of two of the many things he has done: First, his long collaboration and companionship with his dear wife who is as devoted to him in the laboratory as she is in their congenial home. Second, his inspiring association with his former students and associates, many of whom came from far away places — no longer students but as friends — to help him celebrate this significant event in his rich life.

In presenting the EPRA Gold Medal to Franz J. Kallmann, we may say to him with Boris Pasternak: "You and others — this is what you are. Your soul, your immortality, your life in others. . . . You have always been in others. This will be you — the you that enters the future and becomes part of it."

The medal is a replica of our seal, with its Ferret symbolizing research, and with its Eastern Sun symbolizing truth and constantly renewed energy. These symbols very aptly apply to him.

Appendix

CO-SPONSORING ORGANIZATIONS

Academy of Psychosomatic Medicine
American Eugenics Society
American Psychopathological Association
American Society of Human Genetics
Scottish Rite Committee on Research in Schizophrenia

OFFICERS OF EASTERN PSYCHIATRIC RESEARCH ASSOCIATION
1960-61

Charles Buckman, M.D.	President
William Malamud, M. D.	President Elect
Emerick Friedman, M.D.	1st Vice-President
William Furst, M.D.	2nd Vice-President
David J. Impastato, M.D.	Secretary-Treasurer
Albert Browne-Mayers, M.D.	Assistant Secretary-Treasurer

SPONSORING COMMITTEE

Dr. Gilbert R. Barnhart,
  Chief, Division of Research Grants and Demonstrations, Office of Vocational Rehabilitation, U. S. Department of Health, Education, and Welfare
Dr. Lauretta Bender,
  President, American Psychopathological Association
Dr. Francis J. Braceland,
  Psychiatrist-in-Chief, The Institute of Living
Dr. Henry Brill,
  Deputy Commissioner, New York State Department of Mental Hygiene
Dr. Charles Buckman,
  President, Eastern Psychiatric Research Association
Dr. Oskar Diethelm,
  Professor of Psychiatry, Cornell University Medical College
Dr. Theodosius Dobzhansky,
  DaCosta Professor of Zoology, Columbia University
Dr. L. C. Dunn,
  Professor of Zoology, Columbia University
Dr. Robert H. Felix,
  Director, National Institute of Mental Health
Dr. Alfred M. Freedman,
  Professor of Psychiatry, New York Medical College
Dr. H. Bentley Glass,
  Professor of Biology, Johns Hopkins University

Dr. Paul H. Hoch,
New York State Commissioner of Mental Hygiene

Dr. William L. Holt, Jr.,
Professor of Psychiatry, Albany Medical College

Dr. William Horwitz,
Assistant Director, New York State Psychiatric Institute

Dr. David Impastato,
Secretary-Treasurer, Eastern Psychiatric Research Association

Dr. I. Charles Kaufman,
Professor of Psychiatry, State University College of Medicine

Dr. Heinrich Klüver,
Distinguished Service Professor of Biological Psychology, University of Chicago

Dr. Lawrence C. Kolb,
Director, New York State Psychiatric Institute

Dr. Howard Levene,
Professor of Mathematical Statistics and Biometrics, Columbia University

Mr. Adrian Levy,
Assistant Commissioner for Vocational Rehabilitation, New York State Department of Education

Dr. David Levy,
Former Clinical Professor of Psychiatry, Columbia University

Dr. Nolan D. C. Lewis,
Consultant, New Jersey Neuropsychiatric Institute

Dr. William Malamud,
Professional and Research Director, National Association for Mental Health

Dr. H. Houston Merritt,
Dean, College of Physicians and Surgeons, Columbia University

Dr. Robert P. Nenno,
Professor of Psychiatry, Seton Hall College of Medicine

Mr. Frederick Osborn,
Secretary, American Eugenics Society

Dr. Winifred Overholser,
Chairman, Scottish Rite Committee on Research in Schizophrenia

Dr. Howard W. Potter,
Program Director, Letchworth Village Graduate School in Mental Retardation

Dr. Sandor Rado,
Professor of Psychiatry and Dean, The New York School of Psychiatry

Dr. F. C. Redlich,
Professor of Psychiatry, Yale University, School of Medicine

Dr. Milton Rosenbaum
Professor of Psychiatry, Albert Einstein College of Medicine

Dr. Harry Shapiro,
President, American Eugenics Society

Dr. Mary E. Switzer,
> Director, Office of Vocational Rehabilitation, U. S. Department of Health, Education, and Welfare

Dr. S. Bernard Wortis,
> Dean and Professor of Psychiatry, New York University College of Medicine

Dr. Melvin D. Yahr,
> Assistant Dean, College of Physicians and Surgeons, Columbia University

BANQUET PHOTOGRAPHS

Eastern Psychiatric Research Association, October 1961

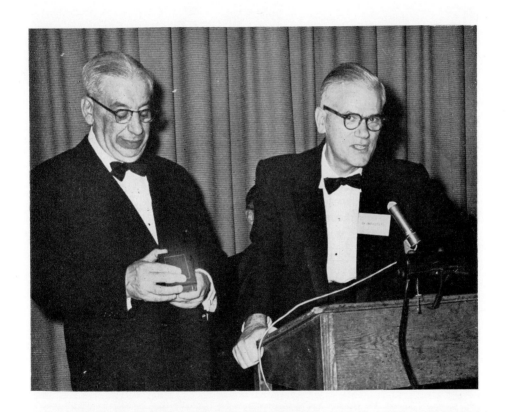

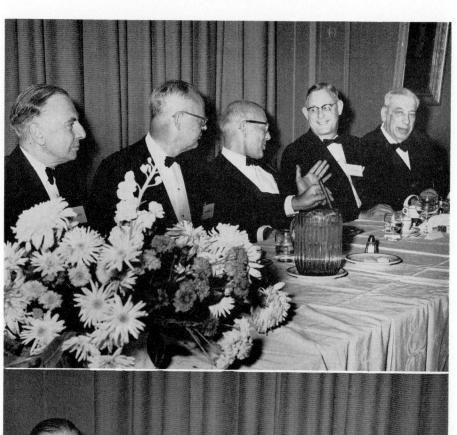

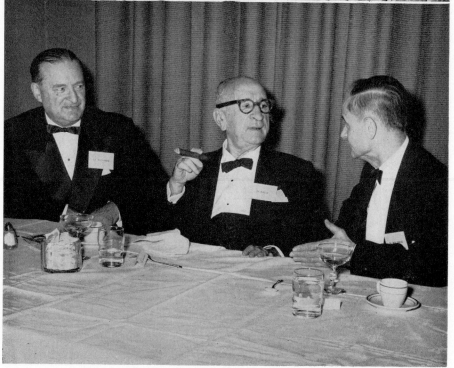

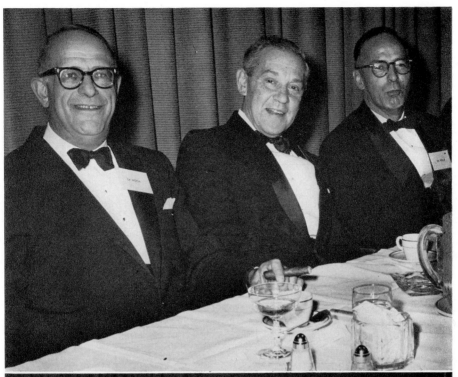

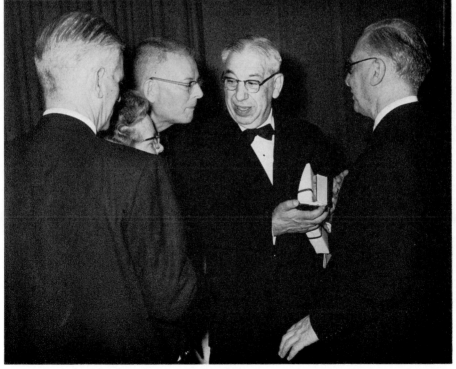

269

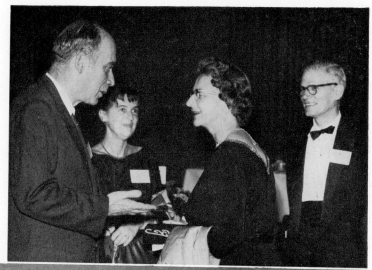

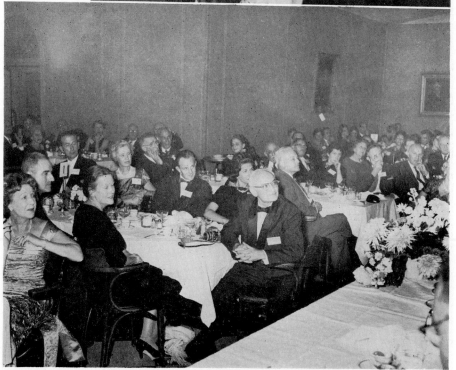

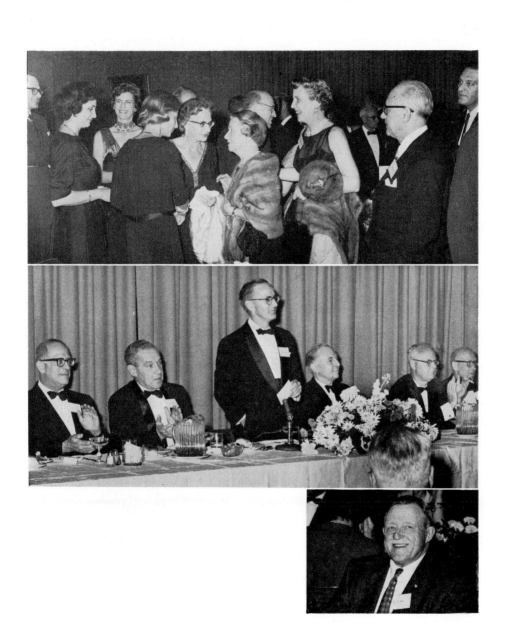

Index

RENEWALS 691-4574

DATE DUE

JAN 0 2		
DEC 1 1		
MAY 0 7		

Demco, Inc. 38-293